DOCTORS' ORDERS

DOCTORS' ORDERS

*The Making of
Status Hierarchies in
an Elite Profession*

TANIA M. JENKINS

Columbia University Press
New York

Columbia University Press gratefully acknowledges the generous support
for this book provided by a member of our Publisher's Circle.

Columbia University Press
Publishers Since 1893
New York   Chichester, West Sussex
cup.columbia.edu
Copyright © 2020 Tania M. Jenkins

Cataloging-in-Publication Data available from the Library of Congress.
ISBN 978-0-231-18934-7 (hardback)
ISBN 978-0-231-18935-4 (trade paper)
ISBN 978-0-231-54829-8 (ebook)
LCCN 2019057510

Cover design: Noah Arlow
Cover image: Getty Images

To Maman Louise

Contents

Preface

In his 2009 novel *Cutting for Stone*, Abraham Verghese tells the story of Marion Stone, an Ethiopian medical student who came to New York City to pursue residency training as a surgeon at Our Lady of Perpetual Succour, a community hospital in the Bronx. One evening it dawned on Marion that only foreign doctors worked at Our Lady. His naïveté provoked laughter from his colleagues. Marion's chief resident gently explained:

"See here," he said, taking a saltshaker and pepper shaker and putting them side by side. "This pepper shaker is *our* kind of hospital. . . . Let's call it an Ellis Island hospital. Such hospitals are always in places where the poor live. The neighborhood is dangerous. Typically such hospitals are *not* part of a medical school. Got it? Now take this saltshaker. This is a Mayflower hospital, a flagship hospital, the teaching hospital for a big medical school. All the medical students and interns are in super white coats with badges that say SUPER MAYFLOWER DOCTOR. Even if they take care of the poor, it's honorable, like being in the Peace Corps, you know? Every American medical student dreams of an internship in a Mayflower hospital. Their worst nightmare is coming to an Ellis Island hospital. Here's the problem—who is going to work in hospitals like ours when there is a bad neighborhood, no medical school, no prestige? . . . Where do you get your interns to fill all these new positions? There are many more internship positions available than there are graduating American medical students. American students have their pick, and let me tell you, they don't want to come and be interns here. Not when they can go to a Mayflower hospital. So every year, Our Lady and all the Ellis Island hospitals look for foreign interns. You are one of hundreds who came as part of this annual migration that keeps hospitals like ours going."[1]

This is a book about a real Mayflower hospital and a real Ellis Island hospital. It explores how their trainees came to be so segregated and how that segregation impacted the residents' education and influenced their career trajectories within the medical profession.

———— ◆ ————

I started doing fieldwork at Legacy Community Hospital through a friend who knew someone who worked there. I was initially interested in studying the medical pecking order, particularly the practice of "pimping"—a pedagogical technique that involves putting subordinates on the spot, often in humiliating ways.[2] Very quickly, however, it became apparent that if I wanted to study hierarchy, Legacy was not the place to do it. I was told as much on my very first day at the hospital when a senior resident explained that where he went to medical school, he could not look his attending physician in the eye. But that wasn't the case at Legacy. After two months of fieldwork, I agreed with him; Legacy was a small, friendly place without much in the way of formal teaching, never mind overt hierarchy or pimping. This prompted me to take a step back and ask myself, What made this hospital different from other hospitals? I realized that as a small community hospital, Legacy was on the lower-status end of the broader spectrum of hospitals. Staring at the roster of internal medicine residents, it dawned on me that hardly any of them were graduates of US allopathic medical schools.[3] In fact, every single resident in Legacy's three-year program had graduated from an international or an osteopathic school.[4] Where were all the US-trained MDs?

As early as my first day in the field—when the Legacy resident told me that if I was looking for hierarchy, I should look elsewhere—I began to entertain the idea of a second field site for comparison. But as my focus shifted from internal institutional hierarchy to broader questions about the sorting of residents and professional status, I had to find a field site that could put my findings from Legacy into perspective. During interviews, residents at Legacy often contrasted "IMG- or DO-friendly" programs (what Verghese called "Ellis Island" programs), which were heavily populated by international medical graduates (IMGs) and osteopathic doctors (DOs), with elite "Mayflower" programs dominated by US-trained MDs (USMDs). Harvey, a US citizen who was an international medical graduate (USIMG), put it this way: "[The] more IMG-friendly programs [are the smaller] community hospitals out in the middle of nowhere. But that makes sense for anything." When I asked him why, he replied: "What do you mean why? Because they are less desirable." He recounted his experience as a medical student rotating in internal medicine (IM): "The program I was at . . . their IM program had a very strong affiliation to [X Medical School], which was a pretty good school in New York, but the thing is, they weren't the *actual* [X Medical School] Hospital IM program, the one based in Manhattan. . . . This was a separate group . . . a satellite hospital that had their own program. It was affiliated with [X Medical School], but that program in Queens where I rotated? That was all foreign grads."

As the dichotomy between "friendly" and "unfriendly" programs became clearer to me, I knew I had to compare my results at Legacy—a friendly program— with those from a more traditional program. Several Legacy residents suggested that I look at Stonewood University Hospital, a local medical center that served as the flagship hospital for a nearby medical school. When I looked up Stonewood's roster of residents, a familiar pattern emerged: the internal medicine program was staffed almost exclusively by USMDs, with only a few exceptions. I took this to be the other half of the puzzle. How did these two programs end up so segregated? How did this segregation affect the trainees' education and career opportunities after graduation? And why would non-USMDs agree to take on positions in less desirable hospitals, as Harvey put it, if they have the same credential (a degree to practice medicine) as USMDs?

To explain how it is that certain hospitals hire only USMDs or non-USMDs, I found it was insufficient to look at the laws or regulations giving USMDs priority for residency because there are none. Instead, I had to look at the unspoken, complex, and sometimes contradictory beliefs and mechanisms that lead to the ordering of US-trained MDs and osteopathic and international medical graduates by their social worth (or status). This is a book about how that ordering works.

Acknowledgments

This book tells the story of the more than 120 residents, attending physicians, and program officials who let me into their lives and hospitals to observe how status works in their profession. They didn't have to let me in. In fact, they had every reason not to, given my inexperience as a new ethnographer, the open-ended nature of my research questions, and the arguably uncomfortable subject I was investigating—status hierarchies. But these respondents did more than tolerate me; they often encouraged my inquisitiveness and vouched for me to their colleagues, opening new opportunities for data collection. I am tremendously grateful to them for allowing me to do this research. Unfortunately, these physicians must remain unnamed, but I truly hope they know how much I appreciate their time, patience, and candor. This book, quite simply, could not have been possible without them.

This book started out as a class project and turned into a dissertation during my doctoral studies at Brown University, and has benefited greatly from my exemplary mentors throughout its almost ten-year lifespan. Phil Brown helped nurture this kernel of a project from the beginning, long before it resembled anything coherent, sitting tirelessly with me and marked-up sets of field notes, offering feedback, wisdom, and encouragement. He taught this skeptic to love the craft of ethnography, with all its pitfalls, uncertainties, and surprises. As a mentor, Susan Short instilled confidence in me as an ethnographer, always offering astute and thought-provoking feedback and consistently encouraging me to think beyond these two cases. I credit her for helping me look for counterfactual explanations for my findings and for always encouraging me to look for puzzles—both theoretical and empirical. Margot Jackson has been a role model for the kind of scholar (and human!) I want to be. I am especially grateful to her for helping me incorporate a life course approach into my ethnography, as well as for helping me think about how my findings speak to larger discussions in social stratification research.

I am also greatly indebted to the scholarly insights I have gleaned from friends and colleagues over the years. Their feedback has helped shape the contours of this book in more ways than I can express. Special thanks to Ann Dill, Greg Elliot, Jose Itzigsohn, Meghan Kallman, Josh Pacewicz, Meredith Pustell, Zhenchao Qian, Mark Suchman, and the Contested Illnesses Research Group at Brown University for their advice and suggestions when this project was in its earliest stages. At the University of Chicago, where I did my postdoctoral work, I am grateful to those who offered me a rich intellectual home in which to grow this project, including John Yoon, David Meltzer and all the folks at the Center for Health and Social Sciences, Andrew Abbott, Marco Garrido, Anna Mueller, Jenny Trinitapoli, Alex Brewer, Katie Hendricks, Andrea Kass, Alicia Riley, and Nora Taplin. Ellen Cohen and Maggie Hassan deserve special recognition for their life-changing support during my postdoctoral studies; for their help I will always be grateful. I am also hugely indebted to Shalini Reddy, internist and collaborator extraordinaire, who provided medical editing for the entire manuscript. Any errors that remain are entirely this sociologist's fault, not hers.

I also want to extend my gratitude to colleagues at Temple University who helped nurture this project during my first two years on the tenure track. I am especially grateful to Josh Klugman for his tireless patience and assistance with statistical analyses, not to mention his sharp wit and vast knowledge of board games. Special thanks to Michael Altimore, Jim Bachmeier, Eugene Chislenko and all the CHAT fellows, Elise Chor, Gretchen Condran, Kim Goyette, Cathy Staples, Alexandra Tate, Rebbeca Tesfai, Bob Wagmiller, Tom Waidzunas, Lu Zhang, and Shanyang Zhao for their friendship, support, and feedback at various points. Judith Levine and Matt Wray were especially helpful with crafting the book proposal and offered strong examples from their own books. I am particularly indebted to my brilliant undergraduate student Grace Franklyn, who helped collect data on all 525 internal medicine programs across the country to measure the extent of segregation in graduate medical education nationwide.

Although I have just recently arrived at my new institution, the University of North Carolina–Chapel Hill, I am incredibly fortunate to be surrounded by such helpful and generous colleagues whose feedback has left an indelible mark on this book, including Howard Aldrich (who introduced me to the myth of success among the unsuccessful), Jacqueline Hagan, Bob Hummer, Ted Mouw, and Andy Perrin. Lisa Pearce and Kate Weisshaar kindly read drafts of chapters and offered insightful feedback that strengthened both my arguments and my prose. I am also grateful to the terrific graduate students in the program from whom I've learned so much already, including Alyssa Rogers Browne and George Hayward, who helped introduce me to the Association of American Medical Colleges' matriculant survey and intergroup contact theory, respectively. Alyssa also provided invaluable editing support in the final stages of the book.

An even greater debt is owed to my peers and other friends in the profession who helped keep momentum going for this project. Sibel Oktay has been an inimitable writing partner and friend throughout this process, always ready with the right words of encouragement (or in especially dire situations, chocolate cookies). Lauren Olsen has offered feedback and fortitude at key moments in this journey. I'm grateful to Ece Özlem Atikcan, Alissa Cordner, Annemarie Jutel, Joanna Kempner, Neda Maghbouleh, and Tyson Smith for helping demystify the book-writing process. Dana Fisher generously offered me desk space at the University of Maryland, where I was a visiting scholar for the year and a half it took me to write the first draft of this book; her friendship and mentorship, however, have continued long after that. Special thanks to Christopher Bethel for his expertise on chemical separation, which helped shape my own concept of status separation. I am continuously energized by the work and support of my colleagues in the Sociology of Health Professions Collective—especially Laura Hirshfield, Kelly Underman, Alexandra Vinson, Barret Michalec, Dan Menchik, Fred Hafferty, Elise Paradis, and Mathieu Albert, all of whom have been champions of this project from its earliest stages. Kelly Underman's vast knowledge of professional socialization was especially helpful in chapter 4. Conversations with Julie Szymczak and her graduate qualitative methods students helped shape several methodological decisions. And big thanks to Liz Chiarello, Johnnie Lotesta, Laura Orrico, Diana Pan, and Laura Senier for their mentorship, guidance, and friendship over this book's long gestation period.

This book has benefited enormously from the terrific team of editorial and production staff at Columbia University Press. Eric Schwartz is an extraordinary editor who does more than just vet manuscripts; he takes pride in helping authors turn their ideas into monographs. He was always available to bounce ideas around or provide helpful feedback whenever I needed it. I can safely say without hyperbole that this is a much better book thanks to his help. I am also thankful to the anonymous reviewers for their apposite and constructive feedback, as well as to Lowell Frye for his tireless efforts behind the scenes as editorial assistant. And special thanks to the production team, especially Ben Kolstad and Marielle Poss, for getting this book press-ready.

This research would not have been possible without the generous financial support of the National Science Foundation, the Social Sciences and Humanities Research Council of Canada, the Office of Research Development at the University of North Carolina–Chapel Hill, Brown University, the Canadian Institutes of Health Research, and the Center for the Humanities at Temple. I am also grateful to the National Residency Matching Program for allowing me to use their Match data and reproduce some of their figures. Portions of the introduction appeared in *Contexts*, while portions of chapter 3 were published in the *Journal of Health and Social Behavior*.

Finally, I want to thank my family and friends who provided a bedrock from which I grew as I wrote this book, especially Andy Fenelon, Caitlin Jones, Lindsay Kuhn, Juyoung Lee, Sibel Oktay, Alexandra Papoutsaki, Heather Randell, Aslı Şahin, Lori Şen, Margaret Taylor, and Moriah Willow. Thanks to my dad, Douglas Jenkins, and my sister, Tricia Jenkins, for always encouraging me to be professionally curious. Special thanks to the newest additions to my family, Emel and Şenel Başar, who are the best in-laws anyone could ask for (really). I especially want to highlight the sacrifices and support of my mom, Louise Leclair, whom I admire tremendously—it is to her that I dedicate this book. Finally, I want to thank my husband, Gökçe Başar, for his patience, love, and unwavering support of me and my work. For years he has had to put up with me talking endlessly about this book, and in the process, he has more than proven himself to be an outstanding physicist-sociologist, friend, and partner.

List of Terms and Acronyms

AAMC	Association of American Medical Colleges
ABIM	American Board of Internal Medicine
ACGME	Accreditation Council for Graduate Medical Education
AMA	American Medical Association
Allopathic medicine	Allopathic is a term used to describe 'mainstream' medicine, often in juxtaposition to osteopathic medicine.
AOA	American Osteopathic Association *or* Alpha Omega Alpha
Attending or attending physician	Senior physician who has completed their medical training
CCU	Cardiac care unit
COMLEX	Comprehensive Osteopathic Medical Licensing Examination, a three-part exam administered by the National Board of Osteopathic Medical Examiners to Doctors of Osteopathic Medicine (DOs) for licensure; similar to the USMLE
DO	Doctor of Osteopathic Medicine
EBM	Evidence-based medicine
ECFMG	Educational Commission for Foreign Medical Graduates
ED	Emergency department
EKG	Electrocardiogram

ERAS	Electronic Residency Application Service
Fellowship	Advanced subspecialty training after residency that can last between one and five years
Housestaff	Collective term for residents at a hospital ("house")
GI	Gastroenterology, the field of medicine focused on the digestive system
ICU	Intensive care unit
IM	Internal medicine
IMG	International medical graduate (non-US citizen)
Intern	First-year resident
ITE	In-Training Examination, a practice exam taken every year during residency to help prepare residents for the American Board of Internal Medicine Certification Examination, which they take after graduating from residency
The Match	National Resident Matching Program® (or The Match®), a nonprofit organization that facilitates the placement of prospective residents and fellows into training programs nationwide through a match algorithm
MCAT	Medical College Admission Test®
MKSAP	Medical Knowledge Self-Assessment Program®
NRMP	National Resident Matching Program
Osteopathic medicine	Compared to a Doctor of Medicine (MD), a Doctor of Osteopathic Medicine (DO) espouses distinct philosophical principles which recognize the body's self-healing abilities. Both types of doctors can practice medicine in the US, but DOs maintain their own medical schools
PCP	Primary care practitioner
PGY	Postgraduate year
Resident	Medical school graduate pursuing 3 or more years of practical specialty training

Scramble	Process whereby unmatched applicants try to match into positions that remain unfilled after The Match through the NRMP's Supplemental Offer and Acceptance Program® (SOAP®)
SES	Socioeconomic status
Solomon Community Hospital	Community hospital program affiliated with Stonewood University that is similar to the program at Legacy because it is staffed totally by non-USMDs
SWU	Stonewood University, the university whose medical school is affiliated with Stonewood University Hospital
Tri-Hospital	A clinical site where Stonewood residents rotated alongside Solomon residents
USIMG	US citizen international medical graduate
USMD	Graduates of US allopathic medical schools
USMLE	US Medical Licensing Examination, a three-step exam that all Doctors of Medicine (MDs), including those trained internationally, must take for licensure in the United States

DOCTORS' ORDERS

Introduction

I met Trevor on his very first day of residency, at the start of three years of practical, on-the-ground training in internal medicine following medical school.[1] He was of medium height with a closely shaven head and a strong build. Trevor was especially fond of white button-down shirts with sleeves rolled up to his elbows, revealing olive-toned forearms. He wore his stethoscope slung over one shoulder—like a purse—and even as a first-year resident (intern), he possessed a quiet calm that was appealing in a doctor.

Trevor had known he wanted to go into medicine from a young age. After going to private elementary and high school in Michigan and graduating from the University of Michigan, he applied to only three medical schools—all in Southeast Asia. It made sense to him financially: "I thought about going to the Caribbean but cost-wise, you know, I was going to be paying US prices. My four years in [Southeast Asia], including housing, tuition, a car, all the miscellaneous costs, it probably cost me in the ballpark of maybe 80K for four years." Tuition and living expenses for medical school in the United States or the Caribbean averaged about three to four times that amount, so Trevor reasoned he had made a sound financial choice.

He was picky, however, about which medical schools he applied to in Southeast Asia. He applied only to programs that would allow him to do clinical rotations in the United States, knowing that he eventually wanted to come back to the United States for residency. "I wanted to have more exposure to the US system, whether it be rotations or just [learning] how medicine is practiced [here]," he explained, adding "I think a lot of [residency] programs—especially for us foreigners—they like it when we have US clinical experience." I remember being startled by his expression: "us foreigners." Trevor was born and raised in

Ann Arbor. When I pointed this out to him, he shrugged and said, "Actually, in terms of residency, everyone is kind of split up by either US grad or foreign grad, so whether I was born here or not, they would still classify me as a foreign grad. . . . [We're American] in every aspect except for how the medical field views us basically."

Every year the United States relies on thousands of medical graduates like Trevor to fill postgraduate residency positions because it does not produce enough doctors to meet its own needs. In 2019, nearly 19,000 American allopathic medical school seniors (USMDs) vied for over 32,000 first-year residency positions.[2] Nearly 94 percent of them were successful, but even if 100 percent had "matched" to a residency, there would still have been more than 13,000 positions left over. That means the United States does not graduate enough MDs by about a third every year. In fact, since the advent of modern residency training in the 1950s, the United States has produced 20 to 45 percent fewer MDs than are needed to staff residency positions nationwide.[3]

To fill the gap, the United States depends on doctors trained in other countries and traditions. In 2019, nearly 10 percent of first-year residency positions were filled by US citizens who were international medical graduates (USIMGs).[4] These are Americans, like Trevor, who take a nontraditional route into medicine by studying overseas (most often in the Caribbean) and coming back to the United States to complete their required residency training. Most USIMGs complete roughly two years of classroom instruction abroad and then finish the last two years of their clinical education in the United States, preparing them for residency positions in the US health care system. Around 55 percent of USIMG applicants successfully matched to residency positions in the United States in 2019.[5]

Another 13 percent of first-year residency positions were filled by international medical graduates who are not US citizens (IMGs).[6] These individuals complete at least undergraduate medical training abroad before deciding to pursue graduate medical education in the United States.[7] Some come to the United States as fully trained, experienced physicians, but all must still complete residency training in the United States before becoming eligible to practice independently.[8] A little more than half (53.4 percent) of all IMG applicants were able to match to a residency program in 2019.[9]

Finally, another 16 percent of first-year residency positions were filled by US-trained osteopathic physicians.[10] Compared to a Doctor of Medicine (MD), a Doctor of Osteopathic Medicine (DO) espouses distinct philosophical principles that emphasize a holistic approach. Both types of doctors can practice medicine in the United States, but DOs maintain their own medical schools and affiliated hospitals. Previously, they also maintained their own residency programs, but as of 2020, all MD and DO programs have merged under a single accreditation system.[11] Despite the previous separation, from the 1990s until 2019, DOs were able to apply to allopathic (or MD-based) residencies for a chance to work in a more diverse set of hospitals and specialties.

While DOs are US-trained doctors, the medical profession often treats them similarly to IMGs because they have taken a nontraditional path to medical school. (I will further describe the history of DO schools later.) Like IMGs, DOs match to residency positions at comparatively lower rates than USMDs do—only 81.5 percent over the past five years compared to 94 percent for USMDs, 55.6 percent for USIMGs, and 53.4 percent for IMGs.[12] Residency therefore is hardly a given for non-USMDs while it is all but guaranteed for USMDs.[13] For these reasons, I refer to all international and osteopathic medical graduates (USIMGs, IMGs, and DOs) jointly as *non-USMDs* in order to contrast them with USMDs.[14] The non-USMDs in each category have distinct histories, trajectories, and perspectives, but what all three groups have in common is this: they are systematically relied upon to fill gaps in the US health care system, yet the medical profession views and treats them differently than USMDs.

Despite representing a sizable chunk of new resident physicians each year, non-USMDs often do not end up in the same specialties as USMDs. Highly prestigious and sought-after fields, such as otolaryngology (also known as ear, nose, and throat) and orthopedic surgery are almost exclusively staffed by USMDs while less prestigious areas like pathology, family medicine, and internal medicine are dominated by non-USMDs.[15]

Even within the specialties that they dominate, non-USMDs often do not match to the same kinds of programs as USMDs,[16] although mean licensing exam scores—one of the biggest predictors of residency placement—are virtually identical between matched USMDs and at least matched international graduates. In fact, on one particularly critical test—Step 1 of the US Medical Licensing Exam (USMLE)—non-US citizen international medical graduates (IMGs) actually outperform US-citizen MDs (i.e., USMDs and USIMGs) and DOs.[17] Furthermore, for the same exact test scores, non-USMDs generally have a much lower probability of matching to their preferred specialty than USMDs do.[18]

Still, USMDs tend to congregate in higher-status hospitals while non-USMDs fill positions in lower-status ones, often in less desirable geographic areas. In some cases, this has resulted in heavily segregated training environments. On the one hand, there are highly prestigious programs staffed mostly by USMDs in university hospitals, which tend to have lower patient-to-nurse ratios, higher procedure volumes, and state-of-the-art equipment and care processes. On the other, there are "DO- or IMG-friendly" programs, as they are known in the blogosphere, which tend to be in smaller community hospitals with lower patient volumes, older technology, and fewer resources than university hospitals.[19] This segregation is so widespread that nationwide, USMDs make up 90 percent or more of the housestaff at over 37 percent of all internal medicine university programs and less than 10 percent of the housestaff at over 51 percent of all internal medicine community programs (see figure I.1).[20] Indeed, the exceptions are the integrated programs, which comprise only about 16 percent of internal medicine residency programs across the country.[21] IMG-friendly programs also have lower American Board of Internal Medicine exam pass rates after graduation compared to USMD-dominated programs, even though international medical graduates have virtually the same average Step 1 scores prior to residency—one of the biggest predictors of Board passage—as USMDs. Thus, not only are USMDs and non-USMDs segregated during residency training; their training may not be equal, at least as measured by Board pass rates.[22]

The distribution of USMDs and non-USMDs need not look this way, however. In fields like computer science, engineering, and physics, where highly skilled foreign workers make up significant proportions of the US workforce, individuals are distributed across specialties and institutions more or less equally, with little concern for citizenship or origin of degree.[23] A survey of graduate programs in science, technology, engineering, and mathematics found that students in some of the nation's most prestigious graduate programs are disproportionately international students.[24] A similar trend exists among university faculty; in natural science and engineering departments, a significantly higher proportion of foreign-born faculty work in high-prestige research (R1 or R2) and doctoral institutions compared to US-born faculty, who are more likely to work in comprehensive or liberal arts colleges.[25]

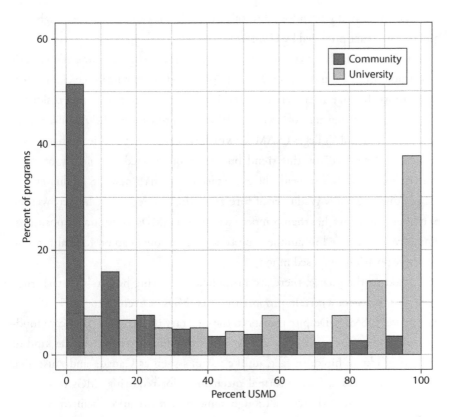

I.1 Distribution of USMD concentration by program type (2017–2018). Proportion of USMDs in community- and university-based internal medicine programs nationwide for 2017–2018.

Source: American Medical Association, Fellowship and Residency Electronic Interactive Database (FREIDA).

These trends beg the question: What is happening in medicine, such that the United States imports nearly one-third of its workforce every year—including some of the world's "best and brightest"[26]—but USMDs do not appear to be competing with these workers (or even with domestically trained DOs) for the most prestigious positions, although such competition is the norm in other fields? After all, whereas law is highly jurisdiction-specific, medicine involves portable skills that should be translatable across contexts; it is what makes organizations like Médecins Sans Frontières possible. Top-notch non-USMDs should be able to compete with USMDs on this basis, especially because after graduation, they have repeatedly been found to offer care that is equal to or even higher in quality than that provided by USMDs.[27]

Yet they decidedly don't compete. In fact, even the slightest hint of competition among USMDs and non-USMDs has provoked alarm within the US medical community. In 2013, nearly six hundred USMDs failed to match to a residency program, prompting talk of a crisis within the profession. The Association of American Medical Colleges (AAMC), which represents US medical schools, was reportedly "troubled" by this trend but never questioned the quality of these unmatched USMDs.[28] Instead, the expectation was that "new US graduates will simply displace many graduates of foreign medical colleges"[29]—who may well be of higher quality—rather than compete with non-USMDs for residency positions, which remain limited in number due to a congressional cap on federal funding for these positions imposed in 1997.[30]

To add to the puzzle, there are no policies requiring hospitals or residency programs to accept a certain proportion of USMDs or even to consider USMDs before non-USMDs. Despite threats to the contrary in the 1980s, Medicare funding, which pays for residency training, still does not vary based on the kind of medical graduate hired. In fact, unlike nations such as Canada and Australia, the United States lacks any formal mechanism for requiring IMGs to *train* in medically underserved areas, although some policies require them to work in such areas for a period of time after graduation.[31] Australia, for example, explicitly requires that internationally trained graduates be given lower priority than domestic medical graduates in awarding residency positions, thereby ensuring that the former will be funneled toward underserved or undesirable areas rather than competing with Australian doctors for the most preferred spots.[32] No such policies exist, however, in the United States. In fact, if they did, it's likely that they would be vigorously opposed by the profession. Professional bodies, like the American Medical Association (AMA), have been very successful at fighting off government interference and would likely balk at efforts to regulate the profession in this way. Besides, the general cultural ethos in the United States is one of meritocracy, where hard work and talent are supposed to be key mechanisms for allocating that opportunity—not policies.[33]

So, on the one hand, the United States relies on non-USMDs to fill much-needed residency positions. On the other, it does not want non-USMDs creating competition for its own medical graduates, even though such competition exists in other high-skilled fields where the United States relies on foreign workers.

How does this work? How does the medical profession ensure that non-USMDs fill undesirable positions without creating additional competition for USMDs? Even US citizens who trained internationally as MDs (USIMGs) or domestically as DOs aren't on an equal footing with USMDs. Recall Trevor's words: "us foreigners." When it comes to trajectories into graduate medical education, the primary deciding characteristic, more than citizenship, seems to be USMD or not.

How do such segregated patterns within graduate medical education emerge? If they're not the result of formal policies, then what are the largely *informal* practices, beliefs, social forces, and prejudices that sustain a system whereby residency programs exclude some of the world's best talent? Officially, The Residency Match promises to be "100 percent objective, 100 percent accurate, and 100 percent committed to a fair and transparent process."[34] Upon closer inspection, however, these patterns of segregation suggest that far more unofficial mechanisms of social stratification are at play. After all, The Match algorithm is only as objective as the inputs it receives from applicants and programs (see the next section, "A Brief History of Graduate Medical Education in the United States," for more on The Match).

This book offers a rare window into those informal mechanisms. It explores how status hierarchies are created among putative equals: trainees within the same specialty, internal medicine. Using ethnographic data from two internal medicine residency programs—one staffed almost exclusively by non-USMDs and the other staffed almost exclusively by USMDs—I explore how this phenomenon of segregation occurs from the residents' and the programs' perspectives. Specifically, I rely on data from in-depth interviews, focus groups, and intensive observations to address four aims: First, I examine how these two programs came to be so segregated, and, second, I trace the impact that segregation has on the residents' training. Third, I follow the trainees longitudinally throughout residency to illustrate how their career trajectories compare at graduation. Finally, I ask how these residents make sense of the status hierarchies among residents from different educational backgrounds, and I consider why non-USMDs would consent to taking on lower-status positions. As one IMG put it, "What the hospitals and the universities here in the States are doing with IMGs is filling the. . . gap." Given this point of view, why would non-USMDs—still members of an elite profession—be willing to serve such a gap-filling function?

I argue that these residents experienced what I call *status separation*, a social process by which those in a seemingly homogenous profession get hierarchically differentiated by pedigree into various strata according to their social worth (status), creating horizontal stratification (or differences in prestige) among trainees in the same specialty. Amidst a widespread and pervasive emphasis on *individual merit* in medicine, I found that largely *structural* advantages and disadvantages, often dating back to childhood differences in social class, are frequently misidentified as differences in individual achievement and motivation among medical graduates, helping USMDs float to the top of the status hierarchy while pushing non-USMDs toward the bottom. I also found that the role of merit is complicated by unequal training structures within the profession. USMDs and non-USMDs are sorted into different training programs—ostensibly on the basis of merit—where they enjoy very different advantages and opportunities. The result is a kind of self-fulfilling prophecy, with USMDs (who are widely assumed to be better from the beginning) becoming stronger residents in large part because of the amount of structural support they receive along the way. In this way, early structural advantages have a way of translating themselves into actual differences in merit and achievement in medicine.

More concretely, I argue that USMDs receive systematic support starting in early life from their parents and eventually from the profession. Once in medical school, they benefit from what I describe as a kind of implicit professional "social contract": in return for successfully "playing the game" of getting into US medical school—involving years of hard work, debt, and deferred gratification—they are nearly guaranteed success in the profession. This social contract makes it almost impossible for USMDs to fail, affording them special "rights" to elite positions within medicine. In this way, USMD leaders elevate those within their ranks and stigmatize those whom they have rejected. In addition to stigma, non-USMDs face systematically harder rules of the game, such that they are often required to do more to reach lower-status (and lower-quality) training positions, even though positions are supposed to be open to everyone equally. And by training in lower-resource environments, non-USMDs, in turn, receive poorer training and less supervision than USMDs, generally making them weaker residents (as measured by pass rates on the American Board of Internal Medicine Certification Examinations and fellowship match rates) compared to USMDs. Still, these non-USMDs consent to such inequality. They readily agree to take on lower-status positions—in part because they feel they have rightfully earned them and in part because they know they are among the lucky few non-USMDs to have matched to residency.

By revealing the subtle, informal, and often unspoken mechanisms that help sustain a myth of uncomplicated meritocracy in medicine, I show how educational institutions—even those at the apex of broader social and professional status hierarchies—can serve to perpetuate broader social processes of inequality along class, race, and nativist lines.[35] This book joins a larger sociological corpus of work that casts doubt on the power of education (even professional education) as a great equalizer,[36] and it illustrates how beliefs in hard work, dedication, and merit, which educational institutions so effectively inculcate into students, can also help make them complicit in their own subordination.[37] That the medical profession is creating an underclass of physicians—and relying on non-USMDs to fill it—suggests that similar processes of othering and subordinating immigrants and minorities, which are found in sectors of the labor force like service and farming, may also be happening in elite professions like medicine. Even the goal is similar: filling jobs Americans don't want. And by studying the inner workings of medicine, I provide insight into similar processes happening in other elite professions—like academia and law—where distinctions are also being drawn between putative equals.

A BRIEF HISTORY OF GRADUATE MEDICAL EDUCATION IN THE UNITED STATES

To understand the current situation in graduate medical education, it is useful to trace how medicine has become both more open and more exclusionary over time as it has balanced the dual goals of protecting its elites and maintaining just the right supply of doctors.

Prior to World War I, postgraduate medical education was uncommon. One-year internships or so-called house pupil or house officer positions were "haphazard," optional, and generally quite rare.[38] After the war, however, hospitals saw growing demand for medical services as advancements in treatments (e.g., antibiotics) and diagnostic equipment (e.g., X-rays) proliferated.[39] Around the same time, private and public sources were investing large amounts of money in hospitals, and specialties began emerging, all of which added to the growing need for round-the-clock staffing in hospitals.[40] In the 1920s and 1930s, internships became more formally distinct from full-fledged (multiyear) residencies and were now mandatory to become a fully licensed physician in any field. Then, in the 1950s, with the advent of specialty certification boards, a multiyear residency became the only acceptable route to specialization, leaving one-year internships for those who preferred to remain generalists. The free-standing internship was eventually abolished in 1975, making a multiyear residency required for all medical graduates.[41] Residency therefore went from being viewed as a *privilege* to effectively becoming a *right* for US physicians, without which they could not practice independently as clinicians.[42]

These changes left the profession with a conundrum: how to increase the supply of physicians in order to meet growing demand while still protecting the profession's inner elite core of USMDs from added competition?

From Sponsored Mobility to Contest Mobility

Prior to 1952, protecting the elite was relatively straightforward, as internship and residency positions were mostly allocated through unofficial "sponsorship" arrangements between applicants and individual clinicians.[43] This was especially true of coveted specialist positions, whereby new recruits would be "directly" sponsored by "one of the inner fraternity" through an apprenticeship model.[44] Elite status in the profession was therefore thought to be a product of "elaborate social machinery rather than . . . a freely competitive milieu"[45] and was transmitted through *sponsored mobility*, whereby trainees for elite positions were chosen "on the basis of whether [elites] judge the candidate to have those qualities they wish to see in fellow members."[46] Unsurprisingly, as a result, the medical elite strongly mirrored the social elite and often excluded women and racial and ethnic minorities.

After World War II, however, as the demand for house officers increased, so did competition between hospitals for good candidates. Students were being asked to make increasingly early commitments to programs (sometimes even on the spot), which prompted much dissatisfaction and stress among trainees.[47] In 1952, that changed with the advent of the National Resident Matching Program (NRMP), better known as The Match—a centralized clearinghouse for residency applications nationwide. The idea was to allow applicants to rank-order their preferences, get hospitals to do the same, and then find a "match," providing the applicant with a single offer from the highest-ranked program that wanted to hire them. The Match was thus designed to level the playing field and do away with both exploding offers and informal sponsorship arrangements, thereby "democratizing" graduate medical education and making it open to any qualified candidate.[48] Traditional barriers based on religion, gender, and race/ethnicity were reduced, and residency positions were distributed more equitably.[49] In this way, The Match theoretically marked an important shift in the medical profession from sponsored to *contest* mobility, whereby "elite status is the prize in an open contest,"[50] with The Match promising "a process that is fair, efficient, transparent, and reliable" and ostensibly open to anyone who is qualified.[51]

Of course, the question of who was qualified was still entirely determined by the profession itself. As much as graduate medical education became more open after the introduction of The Match in the 1950s, the medical profession was still careful about who it allowed into its ranks, using external closure mechanisms like licensure to protect itself from encroachment on its jurisdiction.[52] DOs were a case in point. Despite having made impressive strides in increasing the standards of osteopathic medical education in the 1940s and 1950s, DOs remained shunned by MDs, who maintained formalized control over medical matters. Prior to the 1960s, DOs were prohibited from serving as physicians in the military or holding public health office and were even banned from working in allopathic hospitals in certain states.[53] They were eventually forced to merge into a single (MD) profession in California in 1961, thereby losing their distinctive professional identity.[54] That same year the AMA considered whether to allow "'voluntary' relations of its members with 'osteopaths'" but ultimately decided that "there cannot be two sciences of medicine or two different yet equally valid systems of medical practice."[55] DOs were also prohibited from training in allopathic residency programs, forcing them to form their own parallel graduate medical education system. It wasn't until 1991 that DOs could complete their residency in an allopathic program.[56] Thus, while The Match represented a step forward in terms of "democratizing" the profession, that openness was strategic and mostly reserved for MDs who, once again, viewed residency as their "right."

Balancing Supply and Demand

At the same time, there was still the outstanding problem of a shortage of doctors. The growing demand for trainees still far outweighed the supply of US-trained physicians—a reality that persists to this day (see figures I.2 and I.3). This was particularly true in community hospitals, where some programs struggled to recruit

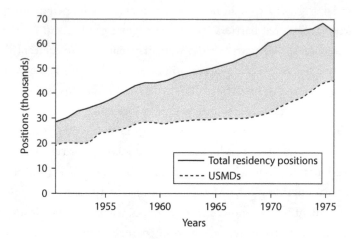

I.2 Number of residency positions and USMD residents nationwide (1950–1977).
Source: Irigoyen and Zambrana (1979).

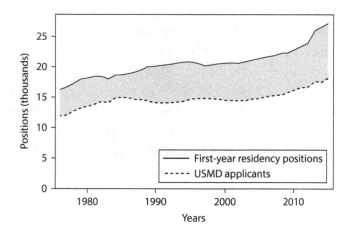

I.3 Number of first-year residency positions and USMD applicants nationwide (1976–2016).
Source: National Resident Matching Program (2016).

even a single intern in some years.[57] The profession could not completely close itself off to outsiders, given the growing demand for medical care.

The solution embraced by many hospitals was to recruit IMGs, effectively opening the nation's doors to the world's best and brightest.[58] Their influx, however, was carefully controlled through centralized governmental policies such as visa restrictions and licensing laws, which helped protect USMDs from competition. Depending on the perceived supply of USMDs at any given moment, policies have either increased or decreased the number of IMGs allowed into the United States to practice medicine.

The first evidence of efforts to regulate the influx of foreign-trained doctors came in 1938, when the AMA required all IMGs to obtain US citizenship prior to being licensed—a rule that was implemented by many state licensing boards until the late 1960s.[59] The increasing specialization of doctors, however, as well as the rising need for medical care, made citizenship an impractical requirement. The Smith-Mundt Act of 1948 extended exchange visitor (J) visas to IMGs for the first time, allowing them to pursue postgraduate training in the United States on the condition that they return to their home country for at least two years prior to applying for legal permanent residency in the United States. The number of eligible IMGs, however, was severely limited. In the 1950s and 1960s, the AMA and the AAMC published a very short list of "acceptable" foreign schools that were believed to operate according to US standards, but this list was highly incomplete and included mostly European schools.[60]

By the early 1960s, the US Department of Labor determined that a doctor shortage was looming, so new laws were passed to waive the two-year home residency requirement for IMGs.[61] By 1965, doctors were exempt from national quotas that limited the number of migrants from certain countries.[62] Preference categories for skilled workers were created in the Immigration and Naturalization Act of 1965, encouraging the immigration of professionals who could help fill gaps in the US economy.[63] By 1970, IMGs could simply exchange their J visas for regular work (H-1B) visas to facilitate their application for permanent residency.[64] Unsurprisingly, the supply of IMGs increased considerably during that period.

Concerns about a shortage of doctors, however, were quickly replaced with fears of an oversupply from the 1970s until the 1990s[65]—fears largely attributed to an overabundance of IMGs.[66] Around this time, offshore medical schools began emerging, raising concerns that USMDs would be crowded out by Caribbean graduates.[67] Because Caribbean graduates were typically US citizens, immigration policies would do little to stem their influx into the United States. USMD numbers were also rising domestically around that time, with a nearly 45 percent increase in the number of medical schools operating during this time period.[68]

Osteopathic medical education was also expanding during this era—a sign of slow, yet growing acceptance of DOs in the profession. In 1968, the AMA finally permitted DOs to become members of the association. By 1973, all fifty states allowed DOs to practice as fully licensed physicians, and as a result of increased public funding, the number of osteopathic medical schools grew from five to fourteen by 1980.[69] Still, DOs were not allowed to train in allopathic residency programs until 1991, which protected USMDs somewhat from osteopathic competition for residency positions.[70]

The result, starting in the early 1970s, was an estimated *surplus* of anywhere from 35,000 to 70,000 doctors.[71] Panic ensued. Scholars wrote about the threat of unemployment for junior doctors and warned of a "grim" outlook awaiting USMDs applying to residency.[72] In response, the government passed the Health Professions Educational Assistance Act of 1976 and the Health Services Extension Act of 1977, which reinstated the two-year foreign residency requirement for J visa holders and required new IMGs to have their visas approved by the US Department of Labor.[73] For its part, the medical profession—much like other elite professions keen on keeping immigrants out[74]—introduced a series of new licensing examination requirements for international graduates, curbing the influx of IMGs by as much as 80 percent.[75]

In the 1980s, there were also (largely unsuccessful) attempts in Congress to limit the number of both IMGs *and* USIMGs allowed to practice in the United States. These included calls for quotas to limit the number of foreign-trained doctors (both IMG and USIMG) that hospitals could hire and threats to cut government funding to any hospital hiring more than the allotted number of IMGs.[76] While these initiatives did not become law, the Higher Education Act of 1992 did manage to restrict federal loans to only a handful of Caribbean schools, thereby limiting government support for USIMGs.[77]

The Current Policy Climate

Based on the policies from the late 1970s to mid-1990s, which aimed to squeeze IMGs out of the health care system, many expected the nation to become less dependent on IMGs over time, eventually preferring to hire US-trained personnel over foreign doctors.[78] Yet self-sufficiency has hardly come to pass. Since the mid-1980s, the proportion of residency positions filled by non-USMDs has risen steadily from 25.5 percent in 1985 to 39.6 percent in 2019, but the *average match rate* for USMDs has remained almost constant (around 93.6 percent).[79] So, while the number of non-USMD trainees has increased, their larger numbers do not seem to be posing additional competition to USMDs, nearly all of whom are still matching to residency, predominantly in their preferred specialties.

These trends are particularly interesting, given the current policy climate, which, compared to the 1970s and 1980s, is relatively open toward noncitizens wanting to practice and stay in the country. Depending on the residency program, IMGs can be sponsored for either H-1B or J visas, with the option of waiving the two-year home residency requirement by working in an underserved area upon graduation. Besides, visa restrictions are ineffective against non-USMDs who are US citizens, such as USIMGs and DOs, whose numbers have increased substantially in recent years, despite the lack of federal loan support for most offshore schools. The number of Caribbean schools catering to US citizens has exploded since the 1970s, with twenty-four new schools built in the early 2000s alone, making a total of around thirty-five universities as of 2014.[80] The number of osteopathic medical schools in the United States has also grown from five in 1968 to thirty-seven in 2013, and the allopathic Accreditation Council for Graduate Medical Education (ACGME) joined forces with the American Osteopathic Association to offer a single graduate medical education accreditation system, overseen by the ACGME, as of 2020.[81]

And even as the formal prerequisites for residency have become more stringent, they have also been applied more uniformly across medical graduates, without specifically disadvantaging non-USMDs. Since 1992, IMGs and USIMGs have been required to take the same USMLEs that USMDs are, not the more difficult exams historically designed to keep IMGs out.[82] All credentials (transcripts and diplomas) must be verified by the Educational Commission for Foreign Medical Graduates (ECFMG) before applying for residency, but the ECFMG's list of approved foreign schools (now contained in the World Directory of Medical Schools) is far more inclusive than the previous list maintained by the AMA and the AAMC in the 1950s and 1960s.[83] Approximately 57.2 percent of all applicants since the mid-1980s have secured ECFMG certification after passing the USMLEs and getting their credentials verified.[84] All this vetting means that only those IMGs who can meet or exceed US standards are permitted to even *apply* for residency.[85]

Residency training itself has also become more uniform in recent years, thanks to centralized efforts to standardize graduate medical education and improve learning outcomes. In the early 2000s, the ACGME moved to evaluate and accredit programs based not only on their structural characteristics (like number of faculty) but also on their residents' abilities to master certain skills and competencies.[86] Thus, by overseeing graduate medical education nationwide, bodies like the ACGME ostensibly help ensure a reasonable degree of standardization across programs—and thus comparability among trainees.

So more than ever, non-USMDs and USMDs *should* be competing on a level playing field as supposed equals in the competition for residency positions. The Match promises contest mobility to ever-larger numbers of non-USMDs. Applicants are objectively assessed and are now largely comparable, thanks to standardized examinations. DOs and MDs are training in accredited programs that ensure minimum quality standards across institutions. And despite failed attempts in the 1980s, there are still no policies requiring hospitals to prioritize USMDs or US citizens. Given these developments, we might expect USMDs and non-USMDs to compete with one another for residency positions, resulting in a heterogeneous distribution of medical graduates in different fields. Instead, what we find is marked segregation along the lines of medical pedigree. How does this happen?

SOCIOLOGY OF THE MEDICAL PROFESSION

Unfortunately, sociological theory about the medical profession does not yet have a good answer to the question of how such segregation arises. With a few notable exceptions, medical sociology has traditionally conceptualized physicians as a largely monolithic group vis-à-vis patients and other professionals, often overlooking informal status distinctions *within* the profession and certainly within specialties. To understand this homogenizing tendency within the discipline, we need to take a historical look at how sociological scholarship on the medical profession has developed by juxtaposing the progression of ideas with macrosocietal changes. This chronological approach is necessary to fully appreciate the evolution of the theories and to understand why they are insufficient today. (Readers less interested in theoretical debates may want to turn to the section entitled "Studying Status Separation.")

A Community of Equals

Early medical sociology had its roots in the functionalist tradition, which sought to understand why professions work and cohere as a unit.[87] Sociologists of that era therefore conceptualized professions as harmonious groups of individuals sharing similar interests, attitudes, and education—"a community of equals."[88]

The so-called golden age of doctoring (1945 to 1965) prompted scholars to consider how medicine became so successfully professionalized that doctors were effectively unopposed when it came to health matters. In *Professional Dominance*, Freidson argued that health services were organized around the dominance of a single profession—physicians—with paramedical workers subordinated not only by a "body of special knowledge and skill" but also by bureaucratic (legal) authority.[89] This legal protection, he argued, was offered to the medical profession in exchange for providing high-quality and esoteric professional services that no one else could offer.

At around the same time, in the 1970s and 1980s, sociologists within the broader discipline were concerned with how to define a profession and how to make sense of professional divisions of labor.[90] Their writings usually looked at how various professionalization projects were used to uphold jurisdictions and boundaries. Abbott, for example, theorized about professions relationally as systems in which dominant factions ruled over subordinate ones, resulting in "jurisdictional disputes."[91] He argued that to understand these disputes, we must look at the work itself and see how it is being "claimed" as part of a jurisdiction. This framing led, for example, to analyses of how psychiatrists—overwhelmed with demands for mental health care—eventually deskilled psychotherapy, yielding its "jurisdiction" to social workers and psychologists.

These studies, however, were rather narrowly focused on how professionals maintained their dominance over intruders—be they governments or other workers. This was partly done for simplicity's sake—i.e., to be able to explain how professions secure power and authority over outsiders.[92] The result, however, was the unintentional obscuring of the medical profession's inner battles for status and power. It also didn't help that most empirical analyses of hospitals and doctors were single-center studies, which only reinforced the impression that the medical profession and medical education were largely uniform.[93]

Only limited work from the 1960s to the early 1980s hinted at stratification within the medical profession. Some scholars distinguished between at least two "lines of authority" within hospitals—administrative and medical—although little was known about how these lines emerged to begin with or how they managed to coexist.[94] Others noted the existence of status hierarchies across specialties[95] or between "town" and "gown" physicians in community and university hospitals.[96] Freidson and Rhea problematized the notion of professions as "companies of equals" by showing that rules, hierarchy, and supervision existed within a clinic to keep fellow physicians (putative equals) in line.[97] For their part, Bucher and Strauss advocated a "process" approach to professions, emphasizing conflicting interests and change. This marked a significant departure from functionalist perspectives, where internal distinctions were considered to be deviations from professional cohesion or to be merely temporary. Bucher and Strauss understood the medical profession to be divided into smaller "segments" that could come into conflict with each other over areas such as the profession's mission, work activities, methodology, and clients. They believed that segments could form across and within specialties, reflecting specific interests, beliefs, and identities, and that each segment had its own missions, organizational forms, and tactics for exerting power, which could create (status) divisions within the profession.[98] Their "process" approach to professions, however, remained marginalized, and sociologists' broader assumption of professional homogeneity persisted until the 1980s.

Professional Decline

As pressure from the state, corporations, and patients began undermining the golden age of doctoring,[99] sociologists became increasingly interested in how professions responded to instability coming from both outside *and* within.[100] The advent of state-sponsored and private insurance meant that corporate and governmental actors came to play an ever-growing role in the dispensation of health care.[101] Sociologists finally began to take notice of "ferment at the core and tensions at the periphery" of medicine as internal fragmentation along specialty lines increased.[102] The community of equals model was no longer tenable.

The eighties saw a flurry of research grappling with the declining status of physicians in society, which threatened the professional dominance perspective. Several competing theories emerged, accompanied by fierce debate. Freidson, the primary proponent of *professional dominance*, maintained that as long as doctors held sole control over their gatekeeping functions (such as deciding who could become a doctor and who should be admitted to a hospital), they would continue to exert dominance over paramedical professionals and patients—despite incursions from nonmedical sources.[103] In response, scholars criticized Freidson for being out of touch with the massive macrosocietal changes happening in the health care system and instead proposed their own theories of professional decline.

One of the more serious challenges to Freidson's professional dominance theory came from the *proletarianization* thesis. Proponents heavily criticized Freidson's contention that the medical profession was impervious to the considerable socioeconomic changes happening around it. These scholars contended that increasing bureaucratization (especially the shift from self-employment to hospital employment) was creating a proletarianized profession, with formerly self-employed practitioners becoming constrained by bureaucratic controls within hospitals.[104] They predicted that, as medical practice became increasingly bureaucratized and specialized, physicians would become mere salaried employees, lose control over the terms and conditions of their professional work, and thereby become proletarianized.

In turn, Freidson strongly criticized proletarianization theorists for overstating physicians' loss of independence.[105] He rejected the notion that simply by joining a bureaucratic organization like a hospital, "[doctors] become mere cogs in a machine of production."[106] He pointed to other professionals, like engineers and professors, who have long worked in bureaucratic organizations without having their knowledge and skill "expropriated" by nonprofessional superiors,[107] and he noted that even with increased government and organizational control, physicians look nothing like typical alienated blue- or white-collar workers.[108]

While there is no doubt that some aspects of proletarianization have materialized (for example, Medicare, rather than physicians, largely dictates reimbursement rates for specific diagnostic codes), for the most part Freidson remains correct that doctors continue to control the processes of entry and the content of their professional work, suggesting that the professional decline forecast by so many sociologists in the 1980s has not come to pass.[109]

A Formal Elite and a Rank and File

The countertheories to professional dominance eventually led Freidson to modify his own theory to account for the persistence of medical dominance *in spite* of growing regulation within medicine. In the twenty years since the end of the golden era, capitation payments emerged, governments began to assume responsibility for the health care costs of the poor and the elderly, private insurance carriers proliferated, and doctors suddenly had to become cost-conscious when making treatment decisions. At the same time, lawyers, judges, and bioethicists were increasingly interfering in medical decision-making as physicians saw their decisions being preemptively questioned in the courts for the first time.[110] Freidson was forced to recognize that these changes posed a considerable threat to medicine's ability to regulate its own affairs, but he also maintained that physicians remained dominant over those affairs—a seemingly paradoxical assertion.

To reconcile these points of view, Freidson proposed a new theory. He argued that the medical profession has had to restructure itself internally, creating a formal elite and a rank and file in order to maintain its dominance in the face of these incursions.[111] This internal reshuffling made it possible for the medical profession to maintain its critical credentialing, gatekeeping, and technical decision-making power in light of external incursions into medicine's core by appointing elites to manage these essential tasks.

Freidson never gave his new theory a name, leaving his contemporaries to generate their own, including *professional subordination*,[112] *reprofessionalization*, *reorganization*,[113] and the more commonly used term *restratification*.[114] Freidson contended that restratification within the profession resulted in three broad categories of physicians: a knowledge elite that creates guidelines, an administrative elite that enforces them, and a rank and file that follows them.[115] He emphasized that these elites were themselves professionals (not outside managers, as predicted by proletarianization theorists) who shared similar basic professional training with the rank and file but who pursued specialized postgraduate training and career trajectories that led them to elite positions where they governed legitimately over the rank and file. Freidson emphasized that the elite and the rank and file were distinguished not merely by a subtle difference in prestige but also by a formal distinction—like that between manager and employee—established through *separate* specialized training for clinician-scientists and physician-managers.[116] Therefore, the profession vested elite practitioners with the bureaucratic authority necessary to establish the standards of medical work, which the rank and file then had to follow.

Freidson, however, also viewed such formal restratification as a potential source of instability within the profession. He predicted that the rank and file might abandon elite professionals due to a lack of shared interests.[117] A decade later Hafferty and Light echoed similar concerns.[118] In this way, restratification theory presents a paradox: on the one hand, these elites are deemed necessary for maintaining professional autonomy, but on the other, the distinction between professional worker and professional leader could potentially lead to a "deep split," or infighting and instability within the profession.[119]

STATUS SEPARATION: A THEORY OF THE INFORMAL ELITE AND THE RANK AND FILE

Formal restratification does not account for the patterns we see today. Yes, the medical profession is experiencing fragmentation due to the rise of the "medical-industrial complex," including the continued gender typing of certain specialties, for example. Still, these formal *vertical* divisions, like those between specialists and generalists, cannot explain the informal *horizontal* status distinctions we find among USMD and non-USMD trainees.[120]

In fact, these informal horizontal patterns more closely resemble the processes of gender inequality in medicine that were documented in the 1980s but were never incorporated into Freidson's contemporaneous theory of formal restratification. In her 1984 book *Women Physicians*, Lorber observed that growing numbers of female physicians were entering medical school with qualifications that were the same as, if not better than, those of their male colleagues and were performing just as well on licensing exams but were often excluded from leadership positions in the upper echelons of the profession.[121] She noted a similar absence of formal discriminatory policies against women and instead urged scholars to look more carefully at the *informal* organization of the profession. She concluded that there was strong evidence of informal sponsorship and patronage structures built into medical education that privileged male physicians, giving them higher status in the profession.

In the nearly four decades since Lorber's work, however, few scholars have continued examining such informal stratifying processes within the profession. Indeed, by focusing so intently on professional autonomy, medical sociologists have tended to overemphasize knowledge-based or role-based divisions of labor rather than more informal status-based distinctions among supposed equals, which are often not the product of established official pathways.[122] The former deal with formal vertical authority over subordinates, while the latter refer to prestige differentials between individuals studying in the same field: horizontal stratification in medical education.[123] Hierarchies in status, defined as collective understandings of social worth or prestige, such as those between USMDs and non-USMDs, remain highly informal, as do the processes for climbing the ranks. In fact, as I will argue, it is precisely this informality and the accompanying belief that anyone can become part of the elite with enough work and dedication that allow such status distinctions to persist.

Furthermore, the "deep split," or instability, that Freidson feared has not come to pass. He and his contemporaries viewed the rise of administrative and knowledge elites as evidence of the increasing rationalization of medicine, which inevitably meant the rank and file would be at odds with elites who increasingly identified with corporate interests. However, these dreaded rifts have not materialized, not even between the formal elite, like physician-executives, and the doctors they manage.[124] Nor have deep tensions emerged between the informal elite and the rank and file, which is especially puzzling. That non-USMDs are willing to take on lower-status positions is evidence that physicians have come to some sort of agreement about how an informal USMD elite can emerge among supposed equals in the absence of formal authority supporting this. This leaves us with two broad questions: How do pedigree-based status distinctions emerge among internal medicine residents, and how are they understood, maintained, and reproduced?

This book picks up where sociologists of the medical profession left off in the 1980s by examining the emergence of informal status differences among USMD and non-USMD internal medicine residents in a process I term *status separation*. Weber coined the term *status order* to describe the distribution of social honor within a community,[125] but little is known about how pedigree determines this distribution in medicine. While prestige differentials between USMDs and non-USMDs may seem obvious, sociologists have yet to theorize about the construction of informal horizontal status distinctions between these different graduates, perhaps because so little has been written in sociology about non-USMDs in the US workforce.[126]

I therefore propose the term *status separation* to describe the informal process by which residents get stratified by pedigree in internal medicine. In chemistry, separation refers to the process of reducing a mixture to its component parts, either through the application of external forces such as centrifuge or via natural processes like gravity (as with oil and water). In this book, I tease out the *social* forces that push USMDs to the top while pushing non-USMDs to the bottom, thereby separating them in status, according to pedigree, within a seemingly homogenous profession. The colloquialism "the cream of the crop" is often used to describe the best of a group, and meritocracy is often assumed to be the process that separates out the elite. I complicate that assumption by showing how informal social forces, such as (1) broader class inequality; (2) sponsorship; (3) status beliefs, bias, and stigma; (4) structural inequality among training programs; and (5) eventual differences in merit resulting from these inequalities, contribute to status separation in medicine.

In so doing, this book engages in a broader conversation with an emerging body of ethnographic work outside of medical sociology that sheds light on the making of elites by similarly showing how structural advantages (often misidentified as merit) can help ensure elite reproduction. Khan's ethnography of St. Paul's, a prestigious boarding school in New Hampshire, explores how an elite education helps groom future generations of elites by instilling in students an "ease of privilege," leading them to assume that their success is a function of what they have accomplished rather than who they are.[127] He argues that this myth is distinctive of a new class of elites who justify their position using meritocracy rather than traditional methods, such as blood or birth order. Similarly, Rivera's ethnography of recruitment in elite professional service firms uncovers analogous processes of structural inequality somewhat later in the elite life course by examining why students from the most elite universities tend to get the most prestigious jobs after graduation when emphasis on equal opportunity in the workplace is at an all-time high.[128]

These books offer rare insights into the social construction of privilege, power, and prestige, but they only detail half of the process—the *elite* half—and thus overlook how an informal professional rank and file simultaneously emerges. By exploring how *both* halves of this process work, we can learn not only how elites rise to the top but also how nonelites are pushed toward the bottom and how they may be unintentionally facilitating the process. As elite professions become increasingly stratified, with the proliferation of temporary lawyers, for example, or the growth of contingent faculty in academia, understanding how status separation mediated through professional education can create an underclass of professionals is of timely importance.[129]

Undercurrents of status separation are found in other social processes of stratification, including biases based on class, gender, minority status, and immigrant status, but none of these classic axes of inequality is sufficient to fully explain the current situation in medicine, where USIMGs, IMGs, and DOs are being subjugated in status to USMDs. Status separation also brings together both structure and agency. For structure, it brings to light the combination of hidden informal mechanisms (such as professional stigma and stereotyping) and more open formal mechanisms (such as institutional policies) that regulate status differences among these actors. For agency, it sheds light on the ways that participants in this field navigate unequal opportunity structures, eventually parlaying structural inequality into individual differences in merit, ability, and achievement. It also involves how they make sense of their status differentiation. Indeed, because so much of status separation is invisible and informal, participants cannot easily identify the underlying operant structures, and, thus, they rely on explanations that tend to focus more on individual shortcomings than on structural considerations. Even for those who merge individual responsibility with a recognition of structural constraints, I will show that there is still a provision of consent, in which participants still buy into the profession and its ways of creating status distinctions.

STUDYING STATUS SEPARATION

This book reveals that segregation and inequality exist between USMDs and non-USMDs, but its primary focus is to examine *how* that inequality gets produced and perceived within the profession. These "process" and "implication" questions require a research method that is well suited to understanding the intricacies and inconsistencies of individuals' beliefs, actions, and decisions as they navigate, produce, and resist broader social structures. Comparative ethnography is ideal for examining these processes because the construction and consequences of status are multiply sited. As I have argued, to examine just one hospital would be to overlook half of this puzzle and potentially obscure broader social structural forces that extend beyond the confines of a single institution.

To this end, this book extends the sociological tradition of hospital ethnography, which was so dominant from the 1960s to 1990s,[130] to compare the internal medicine residency programs in two hospitals in the Northeast: Legacy Community Hospital (a small, DO- and IMG-friendly program) and Stonewood University Hospital (a large, more elite program). I use pseudonyms to refer to these two institutions in the book and will often refer to them as Legacy and Stonewood for short. Internal medicine is the ideal residency for this study because it is composed of nearly equal numbers of USMDs and non-USMDs and offers graduates the opportunity to either remain generalists after residency or sub-specialize in one of nearly a dozen medical specialties.[131] I can therefore gauge the extent to which status inequalities during residency can impact physicians' broader professional trajectories. It is also a residency with roughly equal numbers of men and women, making gender inequality somewhat less of an obvious deter-minant of social status than in other highly masculinized fields, such as surgery.[132]

I rely on a mix of qualitative methods, including participant observation, in-depth interviews, focus groups, and content analysis to capture the infor-mal social processes leading to segregation among residents from 2011 to 2014 (for more detailed reflections on the methods, see the appendix).

SETTINGS

I chose Legacy and Stonewood as field sites because of their status as a commu-nity and a university hospital, respectively, as well as the composition of their internal medicine *housestaff* (a collective term for residents).[133] They are good examples of the broader national trend of segregation in graduate medical educa-tion described at the beginning of this introduction.

As table I.1 shows, the internal medicine residency program at Stonewood University Hospital was three times the size of the program at Legacy, and its three-year (categorical) and primary care track programs were almost exclusively staffed (98 percent) by USMDs.[134] Legacy Community Hospital's internal med-icine residency program, in contrast, had only a small proportion (less than 10 percent) of USMDs, all of whom were "prelims," or interns enrolled in a one-year preliminary program in internal medicine before going on to residencies in spe-cialties like radiology and dermatology. The other 90 percent of Legacy residents were non-USMDs enrolled in the full three-year (categorical) internal medicine program. About 45 percent of Legacy residents were USIMGs, and another 10 percent of its residents were American DOs. Altogether, with the preliminary USMDs, US citizens made up about 65 percent of the housestaff at Legacy. The other 35 percent were IMGs, some of whom had been fully trained as physicians in their home countries prior to moving to the United States.

TABLE I.1 Hospital Characteristics: Internal Medicine Residency Programs

	Legacy Community Hospital	Stonewood University Hospital
Program type	IMG- and DO-friendly	Elite academic
Hospital type	For-profit	Not-for-profit
Number of beds[a]	x	$4.5x$
Patient population	Elderly, Medicare/Medicaid	All ages; safety-net hospital
Attending physician structure	Community-based attendings	Hospital-based attendings
Percentage of non-USMD attendings	55	<5
Number of residents[a]	y	$3y$
Percentage of USMDs[b]	10[c]	98
Percentage of non-USMDs		
USIMGs[b]	45	0
DOs[b]	10	0
IMGs	35	2
Percentage of male residents	66	60
Percentage of nonwhite residents	50	25

[a] To protect the hospitals' identity, I do not disclose the actual number of beds or the size of the housestaff.
[b] US citizens.
[c] All were preliminary (one-year) interns.

Aside from the housestaff, there were other important differences between these two programs. Legacy was a small community hospital catering to a mostly elderly clientele who lived in the surrounding area—a lower-middle-class neighborhood with a high proportion of European immigrants. Patients were generally insured (mostly through Medicare), and many came to the hospital from nursing homes and assisted living facilities. This meant that Legacy dealt primarily with bread-and-butter medicine: congestive heart failure, pneumonia, and chronic obstructive pulmonary disease. Complex cases were few and far between: "There's all sorts of stuff . . . that we can't give our residents experience with here," conceded one Legacy program official. That included exposure to surgical subspecialties such as trauma, OB-GYN, and neurosurgery, as well as some medical subspecialties like interventional cardiology, which is used to treat certain kinds of heart attacks.[135] Patients requiring these types of services were transferred to other hospitals like Stonewood.

As a hospital, Legacy looked and smelled just *ordinary*. A faint odor of sickness hung in the air, usually alongside an unpleasant combination of runny eggs and bodily odors, only mildly diluted by antiseptics. Legacy consisted of a single building with several wings that spanned four floors and were connected by long corridors. The average patient census was generally low, such that it was not uncommon for entire wards of the hospital to be closed off, sometimes for months at a time, as they waited to be filled with people. The general medical wards consisted of several brightly painted hallways of two- to three-person rooms, each with a shared bathroom and beds divided by standard-issue curtains. Private rooms were reserved not for VIPs but for patients needing isolation from infection.

Legacy did not have many of the resources of larger medical centers. Basic infrastructure, such as an in-person translation service for non-English-speaking patients and reliable computer hardware, was lacking.[136] Of the four computers in the residents' lounge, only two reliably had access to the hospital's electronic order entry system. (Legacy did not have a full-fledged electronic health record at the time of my fieldwork, which meant that residents could order labs and medications on the computer but charting was done using old-fashioned pen and paper.) Other computers lacked essential software, like Microsoft Word. As one resident complained angrily one day, without exaggeration, "There's like a 30 percent probability that the computer you choose will work for whatever you need!" The machines bore stickers that read "Donated by [local] University," which hinted at some of the hospital's financial difficulties. Toward the end of my fieldwork, Legacy was acquired by a holdings company, changing its not-for-profit status. When Legacy became a for-profit institution, its trainees lost their eligibility for loan forgiveness from the federal government, but none of them left the program.[137]

Legacy was not always this resource deprived, however. Historically, Legacy was affiliated with Stonewood University (SWU) Medical School, a middle-tier medical school, as was Stonewood University Hospital, and it had a thriving training program that shared resources with the university hospital. Then, around the mid-1990s, Stonewood University Hospital was designated as the primary teaching affiliate for SWU, and there was pressure to abandon Legacy as a satellite hospital. This left Legacy scrambling to find another medical school.

Carter Medical College (located in another state) fit the bill, as it was roughly equally ranked to the SWU Medical School and it offered a degree of prestige to the small community hospital. The relationship between Legacy and Carter Medical College, however, was highly pro forma. Despite wearing badges with the Carter Medical College logo, the Legacy housestaff had virtually no contact with the medical school. Rarely did Carter Medical College physicians come to Legacy for talks or visits. The residents could not easily rotate at the medical school's other affiliated hospitals, and they did not have access to the university's library resources. For most intents and purposes, Legacy was a teaching hospital untethered to a medical school.

The result was an internal medicine residency program that was characterized by a loose structure that prioritized a "humane" residency experience. The low patient census and a relaxed call schedule (Q7, or every seven days) meant that almost everyone described Legacy's program as "laid-back."[138] Even the program leadership was relatively hands-off. This was partly due to the tenure of an interim program leader who agreed to take the job only temporarily after their predecessor was asked to leave due to financial troubles. A permanent replacement was only found four years after the interim program leader had accepted the interim position. "I agreed to do it on an interim basis for one year. And now we're three years later and I'm still doing it," the program leader told me with a shrug one afternoon. Also, the broader program leadership did not work for the program full-time—they had clinical duties of their own, spending three to five half-days per week in private practice. Running the residency program was something they did on a part-time basis.

Stonewood University Hospital, in contrast, was the quintessential academic medical center. It was a massively complex institution, housed on a sprawling urban campus with dozens of buildings. It was so big that when the telltale code bells went off signaling an emergency, the housestaff could sprint for up to ten minutes before reaching the patient's bedside, depending on the location of the emergency. Compared to Legacy, Stonewood's buildings strived to be *extraordinary*, often resembling hotels more than hospitals. Grand lobbies with tasteful art displays awaited patients and visitors, and patients were each assigned private rooms on the teaching floors. Flat-screen televisions dotted the walls, and on the back of the hospital menus distributed to patients before each meal was a list of Stonewood's accomplishments, like being the first hospital to acquire some new scanner. Somehow Stonewood did not even smell like a hospital, even though its patients were often sicker than those at Legacy were.

Stonewood was a safety-net hospital, making it the primary regional care-taker for refugees, the uninsured, and other medically vulnerable populations.[139] Compared to the patients at Legacy, those admitted to Stonewood usually had more complex medical problems requiring coordinated care between medicine and other subspecialties such as neurology and orthopedics. Stonewood's array of offerings included a transplant service, extracorporeal membrane oxygenation, interventional cardiology, and experimental medicine. This made Stonewood a hub for complicated patients transferred from nearby hospitals. Cases were often so complex that residents would frequently recite the mantra "common things being common" to remind themselves to look for proverbial horses, not zebras, when they heard "hoofbeats."[140] Adding to the complexity were the patients' social situations. Patients admitted to the wards came from all walks of life, such that on the same floor one could find a homeless person, a former university president, and a convict awaiting sentencing.

Unlike Legacy, which still relied on paper charts, Stonewood had a full electronic health record available on reliable computers located in every patient room, as well as in common work areas. A laundry service was available to the housestaff, whereas at Legacy a resident whose parents owned a dry-cleaning business would sometimes offer to clean his colleagues' white coats. Even residents' lunches were paid for by Stonewood's Graduate Medical Education Department, which refused corporate sponsorship. In contrast, Legacy relied on lunches purchased by pharmaceutical representatives to make good on its promise of free meals for the housestaff.

Stonewood also had a very stable and dedicated leadership team that main-tained order centrally. The five members of the program directorship worked exclusively on running the program, with only a minority still dabbling in very small private practices. They spent two to three months per year working on the wards to maintain a clinician-educator relationship with their residents. As one program official explained, "As much as I complain about having too much on my plate, I *have* to be on the wards, I *have* to be on the consult service . . . [because] it enables me to understand the challenges that the residents go through" (emphasis in original). They were also actively involved in didactic conferences and one-on-one mentorship with the housestaff. This meant that in comparison to Legacy's program, Stonewood's was both more tightly structured and more intense, with more complex cases and a more demanding call schedule (Q4, or every four days). Unlike Legacy residents, who trained almost exclusively at Legacy Community Hospital, Stonewood residents also rotated at other clinical sites—including community hospitals—as part of their curriculum, but the central leadership headquartered at Stonewood directly oversaw the training at these sites.

Despite the obvious differences between these two hospitals, they still had several important things in common. First, their training programs had a clear clinical focus. Unlike more research-intensive programs, like that at Stanford, which aim to produce clinician-scientists, the programs at both Legacy and Stonewood were in the business of training clinicians. That makes the differences in training approaches between the two programs all the more stark, given that residents in both places were primarily being trained as knowledge *consumers* rather than knowledge *producers*. Also, because both Stonewood and Legacy were affiliated with middle-tier medical schools, they represented neither the very top nor the very bottom of residency programs—in fact, one-fourth of internal medicine residency programs in the country are not even affiliated with a university.[141] They were far more average than that, perhaps making them more comparable than if they were ultraelite or bottom-of-the-barrel programs. As a result, both programs were eminently concerned about their institutional status, with neither one being so entrenched in its status as elite versus nonelite that it was unconcerned by external perceptions.[142] Finally, recall this nationwide comparison: USMDs make up 90 percent or more of the housestaff at over 37 percent of all internal medicine university programs and less than 10 percent of the housestaff at over 51 percent of all internal medicine community programs. Legacy and Stonewood are therefore examples of this much broader phenomenon of segregation in residency training between community and university hospitals nationwide.

PLAN OF THE BOOK

The chapters that follow take the reader through the construction and consequences of professional status distinctions at these two hospitals before, during, and after residency. In chapter 1, I explore how trajectories into residency differed between USMDs and non-USMDs and finds that distinctions among physicians often had their roots in early life. I show how broader social structures sorted individuals into different training pathways by impacting how well they could "play the game" of getting into medical school, which, in turn, determined their opportunity structure within the profession as a whole. I also show that USMDs received far more professional support once they entered medical school, thanks to the "social contract"—an unspoken agreement that the profession would sponsor USMDs through their training toward elite careers.

In chapter 2, I scrutinize the residency recruitment process from the program directors' perspective. I find that segregation in graduate medical education is the result of complex decision-making processes that are deeply imbued with notions of merit, when, in reality, The Match was not an open competition. By contextualizing recruitment practices at these two hospitals within the broader field of residency programs, it becomes apparent that recruitment decisions—and their segregated outcomes—were at least partly shaped by the programs' social positions within that field and by their desire to maximize prestige while minimizing risk.

In the next two chapters, I investigate the impact of segregation on the residents' training. In chapter 3, I examine how approaches to medical education differed between the two hospitals. I find that Legacy's hands-off approach meant that residents were primarily viewed as *laborers* who were expected to get the job done first and then to attend to learning in their considerable spare time. In contrast, the supervisory structure at Stonewood meant that residents were first and foremost considered *trainees* who only secondarily worked for the hospital. I conclude that these differences in education had important implications for both the residents' training and patient care. In chapter 4, I examine how differences in professional development between the two programs can help explain why status hierarchies between USMDs and non-USMDs persist after residency. At Legacy, much of the residents' professional development was contingent upon them forging their own paths rather than upon the program structuring opportunities for them. I argue that this hands-off approach produced residents who were self-starters in some respects but more complacent in others, sometimes leading them to act unprofessionally. In contrast, professional development at Stonewood was an integral part of their approach to residents as trainees (the social contract in action). Thanks to its relative abundance of resources, Stonewood prioritized its residents' success, thereby producing residents who were more motivated but also more smug. In this way, I show that structural inequalities in residency training not only created differences in learning opportunities (chapter 3) but also led to different levels of professionalism. These differences contributed, in turn, to very different postresidency outcomes.

In chapter 5, I trace how USMDs secured choice positions after graduating from residency, thanks to longtime supportive structures that helped make them stronger residents. For their part, non-USMDs were typically excluded from those same positions, both because of differences in merit resulting from the structural inequalities in training and because of stigma and bias associated with their pedigree.

Finally, in chapter 6, I explore how residents made sense of status hierarchies between USMDs and non-USMDs. After examining the belief system underlying status separation within internal medicine, I find that USMDs believed they were more deserving of better opportunities and that non-USMDs often agreed with them—despite clear structural inequalities. Non-USMDs ended up consenting to lower-status positions not only because they feared being replaced by a reserve army of other qualified doctors but also because many believed they *deserved* lower-ranking positions in the profession.

I conclude by summarizing the findings from the previous chapters and offering possible future directions for research. I argue that USMDs rely on non-USMDs to fill less desirable positions within the profession, but in the absence of clear policies directing non-USMDs toward underserved populations and undesirable positions, the profession relies on—and reinforces—*informal* status hierarchies. I theorize about the process of status separation, which helps the US medical profession make good on its promises to USMDs, who have come to expect a certain return on their investment in a medical career. I further find that the absence of formal policies prioritizing USMDs helps secure consent among non-USMDs to fill lower-status positions because it allows for the persistence of American Dream–like beliefs in agency, such that with enough work and dedication, anything is possible. I finally conclude with implications for the medical profession and beyond.

CHAPTER 1

Meet the Residents

You have to start the path in high school, long before you ever should have been forced to decide what you want to do.

A USMD in their first postgraduate year

I t was a crisp autumn afternoon, with the leaves just starting to turn. I entered a large auditorium and took a seat toward the back among a bunch of undergraduates. The health careers advising department at a local university had invited the associate dean of admissions from a nearby medical school to talk about the admissions process. A thin, sprightly man with pointy facial features began to speak into a wireless microphone that continuously rubbed against his suit, producing unpleasant static. "How many of you are going into medicine because you think it's a really good job? C'mon, be honest." Hands started slowly rising as timid undergraduates grinned out of embarrassment. Predictably, the dean soon snapped them out of their reverie: "It's not! Medicine is actually not a good job! The hours are too long, the investment is too high," and he began rattling off reasons to avoid the profession. After a few minutes, however, he returned to his point: "It is a wonderful calling and if you hear that music, there's just no substitute for playing in that orchestra." He continued, "I'm not here to tell you how to apply or give you some magic formula. There's no divine truth." But a few seconds later he added, "The real trick of applying successfully is disclosing something unique about the individual you are."

He then asked the crowd to name some pieces of information that the admissions committee will have about applicants. Someone called out recommendation letters. Another said Medical College Admission Test (MCAT) scores. Someone else volunteered transcripts. The associate dean, now in full performance mode with eyes glinting and hands gesticulating, asked why the student had said transcripts and not grade point average (GPA). He entertained a few responses and then went on to answer his own question: "Have you made progress? We're interested in *trajectory*, the slope of the line—people who improve and grow with the challenges. We want to know a lot more about your academic trajectory than just your GPA." He elaborated: "Choice of major, how much does it matter? Three words: It. Doesn't. Matter! I don't give a damn what you studied; I care that you chose to commit your intellectual energy to something you're passionate about." He asked for more pieces of information. "Activities!" one student called out. The dean nodded: "Activities. You can list up to fifteen and identify the three most meaningful." He continued, "Good applicants tell us about their activities and what they learned about the world. *Great* applicants tell us about their activities and what they learned about themselves."

The associate dean concluded with two final requirements: clinical and research experience. "We need to see that you've cast yourself in the caring role," he trilled after asking students why clinical experience matters. "It's different from shadowing a doctor because you're taking an active role." The second thing is research: "Why do we care? . . . Teamwork! Research is an intensely demanding analytic process—sounds an awful lot like medicine!" Then, in what had become something of a call-and-response, the dean asked, "Does it matter what kind of research?" and the group replied in chorus, "I. Don't. Care." The dean nodded and added that clinical experience and research were not mandatory but that more than 80 percent of those in the current class had research experience and over 90 percent had done clinical work. The mean GPA for the class starting that fall of 2013 was 3.7, and the mean MCAT score was 34.5.[1]

While he may not have intended to set out a "magic formula" for getting into medical school, the associate dean, in essence, did exactly that by hitting on all the major requirements and reminding students that they ultimately have to set themselves apart from thousands of other applicants. This amounts to a process that residents called "playing the game," or checking off the required boxes to get into medical school, which eventually enables them to reach their desired specialty. A group of Stonewood University Hospital residents explained it to me one day:[2]

RESIDENT 1: It's really a pretty straightforward formula. It's just a long, long process. You could fit it all into a page: do well in high school, go to a good college, and then take the easy classes. I feel strongly about that. Your goal is to get a good GPA. [Take] a Kaplan course . . .

RESIDENT 2: Research.

RESIDENT 1: Yeah, research. Study a few months, bust your ass, and knock out a good MCAT score.

RESIDENT 2: Don't act like a douche bag on interviews.

RESIDENT 1: Exactly. Go to a third world country, and do some work.

RESIDENT 3: Yeah, do one thing that's kinda like crazy and . . .

RESIDENT 1: Set up a clinic somewhere in like Haiti or somewhere.

RESIDENT 4: Cure cancer.

RESIDENT 3: Cure cancer [laughs]. Well, it's easy!

Despite what the dean said about there not being a magic formula, these residents understood the game to be highly formulaic, suggesting a type of standardization in the application process: if you check off all the boxes, you'll get in. At the same time, applicants also knew they had to stand out. Successfully playing the game involved differentiating themselves from the rest—an increasingly difficult feat as the proportion of applicants accepted to US allopathic medical schools has steadily decreased from as high as 52.3 percent in 2002 to only 42.6 percent in 2018-2019.[3] In order to check off all those boxes *and* set themselves apart, these undergraduates had to start playing the game long before they sat down in that auditorium. As the epigraph at the beginning of this chapter suggests, the process often starts in high school or earlier, with advantages and disadvantages tending to accumulate over time.[4]

In this chapter, I examine the different trajectories of the residents at Stonewood and Legacy Hospitals and show how they played the game differently. To do so, I draw on two important concepts that will reappear throughout the book. The first has already been introduced: *playing the game*, or the process of gaining admission to medical school and eventually to residency and fellowship.[5] The game begins in early childhood, when ideally one becomes involved in projects and activities that are designed to open doors for the future and that offer early exposure to potential areas of interest. Early socioeconomic privilege associated with graduates of US allopathic medical schools (USMDs) puts them in a position to exercise "planful competence" and allows them to take advantage of further opportunities for support in college and beyond.[6] In this way, the game inherently favors those who are more privileged at the outset.[7]

Early life advantage is not the whole story, however—particularly for graduates of international medical schools, who generally come from very privileged backgrounds but still struggle to get into residency in the United States. Professional and institutional support matters greatly for residency applicants participating in The Match, and as will become clearer, USMDs enjoy far greater professional support in medical school (and beyond) than do non-USMDs of all stripes, making it easier for USMDs to play the game. This support forms a kind of unspoken structural advantage that is often misidentified as a difference in merit, when, in fact, USMDs often informally but systematically receive more help and face fewer barriers in playing the game.

This professional support is integral to the chapter's second key concept: what I call the *social contract* between the US medical profession and USMDs. This professional social contract should not be confused with medicine's social contract with society, whereby physicians are granted status, autonomy, and self-regulation in exchange for competency and altruism.[8] In this context, I define the professional social contract as the unspoken, yet socially agreed-upon inputs and outputs (or benefits) of pursuing an allopathic medical education in the United States. In other words, once individuals put in the work and money to gain admission to a US allopathic medical school, the profession helps ensure that they can attain their professional goals. Some even refer to it as a contract. In the words of one medical school official, "So there is this contract: we'll charge you a lot, but you'll get something out of it." Surprisingly few USMDs flunk out, with nearly 95 percent of matriculated allopathic medical students nationwide graduating within five years.[9] By comparison, nearly one-fifth of matriculated Ph.D. students drop out within five years, and almost 31 percent leave after ten years.[10] Of course, USMD students have undergone a highly selective process and are therefore unlikely to fail, but if and when they do struggle, additional supports (like educational specialists, formal remediation, and special dispensations) help them through. In the end, for the vast majority of USMDs, it is not about *whether* they will match to residency but *where*.[11]

The idea of a social contract among professionals, with its associated inputs and outputs, has its roots in classical sociological theory. In the 1940s, for example, Davis and Moore maintained that in order to be induced to perform certain duties, individuals had to be adequately rewarded—otherwise, no one would willingly choose the work. Regarding medicine in particular, they wrote: "Modern medicine . . . is within the mental capacity of most individuals, but a medical education is so burdensome and expensive that virtually none would undertake it if the position of the MD did not carry a reward commensurate with the sacrifice."[12] The considerable investment inherent to learning medicine therefore engenders expectations of comparably large rewards. Elsewhere, Davis and Moore refer to such rewards as the "*rights* associated with the position," suggesting that professionals come to expect these privileges and benefits as inalienable—much in the same way that USMDs have come to view residency as a *right* more than a privilege.[13] Similarly, Persell and Cookson have written about the "special social rights" afforded to the elite after graduating from elite schools, suggesting that such expected returns play an important role in the making of elites.[14]

To make good on its end of the bargain and deliver these rewards, the medical profession relies on informal sponsorship techniques that help ensure USMDs will become elites. As I mentioned in the introduction, elite status in medicine was historically transmitted via a sponsorship system, whereby new recruits were introduced to the profession by medical elites who inducted them into the "inner fraternity."[15] While the old sponsorship system was replaced by The Match—ostensibly leveling the playing field and replacing sponsored mobility with more meritocratic contest mobility, where "elite status is the prize in an open contest"[16]—I argue that elite reproduction still persists via the informal sponsorship inherent in the social contract, affording USMDs special "rights" or guarantees associated with admission to a US allopathic medical school.[17]

This same social contract, with all its inherent sponsorship, does not extend, however, to those medical students who took alternative paths of entry into the profession, either because they lacked many of the same early life advantages that USMDs had or because they trained in another country or tradition. These non-USMDs not only experience less support than USMDs but also have to contend with the professional stigma of being outsiders in a profession that firmly protects its elite inner core. Non-USMDs also espouse narratives that heavily emphasize agency over structure, which further reifies USMDs' rightful status as elites in the profession. Overall, the experience of these non-USMDs more closely resembles contest mobility, where, rather than benefiting from the buoyancy of informal sponsorship offered exclusively to insiders, they have to sink or swim on their own—a recurring theme for non-USMDs throughout the book.

This chapter traces the trajectories of the four types of medical graduates I studied at Stonewood and Legacy Hospitals (see table 1.1): graduates of US allopathic medical schools (USMDs), American graduates of international

TABLE 1.1 Types of Residents and Their Trajectories

Type of Graduate	Characteristics	Residency Program
Graduates of US allopathic medical schools (USMDs)	Strong support before, during, and after medical school	Stonewood
American graduates of international (usually Caribbean) medical schools (USIMGs)	Low support before, during, and after medical school	Legacy
Graduates of US osteopathic medical schools (DOs)	Mixed support before and during medical school; low support afterward	Legacy
Graduates of international medical schools (IMGs)	Strong support before and during medical school; low support afterward	Legacy

(usually Caribbean) medical schools (USIMGs), graduates of US osteopathic medical schools (DOs), and non-American graduates of international medical schools (IMGs). I present their trajectories separately to highlight how contingent they are on earlier life events and professional support/sponsorship. In so doing, I can reveal how USMDs reproduce their elite status by elevating those within their ranks and by expecting non-USMDs to perform just as well, if not better, with less support. In this way, I shed light on the structural headwinds and tailwinds that lead certain individuals toward certain types of medical schooling, residency programs, and, ultimately, statuses within the same profession.

THE US ALLOPATHIC MEDICAL SCHOOL GRADUATE

Early Life: Support from Parents

The USMDs who participated in this study were typically groomed for success from a very young age, thanks to their social backgrounds. Most came from upper-middle-class, white families and had university-educated parents. These parents had high expectations for their children, assuming they would reach similar levels of professional achievement. Even those USMDs who were born outside of the United States (many of whom were nonwhite) or who came from lower socioeconomic backgrounds were still raised in environments that strongly valued hard work and professional attainment and pushed them to thrive academically. Jack's parents, for example, were recent immigrants who worked odd jobs when they arrived in the United States. Even so, he said, "There was a lot expected from me academically. My mom always had me doing a lot of extracurricular activities, like additional homework," and she would often tell him that "you're gonna be a professional of some sort."

These USMDs also went to school in resource-rich environments with early access to opportunities. For example, a scholarship enabled Ken, a first-generation immigrant, to attend a private school that offered SAT prep courses, helping ensure that he would get into an elite college. Extracurriculars—known for being firmly rooted in social class[18]—also abounded among USMDs and included involvement in volunteer activities, job shadowing, student groups, and research. Long before many USMDs knew they even wanted to go to medical school, their parents and teachers made sure they were playing the game. Many USMDs came from families with the means and motivation to ensure they were well-rounded, like Dale, whose parents would drive him to emergency medical technician classes in the evenings and on weekends: "They were very supportive, and they pushed hard; they challenged me, in a way, to go with it." Sometimes these opportunities were built into the school curriculum, like for Gina, who got involved in biomedical research through a program at her public high school. Others pursued opportunities outside of school that often required considerable resources, like Meredith, whose parents enrolled her in a two-week summer National Youth Leadership Forum on Medicine, which is advertised as "an investment in personal growth and critical skills development that will prepare you for school, college and career success."[19] What it really amounted to was an investment in starting to play the game *early*, if only preemptively, and in nurturing those early indicators of drive and ambition that are so important to admissions committees.

Good guidance in high school also helped these USMDs learn the rules of the game soon enough that they could play it successfully. For Celeste, going to a guidance counselor and finding out the requirements for getting into medical school early was the "obvious" thing to do. She eventually pursued a combined seven-year undergraduate and medical degree right out of high school, allowing her to bypass the MCAT requirement altogether. By knowing how to play competitively early on, she and the six other USMDs I interviewed who pursued seven- or eight-year programs out of high school (roughly 10% of the sample) managed to sidestep an important hurdle—the MCAT—and almost immediately began enjoying the benefits of the social contract, with nearly guaranteed spots in the profession.

College Experience: Support from Peers, Guidance Counselors, and Social Networks

For some, the interest in medicine developed only in college. Several USMDs told me they became drawn to medicine by way of a passion for social change. Others did not know whether medicine was for them, but they knew to keep doors open. As Donald told me, "Freshman year, I signed up for a math class and an English class and a chemistry class just to get started on some of those prerequisites for medical school. . . . I wanted to keep the option open I guess." Keeping options open was a learned, and necessary, strategy for succeeding at the game, as it allowed for maximal (future) choice and minimal constraint. Importantly, it was also the careful product of being groomed for success at an early age—socialization that not everyone received equally.

Much of this socialization came from informal sources, like peers and acquaintances. In fact, a recent survey of matriculating USMDs found that nearly 80 percent of respondents received informal mentoring as an undergraduate.[20] But the degree to which applicants could enact this socialization and play the game successfully was largely contingent on access to other resources, including time. As Leon, a USMD in postgraduate year 2 (PGY-2), recounted:

> At the end of my first semester, there was a panel of students that had just been accepted to medical school and . . . the formula that they were describing to me was that it's not just the grades; it's everything else. These are the same people who are varsity athletes, who have their own businesses. . . . So I realized that you needed that complementary side to it, so I started doing it as much as I could outside of studying.

After that panel, Leon got involved in proteomics research on campus and started playing guitar, practicing karate, and doing international volunteer work during the summers—all of which he could do thanks to the resources (including information and time) at his disposal. Instead of having to work part-time or take care of family members, he could focus on "that complementary side" and take advantage of opportunities, like research, that were available to him on campus.[21]

USMDs also benefited greatly from formal on-campus premed counseling as a guide to playing the game. As one USMD put it, "You get a designated pre-med advisor in college who writes your recommendations, sort of makes sure you submit things on time, makes sure you have all the right things in order." Some elite schools even designate assistant deans and faculty members to assist pre-health career students with their applications. By the same token, a premed counselor could make or break one's application, especially because advisors were known to suggest alternative paths of entry to certain students (as I'll explain later for USIMGs and DOs). Hope described feeling confident about applying to medical school because she had the support of the premed committee:

> If they agree to support you in the application process, you are pretty much— I don't want to say guaranteed to get in—but the idea is that they want to keep it so that . . . they can say we have 100 percent admittance rate into medical school, so they're not going to support an application unless they think that that person is going to get in. So I had full support so I kind of knew [I'd get in].

Premed counselors therefore served as critical gatekeepers, helping students who already showed promise at playing the game succeed even further while steering other students, some of whom perhaps did not have the same early supports in playing the game, toward alternative paths into the profession.

Good guidance was important, but USMDs still had to complete the requirements before applying to medical school. As with most things, they had help. Many studied for the MCAT using expensive prep courses offered by companies like Kaplan and the Princeton Review, with basic packages starting over $1,800.[22] Like the premed counselors, these programs provided the discipline and support needed to succeed on the exam. As Morgan explained, "You just do what they [Kaplan] tell you to." Being able to pay for expensive prep courses gave those applicants a leg up when it came to the MCAT, which many considered the single most rate-limiting step for getting into medical school.

Whenever possible, USMDs also drew on their (or their family's) social networks to help with the applications process. Hope, for example, asked a family friend who was on the medical school's board of directors to make a phone call on her behalf. She admitted, "I don't like telling people because it makes me feel like maybe I wouldn't have gotten in on my own, which I know isn't true." In this way, USMDs mobilized every resource at their disposal to play the game successfully.

While 48 percent of the USMDs I interviewed had gone straight to medical school, another 40 percent took time off to improve their résumés or change careers altogether. Some were wait-listed—or rejected outright—and had to reapply multiple times before gaining admission. Several pursued one- or two-year postbaccalaureate programs to complete the required coursework or improve their academic record. Some postbaccalaureate programs also had linkages to medical schools. Postbaccalaureates were a big help in playing the game; those who could afford the steep tuition also benefited from "wraparound support," including MCAT help, advising, and volunteer opportunities.[23] Regardless of the route they took, USMDs generally had the resources—money, time, and social support—to get the help they needed to try again until they succeeded.

Applying to Medical School: Momentum in the Game and the Runaway Freight Train Especially for those who applied to medical school right after completing their undergraduate degree, every step in the application process—from getting good grades to scoring well on the MCAT to getting involved in extracurricular or research activities—was taken deliberately. Each applicant's goal was to both check off those boxes in the formula *and* set themselves apart from thousands of other applicants, which was the "real trick" for getting into medical school according to the associate dean. Those who played the game exceptionally well described an accumulation of momentum, such that after having opened the necessary doors early on, they could simply coast through when the time came. Barbara, who was accepted to an accelerated six-year BS/MD program straight out of high school, told me that after completing undergrad, "[medicine] wasn't this calling; it wasn't like this was what I've always wanted to do all my life. It just seemed like an appropriate next step."[24]

Barbara's experience was not common, however; more often, applicants reported having to work very hard to get that momentum going. As Collette observed, "If you don't start taking your Chem 101 the first semester of your freshman year, it is going to be very difficult to get everything in by the time you graduate. So you almost have to have an idea that 'I want to do medicine' right

when you come into undergrad. . . . That's part of the mindset of 'just in case.'"
For some, the timing and pressure of the game were too much to bear. Hope, for
example, took a year off to cool down. For others, the momentum described by
Barbara felt more like "a runaway freight train." After getting accepted to a top
medical school, McKayla reacted: "'Oh fuck!' . . . I was just trying to do my best
and see where I'd end up! And then I was like on this whole treadmill where you
couldn't get off." Once you started playing the game (successfully), it was hard to
turn back.

The corollary to the runaway freight train analogy is that once someone gets
into a US allopathic medical school, they are in. Their path is set. Admission
thus represents a critical inflection point in the profession's social contract with
USMDs. As Kyle explained, "Once you get into med school, you can be reasonably sure that if you keep working, you're going to make it through." Unlike
contest mobility, which "tends to delay the final award as long as practicable to
permit a fair race," as Turner puts it, "sponsored mobility tends to place the time
of recruitment as early in life as practicable to insure control over selection and
training."[25] In this way, the "reward" of elite professional status came as early as
admission to medical school for USMDs, when early life support was parlayed
into professional sponsorship. As several residents told me, the hardest part was
getting into medical school. It mattered less how one got there; once inside, the
past had a way of becoming somewhat less important.

Chloe's story is emblematic in this regard. An avid flautist in high school,
she decided late to apply to college after setting aside her dream of becoming
a professional musician. She first went to community college and then transferred
to a four-year college. "Everyone was like, [community college is] the thirteenth
grade and all that kind of stuff." Despite her peers' reactions, she worked hard to
complete her undergraduate degree in four years even though she was a transfer
student. She still struggled with certain elements of the game: her MCAT score
was lower than she would have liked, and her extracurriculars were "the bare
minimum." Even her premed advisor tried to guide her toward DO school:
"He was like, 'Take the MCAT again, take a year off, or [go to] DO school.'"

She ended up applying to MD schools anyway but got many rejections. One
dean of admissions told her, "'Your grades are good, but I can't weigh the A in
chemistry 101 . . . from [a community college] as the same from [a four-year college].'"
When I asked whether the course was a valid prerequisite, Chloe nodded. "Yes, and
it transferred over [from community college], but [the dean said], 'The quality of

the education, the testing, I can't in my book weigh them equally.' " After many rejections, Chloe was eventually accepted to a medical school in the West Indies. But very late in the season, she got an interview at a US allopathic school:

> They were one of those med schools that accepted people with different paths. . . . Not too many people but you would have to have something cool to balance that out. Even *they* have their standards. Had I not been a flautist, they probably wouldn't have taken me. Was I an *active* flautist? No. Did I say that? No. I mean, it's sad but it's true. But at the same time, they were able to look past even a 27 in the MCAT.[26]

Chloe was eventually admitted to that medical school and thrived, ranking at the top of her class. She went on to become a member of the faculty at Stonewood.

Her story captures how getting into a US allopathic medical school represents a key inflection point in the social contract. Despite her struggles, once she was admitted, her trajectory—which had come very close to being that of a Caribbean graduate—changed dramatically, opening opportunities that would have otherwise been inaccessible, like a residency at Stonewood.[27] By getting accepted to a US allopathic medical school, Chloe successfully fulfilled her end of the social contract; now she could reap rewards that would have otherwise been off-limits.

Unlike Chloe, however, few USMDs said they had considered applying to Caribbean or osteopathic schools as a possible plan B. In fact, most fervently advocated against those options when asked what advice they would give to someone who was not admitted to a US allopathic medical school the first time around. Many USMDs shared the common sentiment that attending Caribbean or osteopathic schools was almost a form of cheating—a shortcut that made those who went that route less meritorious because those schools were easier to get into and sometimes did not require the MCAT (see chapter 6 for more on this perspective). This unworthiness, coupled with the knowledge that it would be tougher to match into residency coming from a Caribbean or a DO school, made these alternative paths of entry into the profession especially loathsome to individuals who had, for the most part, been dutifully "opening doors" for decades.

Instead, a surprising proportion (almost 50 percent) of the USMDs I interviewed told me they would have quit medicine altogether if they had not been accepted to medical school the first time around. One USMD shrugged and said, "I remember being like, 'Oh maybe if it doesn't happen, it's just not meant to be.'" While it is impossible to know for sure what these USMDs would have actually done in that situation, their responses suggest there was a lower degree of intrinsic motivation for studying medicine among USMDs compared to other types of medical graduates, many of whom, as I will describe later, viewed medicine as the only thing they ever wanted to do. It also speaks to the ease with which some USMDs could have pivoted to other careers, given how portable embodied cultural capital can be across fields.[28]

Medical School Experience: Support from the Profession

Despite the years of preparation, medical school was still an adjustment for most USMDs. Many likened it to drinking from a gushing fire hydrant of information.[29] However, US allopathic schools did not weed out those who struggled; rather, they helped keep them on track. At Sabrina's school, for example, there was someone with a PhD in education to help students learn how to study. At Zara's school, second-year students would pass on their books to incoming first-year students and check up on them after every exam. USMDs thus benefited from extensive institutional support that helped them get through their medical education—early evidence of the informal sponsorship efforts that allowed the profession to make good on its social contract with USMDs.

At the end of the first two years came the US Medical Licensing Examination (USMLE) Step 1, the first of three examinations that all MDs in the United States must pass to be licensed. USMDs viewed Step 1 as the "great equalizer" because it was an ostensibly objective measure that could be used to mete out residency opportunities. It was also the only data point that was consistently available for all applicants before interview season. As Shelly put it, "[Residency programs] are going to look at that and use it as a way to equate everybody." For those who were undecided about a specialty, Step 1 was again about keeping open as many options as possible. Cassandra, who scored above the 90th percentile on the exam, recounted, "It was really for me more about leaving the door open 'cause I didn't know what I wanted to do yet. . . . We've been taught to leave doors open our whole life, to put a lot of pressure on ourselves. It's not so much what *should* you do—it's what *can* you do."[30] Playing the game thus instilled this pernicious habit of always trying to reach the "top"—which usually involved some form of competitive subspecialty—and constrained those who "just" wanted to do primary care. Women in my interviews were notably more affected by this dilemma, suggesting that gender may complicate the game for female physicians, who traditionally have had to work harder to overcome bias in the profession.[31]

But despite the considerable weight placed on Step 1 (and despite the beliefs about its equalizing power), the stakes were categorically different for USMDs than for non-USMDs, who had to perform extraordinarily well on these exams to match. For most USMDs, simply *passing* Step 1 was essential for getting into an internal medicine residency.[32] One USMD who scored exactly the average shared that "my advisor told me . . . [my score] was good enough, that I wouldn't be excluded from any [internal medicine] residency." USMDs knew they were all but guaranteed a residency position—especially in internal medicine, a relatively uncompetitive specialty—through the unspoken terms of the social contract. In 2019, 93.9 percent of USMD applicants nationwide successfully matched to a residency position (up from an average of 93.4 percent between 1982 and 2018).[33] As one USMD put it, "I mean, for all intents and purposes, once you get into med school you're pretty much assured a residency unless you really screwed things up." Step 1 simply determined where and in what specialty it would be.

They did have to pass, however. When USMDs struggled, most medical schools once again came to their aid by offering prep courses, scheduling advice, and even providing special dispensations—further evidence of the social contract in action. Everything possible was done to keep them on track, and when that failed, personal resources came to the rescue. Greg's story offers a good example: although he failed Step 1 on the first try, his university allowed him to pursue his third-year clerkships as scheduled (while USIMGs were required to pass Step 1 before starting rotations) and offered him time off at the end of the third year to retake Step 1. This time he was not going to take any chances:

> I got in my Toyota Corolla, I drove to Champaign, Illinois, and I went to "Boot Camp for Step 1." . . . It's a place for all of us to isolate [ourselves] in the middle of nowhere and study with a [new] approach to the test. I never knew how to take a test. . . . You had to talk through the questions out loud for an hour three times a week with a tutor. You took practice tests on the weekends and you studied twelve hours a day.

Greg paid $5,000 for four weeks in the guaranteed PASS Program and spent a total of seven weeks studying to retake Step 1.[34] On his second try, he passed with a score that was thirty points higher than his original score but still well below the average. His experience illustrates not only how different the stakes of Step 1 were for USMDs (failing a Step exam would likely have been fatal to the medical career of a non-USMD) but also the degree to which USMDs had the personal, professional, and institutional resources to stay on track.

Applying to Residency: A "Buyer's Market"

Almost all the USMDs I interviewed ended up in internal medicine by *choice* rather than constraint.[35] Many were drawn to the field's cerebral approach. A few especially appreciated that internal medicine kept the door open to subspecialty. And perhaps because it is the residency with the largest number of spots, almost all USMDs described their experience applying to internal medicine residency programs as being "much easier than applying for medical school." The process was exhilarating. For the first time, programs were trying to recruit *them* rather than the other way around. As Gary explained:

> We were kind of ingrained that applying to [internal] medicine was easy. This was a buyer's market—as in, you're an American [allopathic] medical student; odds are you will definitely match somewhere and probably you know at a decent academic [center]. So that thought process was a complete 180 from what I heard when I was an undergrad applying to med school. . . . For me it was just so interesting to have interviews, to be kind of like a hot commodity.

Here Gary emphasized how being a USMD once again represented a critical juncture—"a complete 180"—in playing the game. While applying for residency, he could now reap the benefits of the social contract as a USMD, knowing that he was likely to "definitely match somewhere and probably . . . at a decent academic [center]." To be sure, certain ultraelite options (like Johns Hopkins or Stanford) were probably more likely to be destinations for graduates from top-tier medical schools—evidence that the professional social contract varied somewhat among USMDs from different caliber schools—but for virtually all USMDs, the question was *where*, not *whether*, they would match. As will become clearer in the next chapter, the distinction between USMDs and non-USMDs was far more consequential for residency program directors than any distinctions among USMDs themselves.

USMDs did not apply indiscriminately to residency programs, however. They often received clear guidance about which programs to avoid, including community hospital programs.[36] Ken, for example, described the advice he received from his mentor (a USMD): "So I showed her my list, and she immediately started crossing names off. She was like, 'You don't want to go to UConn [University of Connecticut]; you don't want to go to Bridgeport'—she started crossing them out. . . . A lot of the residents [there] were foreign. Some of them were DOs, same thing for Bridgeport, same thing for Westchester. . . . I think she knew what she was doing." This type of guidance, which promotes a great deal of segregation in training programs, is yet another example of the informal sponsorship that facilitates USMD elite reproduction and enables professional leaders to deliver on their promises to USMD trainees.

Many USMDs told me they were influenced by advisors who told them to avoid applying to programs with high percentages of non-USMDs because this was taken to be a negative indicator regarding the quality of the program. USMDs also strongly preferred university hospitals because they were perceived as more rigorous: "It's just when you have your pick, you might as well be picky," Chloe reasoned. Going to community programs for residency would have also countered the long-standing drive inculcated within USMDs to aim high and keep doors open, so even if they preferred smaller community environments, these were anathema to the very mindset that got them into medical school.[37] Ted, a USMD at Stonewood who matched into a competitive fellowship, explained that by doing a community-based residency, "obviously, you put yourself in a bit of a difficult situation—limiting your options again—because you do make it more difficult to apply for fellowships. Again not impossible, but. . . . " Importantly, both he and Chloe emphasized *agency*, making comments like "when you have *your pick*" and "those who *choose* community programs *put themselves* in a difficult situation when applying for fellowships." These perspectives, however, obscure the structural constraints that prevent many lower-status applicants, like non-USMDs, from "choosing" university-based residencies and that seem to hold them responsible for being unable to achieve the same outcomes in fellowships as USMDs. This belief, in turn, strengthens the elites' perception that their achievements are the product of individual effort rather than systemic advantages designed to ensure their success.[38]

Why Stonewood? Just as with internal medicine, almost every USMD chose Stonewood as either their first or their second choice for residency—not as a fallback option. They were drawn to the program's prestige, friendly personnel, and wide variety of elective tracks. The support they received along the way made it possible for them to choose a place like Stonewood among several other viable alternatives.

Greg's experience, once again, is telling. After failing Step 1 the first time and scoring below the average the second time, he struggled with residency applications. But he was persistent; he played the game effectively by putting in what he called "face time" at Stonewood, doing elective rotations there before applying—a somewhat unusual practice for USMDs, who, unlike non-USMDs, did not have to establish themselves as "known quantities":

> I didn't think I was going to get an interview. I kept calling. So I was "the caller." . . . That's how I got an interview. I kept calling [the coordinator] and telling him how much I loved it here and if I could get an interview, it would be my first choice because I loved it. . . . I told him what it meant to me. He could tell. He was from [the same state as me] so we had [that] connection.

Clearly, elements of both luck and strategy allowed Greg to get his foot in the door at Stonewood, and once he finally was given an interview, his luck continued: "I was interviewed by [an attending who] had failed his [specialty] Boards. So we totally talked about that and how we were not test takers." When I asked Greg how he broached the topic of his failed Step 1 exam, he explained that he did exactly as his mentors had suggested: "Actually *I* brought it up. . . . I wanted to show that it became a strength, you know learning to fail, that I can relate to so many people now." He later found out that before deciding to accept him, the program director called the professor Greg had worked with while putting in "face time" at Stonewood.

When I asked Greg how he made sense of his trajectory into residency at Stonewood, he replied:

> There's no question I had a lot of help getting in. . . . It wasn't just me fighting; this was like *lots* of people on my side. . . . If I didn't have that encouragement, I wouldn't have had the courage to do it really. So it's hard to think about [that support that is] so entrenched in it. And I think I would have been super happy being a gym teacher or elementary school teacher.

Without that support, Greg, by his own admission, probably could not have gone to medical school, much less become a resident at a prestigious institution like Stonewood. This was the pivotal difference between USMDs and everyone else; they were not necessarily smarter or more motivated, but they received the pushes, breaks, and resources they needed along the way to make it to where they wanted to go—from early life into medical school and beyond.

THE CARIBBEAN MEDICAL SCHOOL GRADUATE

Early Life: Humble Beginnings

Compared to USMDs, the majority of Caribbean medical school graduates at Legacy came from more modest backgrounds, which meant their families were less able to offer the same kind of early support that can translate into future opportunities.[39] Around a third were first-generation immigrants to the United States. The rest were born and raised in the United States, with fathers working mostly blue-collar jobs as dry cleaners, contractors, or telephone repairmen and mothers serving as homemakers, nurses, or day care owners. A handful had parents who were physicians, but a much larger percentage of these USIMGs were first-generation college graduates who "didn't really get a lot of pushes," as Adrian put it:

> No one sat down and did homework with me. No, my mom didn't go to PTA meetings; she didn't know about that stuff. I was like lost to everything through high school. . . . A lot of people that I knew who were ahead in the middle and high school stuff, their parents just did a lot for them. Now that's a lot of nurturing.

Adrian recognized the importance of early support and encouragement from parents. Without it, he felt "lost to everything" through high school, which he felt put him at a disadvantage. His experience was quite different from that of the USMDs whose parents drove them to first-aid classes and enrolled them in leadership forums. He was mostly on his own.

Several Caribbean graduates like Adrian developed an early interest in medicine—often in high school—but many of them lacked a plan or the support to pursue that goal from an early age. Harvey told me, "In high school? I had no idea [about how to become a doctor]. . . . I didn't research those things." A few volunteered during high school, but most were just focused on the next immediate step: getting into college.

College Experience: Tracking and Constraints

Despite their more modest upbringings, some Caribbean graduates found a way to attend relatively selective four-year colleges, like the State University of New York, Notre Dame, and Bates. Others, like Adrian, started with community college: "I kind of always wanted to be a doctor, but I didn't think that far ahead," he said, defending his choice of school. Like Chloe (the flautist who was eventually admitted to a US medical school), Adrian was able to transfer successfully into a four-year bachelor's program after a brief stint in community college.

Others opted first for paramedical professions like pharmacy or chiropractic instead of pursuing the MD route right away, in part because some of them lacked the cultural or social capital to aspire to medical school. Consider how Clark, a first-generation immigrant and college graduate, wound up becoming a nurse practitioner (NP):

> I knew I wanted to do something in the medical industry; I wasn't sure what it was. . . . So I went to the local college . . . and I was speaking to an advisor and I told her, "Yeah, I'm interested in being a paramedic, firefighter; you know, I think I like that kind of stuff." And for some reason she said, "Why don't you become a nurse practitioner?" . . . I didn't know what a nurse practitioner was; I'm like, "What is that?" So she gave me some brochures. . . . So I ended up applying to NP school, and I also applied for DO school 'cause I decided, what the heck, why don't I just become a doctor, you know? So I said let's see what happens. The [NP] school granted me the interview first. They really liked me, I liked the school, and I ended up doing that.
>
> [Tania: Were you advised to apply to MD programs?]
>
> Not really. I pretty much did all this on my own 'cause you have to understand, my parents were educated but they weren't *college*-educated. So their aspirations weren't . . . their parents didn't encourage them to go to school, so naturally they don't have that aspiration for their kids either. . . . So all this additional stuff was kind of on my own and I was trying to guide myself.

Tellingly, Clark accounted for his decision to apply only to NP and DO schools by alluding to his family's lower educational attainment and by mentioning how his advisor nudged him toward certain paths. His career planning until that point had been limited, and his aspirations were restricted to those options he was familiar with, like firefighting. His experience was nothing like that of the many USMDs who had been groomed from early childhood to be aware of their options and keep the doors open to get there.

Applying to Medical School: An Uphill Battle

Partly due to their lack of information and support, many USIMGs did not start playing the game as early as USMDs did, which often made for lower grades in college and lower MCAT scores. It also meant fewer of those all-important "meaningful" activities, as the associate dean put it at the beginning of this chapter. Ralph learned this the hard way. He was an atypical Caribbean graduate in that his mother was a medical professional, which helped him land a research assistantship at a hospital one summer. His involvement in varsity sports, however, kept him from dedicating himself wholly to his schoolwork. Sitting in a family room at Legacy one afternoon, Ralph sighed:

> Because I was playing sports all the time, in terms of med school, I was always behind. If you want to go to medical school in the United States, you have to have straight As. You have to have pretty good service; you have to have some element of research. Because there are so many kids who want to do it that they are always looking for something *extra*, because a lot of kids get straight As nowadays, but the difference in somebody's application is the extracurricular activities. . . . So when it was time to apply for med school, I didn't have any of that. The only extracurriculars I had were sports.
>   [TANIA: What about that summer research opportunity?]
>   I had that *one* research gig, but that's not enough. You need more. You're always trying to be better than your competition. It's just like anything in this world. So in that way I was behind the eight ball. I didn't have any of that stuff. . . . There was always research at [my] college too, and I could have done that, but I didn't. [*He goes on to tell me about his younger sister, who was recently admitted to a US medical school.*] If you look at [my résumé] compared to my sister's? Going into medical school, hers was significantly more filled out than mine.

[TANIA: Did she decide earlier on to pursue medicine?]

Yeah, she did. See she did. Oh, it's a huge game, just like with anything. You know, just like getting into residency is a game, and getting into medical school is a game too. And she played it very well. . . . She had the benefit of seeing two older brothers go through it, . . . she knew what was required of her.

Although Ralph had more support than most USIMGs, with a parent in the profession who helped him secure research experience, his story is emblematic of the Caribbean graduate who got a late start playing the game. By his own admission, had he decided to pursue medicine earlier or had he known more about the process like his sister did, he might have made different choices. For these reasons, Ralph was differently situated than other Caribbean graduates like Adrian and Clark—both first-generation college graduates who got a late start because they lacked the resources to play the game strategically. But even *with* those resources, Ralph's experience underlines just how unforgiving the game can be if it is not played in exactly the right way. Ralph was not lazy or undetermined; instead, he dedicated himself to sports in college, which yielded fewer benefits in the game than other activities did. As a result, he was constantly behind others who had strategically begun doing those all-important extracurricular activities from a young age.

This left many applicants at a crossroads: either take more time off to improve their résumé or bypass the game altogether by going the Caribbean route.[40] Most chose the latter—but not necessarily by default or because they had already been rejected by stateside medical schools. About half exclusively targeted offshore schools in their first round of applications. This was especially true of those who had previously worked as paramedical professionals and wanted their prior training to count toward their medical schooling, an advantage offered by several Caribbean schools. Others thought it made financial sense to avoid "the gamble" of applying to stateside medical schools and instead focused on Caribbean options, which were more of a sure thing.[41]

Among those for whom offshore schooling was a backup plan, the decision usually revolved around saving time and/or money. Consider Freddie's story:

I applied to a bunch of American places, at least fifty probably, I guess. . . . It's stressful; I mean it's so competitive. And if you end up having a bad run in a class or something, then it screws you because it just knocks down your GPA, and at that point in time I was young, and I didn't think it mattered and you realize after the fact. . . . So, once I started hearing back a lot of no's [rejections], I said, okay, I either have to figure out what I'm going to do for the next year to give me a better [chance] or just make the plunge. . . . You know, do I take the MCAT a third time? No, I wasn't going to do it 'cause it's time-consuming, it's money-consuming. So I said, okay, screw it. I applied to five of the better [Caribbean] places, and then I started hearing back from those, and I was like, well, I have an option now.

Freddie's story once again highlights the degree of foresight the game requires, as well as how unforgiving the game can be to those without it. It also highlights the critical decision made by many Caribbean grads to either take more time off or go abroad to become a doctor. For many, the desire to practice medicine was more important than the stigma they knew they would face by taking what was seen as a back door into the profession. As Ivy explained, "I knew . . . there would be programs that, when they saw my school, would just toss out my application right away. [But] this is what I wanted to do so badly. . . . I knew this is what I wanted to do, and this is the way I was going to get it done and so I just did it." Ivy's comments highlight just how motivated she was to enter medicine. This represents an important difference in intrinsic motivation between Caribbean graduates like Ivy and USMDs, several of whom said they would have preferred to pursue a different career altogether than to go the Caribbean route.

Medical School Experience: Geographic and Professional Isolation

Once on the islands, Caribbean graduates received far less support in medical school than USMDs did. First, there was the immense isolation of being far away from the usual conveniences and social supports. "It was pretty awful. No, really, it's kind of a hellish place to live," one graduate stated, adding that the paradisiacal nature of the Caribbean wore off rather quickly. Another told me that "at any moment, the running water could go out for no reason, and you could be without it for three hours or for two days; you just didn't know." Then there were the high rates of attrition. Graduates typically spent two years attending classes on the island and then two clinical years doing rotations in the United States. During the first two years, however, up to 50 percent of the students would drop out, depending on the school, such that whatever social support students managed to establish was at risk of dissolving by the week.

Ironically, despite being referred to pejoratively as "backdoor" entryways into the profession,[42] Caribbean schools, with their high attrition rates, are actually most typical of *contest* mobility, which is often considered more meritocratic, as "only a minority of entrants achieve the prize of graduation."[43] In contrast, for all their selectivity and competitiveness, USMD schools are excellent examples of *sponsored* mobility, where elite "selection is supposed to be relatively complete *before* entrance to university" or, in this case, medical school, with roughly 94 percent of matriculants graduating and matching to residency afterward. Yet USMDs were consistently viewed as more deserving and meritorious than Caribbean graduates. Critics point to the alarming attrition rates as bellwethers of quality for Caribbean schools—and their enrollees—but they often ignore the overwhelming odds that successful Caribbean graduates have to overcome in order to match to residency, particularly given how little institutional support they have during medical school.[44]

For example, Caribbean students typically had little to no clinical or research exposure during the first two years. Some USIMGs, like Adrian, believed it was up to the students to surmount these institutional deficiencies: "It would have been great to be at a medical school where your professors are actual doctors in the hospital and they are bringing cases and relating the basic sciences to a case. . . . But they provide you with the information you need to know." Students can succeed, he insisted, "if [they] study, if [they] put the work in and seek out the people who do have experience and ask, well, 'How do I relate this with this? What is important here?'" However, in almost the same breath, Adrian also acknowledged how much easier USMDs had it:

> When you compare it to a US school, they only take a certain amount of spots; they've got 100 seats or 120 seats; they want to keep them filled. That's their roster of people; that's their income, their tuition if you want to look at it like that. They want to do what it takes to keep you. If they see that a student is waning on their grades and they are barely making it, they are going to sign you up for a tutor, they are going to have people come after you. Whereas at an institution that will take a lot of people and the attrition rate is 40 or 50 percent, they figure they can lose a few, you know?

Indeed, therein lay a fundamental difference between USMDs and USIMGs; in the Caribbean, nothing was guaranteed, and success was incumbent on the individual. USMDs, in contrast, were nearly guaranteed safe passage through medical school—thanks to the support and resources offered by those in the profession who did what it took to "keep" them.

When it came time to take the first licensing exam (USMLE Step 1), Caribbean graduates once again found themselves on their own with little help from their medical schools. There were few prep courses like at US institutions and no special arrangements if someone failed (like in Greg's case described earlier). Cameron told me, with some of the old anxiety still visible in his eyes, "So every year you are talking close to $90,000 in racking up debt. So there is a lot of pressure and if you fail this, if you fail that, you know you are screwed . . . and you have to do so well on your USMLEs. So I took all of that to heart." The stakes therefore were high, both financially and professionally. While USMDs were simply required to *pass* their USMLEs to get into prestigious internal medicine programs like Stonewood, USIMGs knew they had to score significantly higher to get into less desirable programs.[45] If they failed to match, their hefty investment in medical school would be for naught.

USIMGs also had a harder time during their third- and fourth-year clinical rotations in the United States, partly because many of their medical schools did not have clinical campuses like US schools did. Some had to pay out-of-pocket for elective rotations. Others had to set up their own rotations without the help of the medical school clerkship coordinators that were available to USMDs. A few even had to rotate at multiple sites across the country, like one graduate who rotated at no fewer than seven hospitals over two years.

Caribbean medical students typically rotated at community hospitals alongside other international or osteopathic students. The few who rotated in mixed settings with USMDs, however, felt judged because of their pedigree. As Allan put it, "They kinda look down on you a little bit. . . . You could tell that there was a difference in the amount of attention that [attending physicians] gave you [as a Caribbean graduate]." Adrian felt he had to defend his right even to be there:

> I heard some guy say to his attending, "These [Caribbean] guys come in and they take our rotations." It's not true because we don't take their rotations, but there is like a sense of [entitlement on behalf of USMDs]. . . . *I* have to fight to get these rotations. *I* have to call program directors from every

hospital to set these things up. *I* have to kill myself while you got it good. But at the same time, they put themselves in a position to have an easier time than me. I set myself up to have a harder path, y'know? (emphasis in original)

Adrian's comments highlight how much harder USIMGs had to work to get the same rotations as USMDs. Several Caribbean graduates pointed out that their training was similar to that of USMDs because they did their clinical rotations in the United States. Many of them took the same National Board of Medical Examiners (NBME) exams as their US-trained counterparts, and some of them rotated at the same hospitals. Yet they still held themselves responsible for having a harder path. That extra work, they reasoned, was the cost of going to the Caribbean.

To sum up, Caribbean graduates often had to navigate more uncertain career trajectories with less help than USMDs received, ending up in stigmatized "backdoor" entryway schools with predatory admissions policies and considerably less institutional support. By almost all accounts, they had to do more with less to get into residency, as is typical of contest mobility, but they consistently blamed themselves for their lot, readily buying into the myth that USMDs were better because they had worked harder—a myth that handily justified USMDs' elite status while obscuring the systematic advantages that all but guaranteed that status.

Applying to Residency: Constraint Over Choice

Most USIMGs I spoke to ended up in internal medicine, although less by choice than by constraint. First, unlike USMDs, USIMGs were far from guaranteed that they would match into residency, with only 59 percent of these applicants securing positions in 2019 (up from an average of 50.6 percent from 1982 to 2017).[46] Second, USIMGs understood certain competitive residencies to be almost off-limits, particularly the "ROAD to Success" specialties: Radiology, Ophthalmology, Anesthesia, and Dermatology. "The things that are easy to get," Georgina explained, "are internal medicine, psychiatry; OB-GYN [is] hit or miss, but you can get it."[47] Despite these limitations, however, several USIMGs believed that nothing was impossible if they worked hard enough. Harvey explained that to match into a field "like ophthalmology . . . [y]ou're going to [have to] be top of your class, do tons of research in medical school from the very beginning and

maybe know someone. . . . That's how you get something more competitive."
The stigma of a Caribbean medical degree, it seemed, could be managed with
the right amount of effort.

Working hard had its limits, however, in light of the considerable structural
barriers facing USIMGs. Consider Allan's experience with anesthesia:

> See, the thing is they didn't really have an anesthesia residency program where
> I [rotated]. It was a community-based program, but I worked with this young
> anesthesiologist who just graduated and he started working in the area. And
> I had to rotate with him; he taught me a lot. I got pretty good at it, so I did
> a few more rotations elsewhere, and I impressed everywhere I went. But my
> grades weren't good enough to get into an anesthesia program, you know,
> which was a shame.
>
> [TANIA: But you said earlier that you graduated with the highest honors?]
>
> Yeah, but still, the highest honors from [the Caribbean] unfortunately still
> is not good enough in a lot of places.

Despite earning the highest honors at his school, Allan could not help the fact
that his rotations were at community hospitals without anesthesiology residency
programs instead of at university programs where he could have caught the eye of
a program director. That structural reality, combined with the stigma of studying
in the Caribbean, meant that he would probably never be deemed as good as a
USMD, no matter how high his grades were.

Many USIMGs therefore strategically selected out of competitive residencies
and ended up in internal medicine because it was more feasible. This meant,
however, that more than one Caribbean graduate had to relinquish their dream
of becoming a surgeon, radiologist, or anesthesiologist. Harvey, like Allan, also
had a strong interest in anesthesiology but was unable to match. "So I felt like I
made the right choice in the end," he said about ending up at Legacy, his third-
choice program. "Even though I feel like my heart was with anesthesiology.
I really loved it. . . . I probably should have done better [in school]." Harvey
blamed himself for not getting the scores needed to get into anesthesiology, but,
interestingly, he referred to having made the right *choice* to pursue internal medicine. In this way, Caribbean graduates repeatedly invoked "choice" and (over)
emphasized agency, rather than underscoring the constraints they faced, when
making sense of their residency positions—much like the USMDs who were

quoted earlier discussing fellowship options for those who "choose" community training programs.

Why Legacy? Knowing they faced an uphill battle, most Caribbean graduates didn't bother applying to "unfriendly" programs (like Stonewood) that had few international graduates on the housestaff. As Ralph told me, "I applied to programs that I knew I could get into," which typically meant community hospitals. But he also added, "Because I went to a Caribbean medical school, I applied everywhere." USIMGs applied to anywhere between 40 and 250 programs—far more than USMDs, who usually limited themselves to 10–15 places.[48]

Legacy was a safer bet for Caribbean grads. But like the selection of internal medicine, the decision to apply to Legacy was more the result of constraint than choice. As respondents explained, it was difficult to *choose* something when there were few or no other options on the table. Most Caribbean graduates prematched into Legacy (meaning they were offered a binding contract before The Match), which at least guaranteed them a residency position, even if it wasn't the one they really wanted.[49] Adrian's story once again is telling in this regard. He initially wanted to pursue surgery:

> I was supposed to do a formal interview [at a surgical program] late in the season because they interview only US[MD] students. I was going to be their only Caribbean student. I had a big talk with the chief of surgery, and . . . he said, "If you don't have something [special]. . . . These guys, our US students, *they have worked all their life*; they're doing research; they're going to teach me stuff. What are you going to teach me?" I said, "Honestly, I don't know what I'm going to teach you, but this is what I want to do; this is what I picture myself doing. I love being in the OR." He talked for most of the time and said, "We don't prematch. I think we can set you up with a preliminary [one-year] spot, and you can earn a way into a categorical [five-year] position." . . . At the same time, I was debating about the whole marriage/family thing, and I came [to interview at Legacy]. It seemed good. I was exploring my options. [Legacy] offered me the prematch. I had to sign it by December, before I could do my official interview [at the surgical program]. I took [the prematch], and it took me off the market. A bird in the hand is worth a hundred in the bush, especially if that hundred in the bush isn't something you're sure you want to do anymore. (emphasis added)

Like other USIMGs, Adrian ended up choosing the certainty of a prematch offer at a less prestigious program over the risk of not matching into a more prestigious specialty or program. But he also internalized the unforgiving and stigmatizing belief, reinforced by the chief of surgery, as well as by the majority of USMDs (I will return to this in chapter 6), that he had not worked all his life for this and was thus less deserving. As Adrian said earlier, "I set myself up to have a harder path," even though he was a first-generation college graduate who faced more challenges with fewer resources than most USMDs did. For USIMGs, consistently lower support during early life, college, and medical school led to limited choices when it came to residency. Yet they continuously (over)emphasized agency—and its corollary, self-blame—and in the process helped obscure the structural obstacles that constrained their trajectories.

THE US OSTEOPATHIC MEDICAL SCHOOL GRADUATE

Early Life and College Experience: Mixed Support

The DOs I interviewed at Legacy exhibited characteristics of both USMDs and USIMGs: like USMDs, they enjoyed early life advantages, but like USIMGs, they lacked support from the profession during medical school and when applying to residency. Compared to Caribbean graduates, most DOs were raised in higher socioeconomic status (SES) homes and received more nurturing growing up. A little under half the DOs I interviewed had parents who were physicians. Others' fathers were small business owners or high school science teachers. Several had mothers who were nurses. Having academically inclined parents helped prepare young would-be DOs for the game. Ashley, for example, wasn't sure that she wanted to pursue medicine in high school, but she knew from her parents (also medical professionals) that she should keep doors open, so she volunteered throughout high school, which came in handy when she eventually applied to medical school.

Several DOs took a more traditional route to medical school, pursuing a standard premed major in college. Like many USMDs, others took time off after college before proceeding to medical school. Edward, for example, took postbaccalaureate courses through a program that linked directly to an osteopathic medical school: "I was accepted into med school before I finished the [postbaccalaureate] program—before I even took my MCATs." In this way, Edward played the game strategically; the postbaccalaureate eliminated the uncertainties of applying the traditional way—an approach seldom taken by the USIMGs I interviewed, perhaps because of the time and cost involved.

Applying to Medical School: Why Become a DO?

When it came to choosing the DO versus the MD route, about half chose osteopathic medicine a priori—i.e., they embraced the osteopathic approach to medicine—and half ended up in DO school as a fallback option. Olivia was a good example of the former; her mother was a DO, and she admired the way she interacted with patients: "I only applied to osteopathic schools 'cause I liked the idea of approaching it as a whole patient and having another tool, like manipulation, to treat a patient." Others, like Margaret and Jacob, applied to both osteopathic and allopathic programs simultaneously. Like some USIMGs, Margaret applied only to less competitive DO and Caribbean programs because she felt her application profile was weaker than that of others. Despite having been accepted to Caribbean schools, however, Margaret preferred the DO route, viewing osteopathic manipulation as a kind of bonus: "Going to a DO school, you learn manipulation, you learn other skills, and they are more patient-oriented, more clinically oriented, and I felt like that was better for me." Jacob, in contrast, who applied to seven- and eight-year programs out of high school, ended up in a DO school because it was his only option at the time: "The first seven-year program that actually contacted me I said, 'Hey, let's go,' and I hopped on the bandwagon and took it from there." Jacob felt he played the game strategically by choosing the first option available out of high school because, in his own words, his "whole vision was basically to finish as soon as possible so I could start my life."

Only a minority chose DO school somewhat begrudgingly, after several failed attempts at getting into allopathic schools. After three rounds of applying to MD schools with lower-than-desirable MCAT scores, Ashley finally applied to osteopathic school at the behest of her advisor at Colby College, who was "really talking up [DO school]." Like Clark, who was nudged toward a nurse practitioner career, Ashley was ushered into an alternative track (or "cooled out," as Goffman would put it[50]) by counselors at Colby College, where in 2014 their website advertised that medical school admission statistics hovered between 85 and 100 percent.[51] Pushing students like Ashley toward DO school helped keep those percentages high (because colleges do not distinguish between DO and MD schools in their statistics), thereby shaping individual students' trajectories through the maintenance of the college's elite status.

Graduates were well aware of the professional stigma they would face by becoming DOs. They knew they would have a harder time than their allopathic counterparts, who enjoyed professional sponsorship from USMD elites. Still, some felt that training in the United States—albeit at an osteopathic school— was better than going abroad in terms of opportunities for residency; as one DO opined, "At the end of the day, I would rather go to an American school if I wanted to practice in the United States as opposed to going to the Caribbean regardless of how connected [the school is]." Several also invoked their ultimate goal—being a doctor—as being more important than whatever stigma may be attached to their degree. Recall that the same was true of many USIMGs, possibly indicating a higher level of intrinsic motivation than that of some USMDs who said they would have quit medicine rather than pursue alternative paths of entry. Several DOs bemoaned society's poor understanding of the differences between DOs and MDs and the assumption that the former are inferior. Many DOs pointed out that their training was equal to, if not more advanced than, allopathic training: "It honestly [gives] you 200-300 more hours of schooling just in osteopathy, manipulation—basically chiropractic stuff and on top of that you have medicine. . . . It's medicine and *then* some," argued Jacob.

Medical School Experience: Mixed Support

As Jacob pointed out, the osteopathic and allopathic undergraduate medical curricula are very similar except that the former requires students to learn osteopathic manipulation alongside regular anatomy and pathophysiology. Correspondingly, DOs have their own three-step examination, known as the COMLEX (or Comprehensive Osteopathic Medical Licensing Examination), which is akin to the USMLE for allopathic graduates, and at the time of my research, they also had their own separate residency programs accredited by the American Osteopathic Association (AOA). Some DOs took the USMLE Step 1 in addition to the COMLEX to be eligible for allopathic residency programs, which increased their chances of matching into more-competitive specialties. Those who did so, however, had to do without the institutional support (such as prep courses and time off to prepare) that USMDs received from their schools—think back to Greg's experience described earlier. Other DOs, like Jacob, refused to take the USMLE out of principle: "I said, you know what? I am an osteopath, I'm proud of being an osteopath, [and] I am going to take my own Boards [and] test my knowledge that way."

The problem was that many allopathic residency programs refused to consider applicants without USMLE scores.[52] This represented an important hurdle and dilemma for some DOs: either take the USMLE (which was costly and risky, as they had been not been trained to take the allopathic exams) or face limited opportunities for residency. One study found that nearly half of DOs chose not to take the USMLE, and among those, approximately 36 percent reported experiencing discrimination for not having taken it.[53] Margaret pointed out that this struggle has profound implications for the osteopathic profession, which endeavors to maintain a separate identity from MDs: "You know, if we keep taking the USMLEs, then what are we saying? . . . What's the point of going to DO school? You're not separating [the professions]; you're not showing that you can do it yourself."

While DOs were still struggling to establish their legitimacy as a profession after decades of formal subordination by USMDs (see the introduction), DO trainees also had more-limited opportunities during medical school, which influenced their ability to apply to more competitive residency positions. Some DOs, for example, struggled to get adequate clinical exposure during their third and four years of medical school. Stand-alone osteopathic hospitals have been rapidly closing over the last few decades; for instance, in 1988, Texas had thirty-five such hospitals, and as of 2004, it had none.[54] The result is that osteopathic schools must vie for training opportunities in hospitals that are not already affiliated with major allopathic schools—namely, community hospitals. This can sometimes limit DOs' exposure to certain types of medicine such as inpatient pediatrics because children's hospitals tend to be university hospitals already affiliated with allopathic medical schools. One DO told me that students from the local osteopathic medical school were prohibited from rotating at the inpatient children's hospital affiliated with Stonewood University for "political reasons." (For more details about restrictions on clinical rotations at Stonewood, see chapter 2.) Also, by rotating in community hospitals, DOs often work alongside allopathic physicians who are ill-equipped to supervise them while they practice osteopathic manipulative techniques.

The decline of osteopathic hospitals has meant that DOs are training in allopathic community settings and do not receive the professional support and sponsorship they need to have the same training opportunities as allopathic graduates, thereby putting them at a systematic disadvantage when applying for residency positions. These professional-level deficits, however—the result of decades of subjugation by allopathic elites—were often misidentified as individual-level inadequacies, with DOs being labeled and stigmatized as inferior to MDs (see chapter 2), when, in fact, DOs had to succeed *in spite* of training with fewer supports than USMDs had. As is typical of contest mobility systems, "[v]ictory [had to] be won solely by one's own efforts," with DOs having to do more to prove themselves with less help than USMDs have.[55]

Applying to Residency: Professional Isolation

Only about a third of the DOs I interviewed at Legacy were in the categorical (three-year) residency program, and they selected allopathic internal medicine residencies because they believed they opened more doors for subspecialty training. Another third of DOs were preliminary (one-year) interns going on to pursue physical medicine and rehabilitation (PM&R) afterward—a common specialty for osteopathic physicians, who, after all, specialize in the musculo-skeletal system. The rest were medical students rotating at Legacy. One preliminary DO said he specifically chose osteopathic medicine because he knew it would not count against him when applying for PM&R residencies. He added the following caveat, however:

> That's not the case for more competitive, allopathic-based residency programs like dermatology or general surgery. . . . The AOA does have their own [programs], but there are only one or two [programs per specialty], and they take two people a year, you know . . . versus the number [of programs] that MDs have.[56] So [DOs] will end up giving up on it and saying "Well, I'll just do [internal medicine] instead."

Thus, like USIMGs, many DOs defaulted to internal medicine because it was reasonably within reach. In 2019, approximately 84.6 percent of DO applicants successfully matched to an allopathic residency (up from 74.8 percent in 2013 around the time of my fieldwork), and among those who matched, 24 percent went into internal medicine—the most common specialty choice for DOs.[57]

Why Legacy? Several DOs suspected they faced discrimination due to the stigma of their degree when applying to residency programs. Ashley, a DO student who wanted to become an orthopedist, confided, "Especially at the [elite] schools, they'll just be like, well she's a DO . . . and just write [her] off, and so even though [the DO has] done really well, they're not going to get into a residency [because] of the letters behind their name." Like USIMGs, many DOs accepted this stigma as a natural (if unfortunate) part of having chosen an alternative trajectory into the profession. As Jacob reasoned, "There is a tougher road for different paths."

Like USIMGs, DOs learned through online forums and word of mouth which programs were "friendly." Legacy accepted the COMLEX and was appealing because of its more laid-back approach to training. One DO accepted a prematch offer from Legacy (their second-choice program) partly to bypass the uncertainty of The Match: "My number two [program] was offering me prematch. It's the dumbest thing ever if I do not take my prematch and get out of The Match. . . . I took it because you just never know."

In sum, while DOs typically experienced more support in early life than USIMGs did, the stigma associated with their degree, combined with less support from a weaker profession, meant that their trajectories were more constrained than those of USMDs. Still, they had pride in their status, more than USIMGs had, even though some, like Jacob, accepted that taking an alternative route came with professional consequences. Choosing an allopathic residency opened more options for subspecialty, but it also meant having to fight an uphill battle among MDs who generally did not view DOs as equals. They faced perceived discrimination because of their degree, as well as more explicit barriers like the USMLEs. But like their Caribbean counterparts, many DOs internalized the belief that this was the price of having chosen an alternative path of entry into the profession. They came to expect very different things from their profession, reflecting more of a contested than a sponsored trajectory into medicine.

THE INTERNATIONAL MEDICAL SCHOOL GRADUATE

Early Life: Strong Support

Finally, we come to the IMGs, whose trajectories looked most similar to those of USMDs until they applied for residency—where the stigma associated with their pedigree required them to overcome additional barriers *and* outperform USMDs to compete for less prestigious residency positions. Like many USMDs, IMGs typically grew up in high-SES families. Their fathers were typically high-ranking executives or scientists in universities, corporations, and the military while their mothers were engineers or housewives. Only one was a first-generation college graduate. Hailing from Europe, the Middle East, and Asia, almost all IMGs went to private high school, affording them many of the same privileges as USMDs growing up.

Several IMGs were driven to careers in medicine at the suggestion of their families. In some cases, it was the result of parents living vicariously through their children. Others had more intrinsic motivations for studying medicine. For Yasmin, it was a mix of genuine interest and encouragement in school: "So I just remember that I wanted to be a doctor for some reason since I was younger, but then when I was in high school, . . . if you have good grades in biology and stuff, they would encourage you—'Oh, you should go into the medical field'—and that forced me to focus on that." IMGs therefore received the early pushes they needed to achieve their goals, much like USMDs did.

Applying to Medical School: Standardized Testing

The game for getting into medical school looked quite different for IMGs than for Americans. In other countries, medicine is usually an undergraduate degree lasting six to seven years (instead of being a four-year postgraduate degree, as in the United States). Also, unlike in the United States, where applicants need to list up to fifteen research, clinical, and volunteer activities to be considered for admission—like "curing cancer," as residents joked at the beginning of this chapter—the only requirement for getting into medical school for most IMGs is passing a national university entrance exam. As Kamal explained, "If you get the grade, you go to that school." Unsurprisingly, many spent years studying for the entrance exam. Joe took five additional hours of classes every day for three years to prepare. When I expressed surprise at how long he spent studying, he shook his head and said simply, "I had to sacrifice before getting a position in medical school." Like many USMDs, Joe was also fortunate enough to have parents who could afford these extra lessons. Eventually, the IMGs' investment paid off, as they all scored high enough on their entrance exams to get admitted, often to their first-choice schools.

Medical School Experience: Extensive Clinical Experience

IMGs were typically strong academic performers throughout medical school. Esra, who scored in the top 10 percent nationwide out of high school, remained in the top 10 percent of students throughout her medical training. Joe, who was class president for two years, was fourth in his class of 120. Aziz was second out of 650 students. They also accumulated extensive clinical experience. As part of their six- or seven-year degrees, several IMGs had to do a rural year or rotation, which often meant they were the only doctor for miles in remote regions, practicing as semiautonomous clinicians. After graduation, some IMGs accrued additional years of clinical experience prior to coming to the United States. After completing ten years of training, which included earning a PhD, Lin practiced as an attending physician for three years. Similarly, Joe worked as a generalist for two years and then was appointed deputy medical director of a hospital. He also opened his own clinic with colleagues—all before the age of forty. Others completed residency training before coming to the United States, as was the case for one European graduate who was a fully trained surgical sub-specialist. In this way, IMGs at Legacy were not simply academically accomplished. Many also had significant clinical experience under their belt compared to newly minted USMDs.

Many came to the United States for professional advancement: "It's like the best place in the world to practice medicine," Esra said matter-of-factly. Yasmin explained further: "All the studies, the trials are done here." Still others were intent on leaving their home countries for political or economic reasons. Kamal's father initially wanted him to stay to run the family business, but sensing political unrest, Kamal came to the United States and now says, "[My father] is calling me and saying 'So what are the chances of me coming?' He's talking like that because the country is very ugly right now." A combination of push and pull factors therefore led IMGs to seek professional opportunities in the United States.

Applying to Residency: Added Barriers

Until now, like USMDs, IMGs enjoyed relatively high levels of support and advantage both before and during medical school. But because they trained in other countries and health care systems, IMGs were probably the most "unknown quantity" of all the non-USMDs, especially regarding cultural "fit" with American patients, making them less attractive candidates for residency positions (as I'll explain in chapter 2). These unknowns gave way to assumptions about cultural incompetence, which eventually led to a highly intractable stigma associated with being an IMG—a stigma that indisputably benefited USMDs.

On top of the stigma, IMGs lacked the support given to USMDs by local advisors who guided them through the system. IMGs had to sink or swim on their own, as is expected in contest mobility. To overcome some of these barriers, many IMGs came to the United States to do "audition" rotations, which increased their familiarity with the US health care system and helped them develop relationships with local physicians. As foreigners, however, many IMGs could only *observe* during these rotations, not take on their own patients like US students could, which limited the extent to which IMGs could impress potential employers with their advanced clinical skills. In addition to paying for room and board, visiting international students also had to pay several hundred to several thousand dollars to hospitals for observerships. This meant that getting a US residency position was a costly and time-consuming endeavor for IMGs, several of whom spent over $10,000 on observerships alone.

Then there was the cost of the exams. IMGs had to take the same USMLEs as US students before applying to residency, but these exams carried added expenses for IMGs. In addition to the cost of the tests themselves and the associated surcharges for taking them internationally, there were steep travel expenses associated with the clinical skills portion of Step 2. That portion of the exam, which relies on standardized patients to assess applicants' clinical and communication skills, is administered in only five cities across the United States. IMGs can request a location but are not guaranteed to get their choice. This made it more difficult for some IMGs to complete the licensing exams in a timely fashion, often delaying their applications to residency.

Furthermore, IMGs did not just have to *pass* their Step exams; like USIMGs and DOs, they understood that they had to score even higher than USMDs on the same tests to be considered for less prestigious residency positions. Ali, a graduate from the Middle East, explained, "[For] Step 1, I scored [in the] 95th percentile. And for my Step 2, I was [in the] 99th percentile. . . . This is the difference between us who are coming from outside of the [United States]—[we] must have high scores because [we] have less privilege. . . . So, for us, if I am getting 99 and a US citizen [gets] like 80, they will prefer maybe to take that 80." Of the twelve IMGs I interviewed, five of them shared their USMLE Step 1 and

2 scores with me; none of them was below the 90th percentile. These findings echo national trends, such that those IMGs who match to internal medicine as their preferred specialty have significantly higher USMLE Step 1 scores than matched USMDs have.[58]

Yet despite their strong performance in medical school and considerable clinical training and experience, IMGs still faced significant barriers when applying for US residencies. They lacked the benefits of sponsorship from the profession in *this* country, which meant that matching was far from guaranteed, with only 58.6 percent of IMG applicants nationwide getting a residency position in 2019, up from an average of 44.1 percent between 1982 and 2017.[59] And much like the Caribbean and osteopathic graduates, who also lacked professional support, IMGs were quite limited in the range of subspecialties to which they felt they could apply. This meant that very few ended up in internal medicine by choice. Rather, it was what they felt was attainable. Yasmin, for example, was originally interested in dermatology but did not bother applying because it was too competitive. When I asked how she could not be a competitive candidate, having scored in the 99th percentile on Steps 1 and 2, she shook her head and replied: "Yeah, but the thing is for IMGs. . . . This is why we *have* to have double 99s and like other stuff, but that doesn't make us equal to US graduates or people who are from here. So they get better chances, even if they don't have double 99s." Even with the highest possible scores on the USMLE, this IMG suspected she would not be evaluated objectively compared to a (lower-scoring) USMD. As a result, she and other IMGs self-selected out of more competitive fields.

Why Legacy? Much like DOs and USIMGs, many IMGs specifically applied to internal medicine programs that were likely to accept them. They typically relied on internet forums, like matcharesident.com, to get a sense of which programs were "friendly." For a price, these websites generate personalized lists of suitable programs based on an applicant's scores, geographic specifications, and nationality. Then it is up to the applicant to decide which programs they prefer. Also like USIMGs, most IMGs applied to hundreds of programs at considerable expense. Faisal, who was from the Middle East, told me, "I applied everywhere. I think 120, 130 [programs]. I remember it [cost me] around $3,000."[60] By comparison, sending forty applications was considered excessive for USMDs.[61] To play the game successfully, IMGs therefore require substantial resources in order to overcome the odds, which are stacked against them.

Like many of the non-USMDs, IMGs often ended up at Legacy more out of constraint than by choice after accepting a prematch offer. Tellingly, when I asked Kamal why he chose Legacy for his residency (after applying to over two hundred programs), he replied, "So when I was doing my research, I knew this hospital was very nice. And when you say 'choose,' I didn't really have a choice. I got five interview invitations. [Legacy] was the first one. I was offered a prematch, so I was like, 'This is a prematch contract. What should I do? Take it or wait?' And then it literally took me a few hours, and I'm like, 'I'll take it, no chances, I need a job.'" Like many other non-USMDs at Legacy, Kamal preferred the certainty of a residency contract over the possibility of not matching at all, though he made it clear that he was constrained in his decision-making.

For most IMGs who trained in large university settings back home, Legacy was not their first-choice institution. The few who went through The Match (rather than accepting a prematch offer) expressed surprise when they found out they had matched to Legacy. As one resident shared, "I wanted to go into a bigger academic university hospital, and I interviewed at a few actually. . . . [When I found out I matched at Legacy,] I went home, and I started crying. I wasn't happy at all. . . . [Legacy] was the last one on my list." In some ways, this resident's experience was emblematic of the IMGs' constraints: despite growing up with backgrounds similar to those of USMDs, they lacked the professional support and pedigree needed to match with their specialty and residency program of choice. Instead, they had to achieve the highest scores and incur considerable expenses in hopes of securing some of the least prestigious residency positions in the United States.

CONCLUSION

In sum, I find that structural advantages starting early in life can carry forward into medical training, leading to distinct trajectories into medicine. Of course, it took hard work and intelligence for all applicants to get into medical school, but USMDs consistently had more help along the way, which complicates prevailing views about meritocracy in medicine. Instead, I found that medical education is deeply embroiled in, and often reproduces, broader social relations and hierarchies.[62] US allopathic graduates consistently accumulated advantages from childhood, where they grew up in households that strongly valued education, through college, where they had dedicated premed advisors who kept them on track when playing the game. Then, in return for having completed their part of the social contract, USMDs were sponsored by the profession upon entry into medical school—getting support with everything from studying for exams to scheduling rotations to completing the residency application process—thereby nearly guaranteeing their safe passage through the MD degree toward an eventual match to their residency program of choice. While formal sponsorship arrangements may no longer exist as official path-ways into residency,[63] I found that this process very much continues informally as the profession fulfills its implicit "social contract" with USMD trainees by shepherding them toward elite positions.[64] Importantly, I also found that USMDs repeatedly pointed to their own efforts, rather than the profession's, to account for their success.

In comparison, I found that USIMGs, DOs, and IMGs at Legacy had com-paratively fewer financial, educational, and professional resources than USMDs did, thereby putting them at an important disadvantage when playing the game. They had to overcome more barriers, including powerful professional stigmas, with fewer resources than USMDs while competing in an ostensibly open con-test for elite residency positions, when, in fact, elite status was all but reserved for sponsored USMDs within the profession. I found that the result was two tracks—one marked by sponsored mobility for USMDs, where matching to residency was virtually preordained, and the other marked by contest mobility, where stigmatized non-USMDs had to compete fiercely with less help so that a fraction of them could fill lower-status positions. Thus, compared to the USMDs at Stonewood, the applicants who matched to Legacy residencies were far more constrained in their options, often preferring a more certain path toward a career in medicine (by accepting a prematch offer at Legacy) over the unfavorable odds they faced in The Match. These constraints were also often misidentified as fully agentic decisions, sometimes leading to self-blame, especially among the USIMGs—a finding that begins to foreshadow why non-USMDs consent so enthusiastically to lower-status positions (see chapter 6).[65]

Importantly, despite initial variations in the individual trajectories of each type of graduate, these dissimilarities became less consequential once they got into medical school, signaling just how important USMD/non-USMD status is for determining opportunity and mobility within the profession. That Chloe (a USMD) attended community college prior to med school, for example, was insignificant for her prospects in residency, as was the fact that Ralph (a USIMG) had a mother who was a physician. They were now, respectively, American and Caribbean graduates, and whatever came before was far less relevant for residency than where they went to medical school.

Indeed, if the game was truly meritocratic and if the playing field was actually level, where one went to medical school should have been largely immaterial for getting into residency. Except for DOs, all applicants shared the same degree (MD), and, importantly, they took the same licensing examinations. Despite these equalizing factors, graduates perceived that the informal rules of the game differed depending on who was applying. An average Step 1 score did not seem to have the same implications for a USMD as for a non-USMD. Graduating with the highest honors from a Caribbean medical school was not worth as much as doing the same from any US medical school. Even those with extensive prior clinical experience, like IMGs, were viewed as subpar compared to USMDs.

As it turns out, the unspoken rules of the game *were* indeed different depending on the applicant, and in the next chapter, I will illustrate how these perceptions shaped the recruitment process into residency from the perspective of the program directors.

CHAPTER 2

The Match List

E very year Stonewood University Hospital and Legacy Community Hospital each received thousands of applications for their internal medicine residency programs. The criteria on both programs' websites were quite basic. Stonewood required that applicants score 192 (the passing grade) or above on Steps 1 and 2 of the US Medical Licensing Examination (USMLE), which students take before graduating from medical school. For the benefit of international medical graduate (IMG) applicants, the website also noted that US clinical experience was preferred and that the program was unable to sponsor H-1 visas for non-US residents (implying that Stonewood sponsored only the less desirable J-1 exchange visitor visas).[1] Legacy's criteria were even more stringent, not only requiring passing grades on the USMLE but also, for IMG applicants, indicating a preference for those who had completed a full year of US clinical experience and graduated within the past five years. Legacy, too, sponsored only J-1 visas. Importantly, international and osteopathic applicants were not discouraged from applying to either program.

Consequently, Legacy and Stonewood received scores of applications from both graduates of US allopathic medical schools (USMDs) and non-USMDs. Despite being widely perceived as a less desirable workplace for USMDs, Legacy still received hundreds of applications from USMDs while more than two-thirds of the applications to Stonewood were from US-trained osteopathic graduates (DOs), US citizen international medical graduates (USIMGs), and IMGs. Yet these two programs remained highly segregated, such that Legacy exclusively matched with non-USMDs for its three-year categorical program and Stonewood maintained a housestaff in which nearly 100 percent of the residents were USMDs.

Self-selection alone therefore cannot explain how or why both Legacy and Stonewood had such segregated housestaffs. How then did program officials decide whom to interview among thousands of applications? How did they end up so segregated, with Stonewood recruiting almost exclusively USMDs and Legacy recruiting almost exclusively non-USMDs? And how did program officials justify their decisions?

In the previous chapter, I traced the pathways of different medical graduates into residency to better understand why certain individuals ended up at either Stonewood or Legacy. As the name implies, however, The Match involves reconciling the preferences of a second set of actors—program officials, who rank-order applicants after interviewing them—with the applicants' preferences, resulting in matches of applicants and programs based on mutual preference.[2] At the beginning of their fourth year of medical school, students apply to their desired residency programs nationwide, which, in turn, decide whom to interview. After the interview period, applicants and programs produce what is known as a rank list. For programs, this means rank-ordering interviewees from most to least preferred; for applicants, it means doing the same with the programs where they interviewed. Then the National Resident Matching Program algorithm uses game theory to reconcile the applicants' rank-ordered choices with the programs' candidate rankings.[3] Accordingly, on Match Day in March, applicants receive an offer from a single residency program, which, once signed, becomes legally binding.[4]

So how did this routinized matching process yield such polarized results at Legacy and Stonewood? In this chapter, I offer a rare glimpse into the process of residency recruitment from the program leadership's perspective at each hospital, examining the decision makers' stated rationales—and their underlying biases—that resulted in nearly perfect segregation among these two residency programs.[5] Program officials defended their recruitment practices by drawing on different meritocratic logics of objectivity and risk aversion, when, in reality, I found that The Match was not an open competition at these two hospitals. By contextualizing these recruitment practices within the broader hierarchical field of residency programs, it becomes clear that these recruitment decisions—and their segregated outcomes—were strongly shaped by the programs' social positions within that field and by the program officials' desire to maximize prestige while minimizing risk.[6]

THE HIERARCHICAL FIELD OF RESIDENCY PROGRAMS

Most respondents understood residency programs to be broadly divided into three informal tiers based on status. While medical schools and hospitals are given official rankings, residency programs are not,[7] so reputation is one of the only ways to distinguish a program's caliber.[8] As one Stonewood resident put it, "It's all word of mouth. . . . There's no tangible number you put on it." Still, there were rules of thumb for differentiating between programs of different stature. Top-tier programs were places like Johns Hopkins and Stanford: "big, massive, research-oriented, driving-the-bus-of-medicine-forward-type-institutions," explained one Stonewood attending physician. Middle-tier programs were the more clinically driven programs, places like Jefferson and Temple, with less of a focus on research but a strong clinical curriculum. Finally, bottom-tier programs were typically characterized as community programs with low pass rates on American Board of Internal Medicine Certification Examinations (Boards) and high proportions of non-USMDs. As one Stonewood chief resident put it, "[A bottom-tier program is located in] Anywhere, USA. It doesn't fill the rank list; it's full of foreign medical grads. Lots of failures on the Boards." When I asked another Stonewood resident what a lower-tier program looked like to them, they responded, "I don't want to sound racial or anything but . . . having more foreign medical graduates in the program." Non-USMDs were clearly perceived as having a lower status within the profession, and programs that accepted them were, by extension, also considered to have a lower status.

There was consensus at both hospitals that Stonewood and Legacy belonged to different tiers. According to Stonewood officials, the Stonewood program fell squarely in the top third of all residencies in the United States. Stonewood residents, for their part, viewed it more as a high-middle-tier program. As one resident put it, "[Tier one programs are] ahead of the game; they're the trendsetters, and we [at Stonewood] are trend followers." Stonewood was decidedly more clinically oriented than research oriented, which was consistent with programs in the middle tier, but its trainees were almost exclusively USMDs, putting it toward the top of that tier. Legacy, in contrast, was widely perceived to be a bottom-tier program, even by its own residents. As Raoul, a resident in his third postgraduate year (PGY-3) at Legacy, admitted to me, "I think it's tier three or so.

I don't think this is a good program." As evidence, he pointed to Legacy's low Board passage rates (which hovered at about one standard deviation below the national mean in 2012–2014), but the hospital's status as a for-profit community hospital staffed almost exclusively by non-USMDs would likely have been enough by itself to earn its program a spot in the bottom tier.[9] At the same time, the program was affiliated with a reasonably well-known medical school, which put it toward the top of that bottom tier.

Despite occupying very different social locations, both Legacy and Stonewood were keen on climbing the ranks, which they did, in part, through The Match. Because there are "no tangible number[s]" formally ranking residency programs, recruitment is a key factor that shapes program reputation. Aside from faculty profiles, the lists resulting from The Match ("Match Lists") are one of the only highly visible signals of a program's competitiveness within the field, and they assume central importance for program leadership precisely for this reason. Every year on Match Day, officials from both hospitals would post the names of newly matched residents alongside their medical schools of origin on the wall for everyone to see. That list would eventually make its way onto each program's website, where current residents appeared alongside their pedigree. The perceived competitiveness of the new cohort of residents (and, by extension, the program itself) would then be assessed by various internal stakeholders, including current residents, faculty, medical school officials, graduate medical education officers, other residency programs in the hospital, and the chief of medicine.[10] It would also be analyzed by external stakeholders, such as rival programs, alumni, fellowship directors, employers, and future applicants, who would carefully scrutinize achievements in recruitment for signs about the program's overall worth.[11] In fact, when I asked a program leader how they would define what they called "higher-pedigree" programs, they pointed to the "baseline standard of the other housestaff," highlighting how the perceived caliber of the residents, as portrayed on these publicized lists, could shape a program's reputation. While residency programs also rely on other signals to boost their reputations, such as residents' Fellowship Match results and Board certification rates, almost all of these signals are contingent on recruiting high-quality residents from the outset.

Program officials also pored over other programs' Match lists, being sure to look left, right, up, and down at their competition to see how they fared in comparison. Stonewood, for instance, surveyed the hundreds of medical students it interviewed to see where they eventually matched and thus where their competition lay. During one noontime meeting, the top brass at Stonewood huddled around the results of the in-house survey, saying "These are all our usual folks," referring to the schools from which the newly matched residents were coming. "Still not getting Ivy League graduates," announced one official with a furrowed brow. Another asked, "Where do the rest in the top [half] go [if they don't match to Stonewood]?" Someone began listing large, research-intensive programs in the Northeast and on the West Coast. "You have to believe some of it's geographic," said someone else, who pointed to a program that was perceived to be lower in status than Stonewood but to be in a better location. Another concluded, "I think we got the right schools as competitors."

The Match list was thus a beacon for program reputation. It both signaled *and* shaped a program's status. That is why pressures to increase the programs' prestige so heavily influenced the programs' approaches to recruitment. One Stonewood University official explained the homogeneity of Stonewood's and Legacy's residency programs by observing:

> I think it has an awful lot to do with perceived prestige of a program. So one way that you increase [it] . . . is to eliminate international medical grads. So it winds up being a dynamic that promotes complete polarization. If at the start a place has one quarter international grads and another place has three quarters, then US grads don't want to go to the place with three quarters, so they're more likely to go to the place with one quarter. So you wind up with all or none.

Another faculty member at Stonewood offered a similar explanation about the absence of DOs from the Stonewood housestaff: "I think part of this is maybe game playing and [the leadership factoring in] what outsiders looking in, grading the program, might think."[12] Status segregation was thus at least partly the product of efforts to increase program prestige and attractiveness. So how did these efforts play out at Legacy and Stonewood? What justifications did program leaders offer for recruiting such segregated housestaffs? And how did program prestige factor in as an implicit motivation?

LEGACY

Justifications: An "Unbiased" Selection Process

While there may have been widespread agreement that Legacy was a bottom-tier program, in 2012 new leadership was brought in to help improve the program's standing, which they did partly through residency recruitment. Previously, Legacy relied on the chief resident to whittle down more than two thousand applications to several hundred interview candidates. The new leadership, however, heralded major changes to the selection process, making screening conditions, in their words, more "explicit" and "objective" and therefore more meritocratic—qualities that program officials made sure to emphasize early and often. First, an initial review of applications weeded out candidates who were deemed unacceptable (e.g., those with a history of disciplinary actions or failure on the USMLE). This brought down the pool of candidates to approximately fifteen hundred. The remaining applicants were then split into five pools: (1) US students at US medical schools (USMDs and DOs), (2) US students at foreign medical schools (USIMGs), (3) foreign students at schools with US affiliations (e.g., Ben-Gurion Medical School in Israel, affiliated with Columbia University Medical Center), (4) foreign students at foreign medical schools (IMGs), and (5) foreign students at US medical schools. These pools represented a more open and inclusive approach for Legacy: "This is new . . . because in the past, we said, oops, we only interviewed [USIMGs], and that's not cool," explained one high-ranking member of the program leadership, adding that the program should not limit itself unnecessarily to international graduates. Interviewing USMDs meant that Legacy was now (at least partly) in direct competition with Stonewood.

After dividing up the applicants, program leaders then considered additional criteria in deciding whom to interview: "We had a targeting strategy with five *objective* criteria," the senior official explained, emphasizing the rigor of the selection process: "(1) undergrad GPA [grade point average], including undergrad school . . . a-GPA-whatever at Princeton is different from a 4.0 GPA at wherever-[University]; (2) medical school GPA or equivalent scoring in foreign medical schools; (3) standardized test scores [USMLE]; (4) formal letters from the dean and program directors, which we ranked; and (5) outside, external references and personal statements." The official made sure to add, "We weighed the scores more heavily than the letters because the latter were more subjective," once again emphasizing objectivity in the process.

An important part of the revitalized selection process was the establishment of a Resident Selection Committee that would meet weekly to discuss interviewees and rank them against the other applicants. As the same official explained, "My aim was to create a situation with multidisciplinary and multidemographic inputs . . . and also remove any bias." Here again the absence of bias was emphasized voluntarily by Legacy decision makers. Each applicant was interviewed by at least three faculty members, and each interviewer filled out the same evaluation form "so we had some objectivity there again," repeated the official.

Program leaders were also adamant about rejecting what they described as "subjective" influences. As one program leader grumbled, "I [get] piles of personal letters and phone calls from physicians in the community who want me to interview their relative or their friend or . . . somebody they worked with and we have to sort all that out." The leader continued, "[A colleague] wanted us to interview his niece. I'm sure she's a wonderful person, but she's failed three different tests, and her medical school scores were mediocre at best, and we just had to say, 'We just aren't going to take you.' " Legacy even developed an informal policy against "leaks," as another high-ranking official called them: "I told the committee; I actually wrote it down and scripted it for them: the answer is 'I can't do that because it would be unfair to all the other people'. . . . A close friend of mine wanted me to get his daughter an interview, and I told him no. He's still upset at me for that."

In line with Legacy's "objective" approach, there was also a stated emphasis on evaluating candidates for their individual merits rather than their medical pedigree. The Legacy leadership even invested time in learning more about international medical schools to develop trust with these institutions. The senior official told me, "We did a lot of due diligence with the foreign schools this year. I said, 'Let's learn five to ten [of them] and get to know them really well so they don't try to trick us.' " As they put it, "We're guarding correctly against introducing bias."[13] When I asked what kind of bias they were referring to, the official replied, "You know, [like bias against] a foreign student at a US medical school. . . . Or a Middle Eastern med student at a Middle Eastern school," which would involve relying on medical school pedigree as a heuristic for assessing the student's merit. Another faculty member reasoned, "It's [about] just allowing the individual to prove themselves, not necessarily on the school name but on what their grades are and what their academic scores are, what their rotations have been like."

Consequently, the Legacy leadership often disputed claims that USMDs were better doctors than non-USMDs. As the senior official put it, "You'd be hard-pressed, in my opinion, to say that one's better than the other," referring to USMDs and non-USMDs. "These people [non-USMDs] are very, very good, and they need to work really, really hard [to get into residency]. I have a lot of respect for people who have gone that route. It's even harder for people who are foreigners because there's the language issue. You gotta admire that grit. . . . So I've come to the conclusion that you've gotta go with the talent." Some leaders even noted that non-USMDs may be stronger in some areas, such as infectious diseases, than USMDs. As one junior faculty member noted, "People [who] trained back in India or in Southeast Asia, they have different disease populations so they might have more knowledge on that subject, which is great because they can share whatever they know." This faculty member also added, "Non-US grads . . . might have higher [exam] scores because they try hard to get into good programs."

Legacy officials also insisted that their recruitment methods were better and more fair than the ones used at Stonewood, the biggest competitor in town. It was widely known that Stonewood excluded non-USMDs from consideration for residency, which prompted Legacy leaders to distinguish themselves as being less biased and thus better able to ferret out good talent, regardless of medical pedigree. For example, one Legacy official distinguished their institution from Stonewood by saying "I think the way we do it here is the right way. The way that works." Another described Stonewood's approach more bluntly: "I would call it discrimination. . . . [Stonewood is] automatically excluding people who may well be as qualified as the people [they] are taking; it's just that [they] don't want to hear about it." Decision makers at Legacy described going to great lengths to minimize bias wherever possible in the selection process, thereby emphasizing how objective and meritocratic their decisions were.

Motivations: Protecting the Program's Status

For all that program leaders claimed to objectively "go with the talent," regardless of medical pedigree, however, many Legacy officials also admitted to giving USMDs preference over non-USMDs, *even* when they disputed claims that USMDs were better doctors. As one program official explained:

> I tried to focus more on the US medical grads first, for the first [part] of interview [season]. . . . Coming from such a small program, it's less likely for

the US grads to come here because they are looking for . . . bigger university hospitals. So we are trying to invite more US grads early in the season to gauge if they are good, if they're going to come here or not.

When I asked what they meant by "focus more" on USMDs, the official replied that, given candidates with the same scores, they would interview the US grad first. Another program leader went even further: "If [a USMD applicant is] average and you're comparing them to somebody [a non-USMD] that's probably above-average, [the average USMD] will probably get ranked higher. Typically, they'll be ranked higher." This leader went on to explain their reasoning: "Because it's a name [thing]. Do you want somebody on your list that's from UPenn [University of Pennsylvania], or do you want somebody that's from [*laughs*] St. Kitts and Nevis, you know? Nobody knows what that individual from the Caribbean has accomplished, but they do know that if you got into UPenn, well then you must have been a stellar student." Tellingly, this program leader empha- sized the "name" thing—or the symbolic capital associated with an Ivy League pedigree—more than the candidates' individual merits. Symbolic capital is an intangible property, like prestige, that can exert "a sort of magical power" upon others who recognize this property from a distance.[14] In this case, Legacy would look more competitive to prospective applicants, patients, and peer programs if it attracted *a* student—any student—from a USMD school, rather than even a top student from a non-USMD school, because of the prestige associated with USMDs. Even low-performing USMDs were essentially guaranteed a residency position *somewhere* because (in addition to benefiting from the sponsorship detailed in chapter 1) they had symbolic capital in the form of the prestige that they could bring to lower-tier programs. To wit, it did not seem to matter which US medical schools Legacy recruited from as long as they were US allopathic schools. When I sought to clarify with the official who admitted to focusing more on USMDs whether they preferred US grads from top schools, they shook their head: "No, it didn't matter. Whoever applies to this program." In this way, all USMDs were viewed equally favorably at Legacy, whether they graduated from Harvard or Hofstra.

Thus, as much as Legacy claimed that its process was less biased and more meritocratic than Stonewood's, program leaders still immediately divided up applicants into pools based on their medical school pedigree and still preferred USMDs over non-USMDs because they represented a boon to the residency program's reputation. As many as half of all interviews at Legacy were granted to

USMDs, which notably distinguished Legacy from other IMG- or DO-friendly community hospitals in the area that almost exclusively interviewed non-USMDs.[15] But being a bottom-tier community program, Legacy struggled to recruit these high-prestige USMDs through The Match, no matter how highly program officials ranked them. As one official put it, "We want them. It's that they don't want us. We put a bunch of them on our [Match] list every year," implying that USMDs do not rank Legacy high enough on their *own* Match lists to match there. So to avoid putting its program in a position where it would *lose* status by not filling all of its residency spots and would leave the hospital understaffed, Legacy had to prioritize applicants who were more likely to rank Legacy highly: non-USMDs.[16] As a senior Legacy official noted, "[The Match] is all about likelihoods and probabilities, and we want to contribute to our probability of matching."

In reality, Legacy faced even bigger problems than just losing status—it could lose its accreditation altogether if it wasn't careful with recruitment. As a senior member of the program leadership disclosed:

> I'm acutely aware of the fact that the ACGME [Accreditation Council for Graduate Medical Education] keeps track of our Board pass rates [which have been below the national mean], . . . and I know that the ability to do well on tests is predicted by your former test performance. I have found myself having to take the position that we need people who are going to take the tests. Because our program won't get accredited if we don't produce people who can pass the Board tests. . . . So we need to attract and rank people who have a history of being able to do well in tests and we need to teach them well.

These concerns complicated Legacy's hopes of attracting USMDs to improve the program's reputation. They made high-scoring non-USMDs comparatively more appealing than bottom-of-the-barrel USMDs, who may have raised the program's prestige in the short run but could ultimately have endangered Legacy's reputation in the long run by bringing down Board pass rates. This official continued, "There are residents from US medical schools who we don't want actually because they haven't done that well in medical school or they've had behavioral problems." They went on to give an example of a (rare) former USMD resident who did not succeed at Legacy, which hurt the program's reputation. These concerns ironically lent support to all the emphasis program officials placed on meritocracy because the program could justify matching with high-performing non-USMDs with exemplary USMLE scores rather than prestige-boosting USMDs.

Besides, they could still try to Americanize the housestaff in the process. A Caribbean-trained chief resident tuned program officials into an untapped resource: USIMGs, mostly from Caribbean schools. Focusing recruitment on this pool provided Legacy a way to make the housestaff more American without necessarily recruiting tough-to-get USMDs. A program official reflected:

> Previously we favored [non-US] medical students who graduated from foreign schools, I mean after US medical schools. . . . Now we take American [USIMGs] who don't have to overcome the hurdles of [acculturation] and stuff that these other people—the foreign medical graduates—do. It has made things, I think, easier for patients and easier for us and *made the program more attractive to other Americans.* And I think that's generally been a good thing. (emphasis added)

Legacy therefore tried to improve its stature by reducing the number of IMGs it recruited. These efforts were not lost on some Legacy residents who noticed that higher-ups were intent on hiring more USIMGs to make the program more appealing to Americans. One evening some international residents were discussing the likely pick for next year's chief resident. "They don't want a chief with an accent," one of them said. Another talked about efforts to improve the "quality of applicants" by prioritizing US citizens: "If the chief was Indian or Arabic, US citizens wouldn't come," said the resident. The next chief resident was indeed a Caribbean graduate, and the following class of interns contained only two IMGs. Knowing it could not recruit enough USMDs to stop hiring non-USMDs altogether, Legacy seemed to focus its efforts on attracting the next best thing: Americans who trained abroad.

Legacy's Match List: Maintaining the Status Quo

On Match Day 2012, a Legacy official came to noon conference to announce the results to the housestaff: "We matched fully this year. We did very well. We're very delighted with the results of The Match." Importantly, his first words emphasized that Legacy filled all its positions. Maintaining the program's status by filling all its positions was one of Legacy's basic priorities. That year Legacy filled over half of its positions using "prematch" offers, which was less risky than going through The Match. Prior to 2013, programs could allocate residency positions through (1) prematch contracts, whereby programs extended residency offers to interviewees on the spot before The Match occurred; (2) The Match; or (3) some combination thereof. The catch was that prematch contracts were available only to non-USMDs; all USMDs had to go through The Match.

The official continued, "We were very competitive this year in every pool." Regarding the preliminary interns who would spend only a year at Legacy, he said, "We got five exceptionally good people—five of our top choices." When describing the categorical interns who would pursue the full three-year program, he added, "We made [a number of] prematch offers, and they were all accepted, which is exceptional. [About half] of them are very strong; the rest are within the middle of our matching range."

For the new intern class of 2012, approximately 25 percent were IMGs, 50 percent were USIMGs, 5 percent were DOs, and roughly 20 percent were USMDs. There was not a single USMD in the three-year categorical program. The USMDs were all preliminary interns who would do a year at Legacy before pursuing competitive residencies in select specialties at more prestigious hospitals.

In 2013, the National Resident Matching Program's All In Policy changed the rules regarding prematches. Programs were now required either to put all their positions in The Match (or another national matching plan) or to exclusively recruit candidates via prematches, thereby forcing most hospitals to forego prematches altogether.[17] In order to remain competitive among USMDs, who were not eligible for prematch offers, most programs, including Legacy, opted to go "All In," thereby eliminating prematches.

With fewer guarantees via prematches and in line with efforts to recruit a more "Americanized" housestaff, the 2013 Legacy Match list prioritized USIMGs. In the new cohort of interns, 12 percent were IMGs (down from roughly 25 percent the year before), nearly 60 percent were USIMGs (up from 50 percent previously), and around 20 percent were USMDs and 5 percent were DOs, who exclusively filled spots as preliminary interns. The leadership was quite proud of that Match list: "This year we didn't go above 30 [in our rank list]. Historically, it was [closer to] 50," said one leader, referring to the fact that candidates ranked as high as around the fiftieth position would match in previous years. This was a marker of success for Legacy. In the first year of the All In Policy, at least Legacy did not lose status, and, in fact, it may have gained a little by matching with more USIMGs.

In this way, Legacy officials made recruitment decisions with an eye toward the program's social standing. They may have emphasized a highly meritocratic approach that supposedly distinguished them from Stonewood, but they also openly admitted to preferring (even lower-performing) USMDs. To smooth over these contradictions and justify an all-non-USMD housestaff, Legacy officials strongly emphasized a rhetoric of objectivity that helped eclipse their preference for prestige-boosting USMDs, whom they could not successfully recruit. In so doing, Legacy officials were careful to maximize program prestige while minimizing risk. Pouring all of their resources into recruiting USMDs would have been a high-reward but also a very high-risk endeavor, especially given the ultimate risks of not filling the program or, worse, losing accreditation. So Legacy compromised by recruiting mostly USIMGs, resulting in an internal medicine housestaff without a single USMD past their intern year.

STONEWOOD

Justifications: A "Risk-Averse" Selection Process

Like Legacy, Stonewood had to sort through thousands of applications to decide on several hundred interviewees. Also, like their Legacy counterparts, Stonewood leaders described their process as meritocratic, allocating interviews on the basis of individuals' talent and achievements, such as high Board scores and honor society memberships. As one senior Stonewood program leader said, "You are trying to match with what you perceive as the best students," a sentiment that was echoed by several Stonewood officials. Another faculty member explained, "We have an obligation to our patients to make sure that we give them the best possible doctors to take care of them. Any time you take a chance on a resident, you're potentially taking a chance on a patient." Assessing talent and ability among applicants was therefore viewed not only as important for hiring good workers but also as critical for providing the best patient care at Stonewood, which considerably raised the stakes.

But with thousands of applications, how did the program leadership distinguish the best from the rest? A senior program official explained that because of the rise in the number of applications each year, the percentage of applicants invited for an interview decreased from 60 to 70 percent in previous years to roughly 50 percent that year. Knowing that Stonewood received over three thousand applications and interviewed only several hundred individuals (a proportion closer to 15 percent of all applicants), I was puzzled. So I asked what happened to the applications from DOs, IMGs, and USIMGs. The program official replied slowly, choosing their words carefully:[18] "So those, those are the ones that [we] look at. We look for people . . . we know, if they've done rotations here, if someone on the faculty has advocated for them . . . that is very meaningful, so that's a few. We look at schools that we've had some track record with. . . . There's probably *a half dozen to a dozen international graduates* that we invite" (emphasis added). When I asked what percentage of those international graduates were USIMGs from the Caribbean, the official replied after a very long pause, "It's too small a number to really quantify. But it's pretty small." Of the three thousand applications received yearly at Stonewood, around a third were from USMDs, and the remaining two-thirds were from non-USMDs, of which only six to twelve received interviews. Thus, when this official said earlier that they interviewed around 50 percent of applicants, they were really referring only to USMD applicants. Without something to distinguish non-USMDs, their applications were simply discarded without review. As another high-ranking official confirmed, "The only way [a non-USMD] will be put on the list for consideration is that they may know someone who currently is an attending physician here . . . otherwise they'll get filtered out".

Unlike Legacy, Stonewood nearly exclusively interviewed USMDs, with only around 2 percent of interviews accorded to non-USMDs. When asked about the lack of non-USMDs on the housestaff, one senior official at Stonewood responded that this was by design: "That's a conscious—well, it's not no foreign grads; every year . . . there's always somebody who is some kind of exception. That's a highly workable decision about what we *prefer*. I've never heard us discuss that, but they're clearly, they must be tiered that way, like it's better to be a US allopathic candidate than it is not" (emphasis added). The unspoken yet agreed-upon preference for USMDs translated into the nearly categorical rejection of non-USMDs. This was particularly true of USIMGs trained in the Caribbean; when asked about the chances of a Caribbean graduate matching at Stonewood, one official replied bluntly, "Probably as close to zero as you can get. I don't even know if we have ever even interviewed someone."

Stonewood officials therefore made few real attempts to actually assess the merits of non-USMD applicants, usually discarding them without review. Part of the reason, they said, had to do with high applicant volumes and limited time. Going through the hundreds of USMD applications alone was time consuming enough without having to consider the thousands of non-USMD applicants. As one senior official told me, "When you have [nearly one thousand USMD] applicants or so, you've got to sort of cut it off somewhere." Thus, because of limited resources, the program leaders relied on pedigree (USMD versus non-USMD) as a time-saving heuristic to help them decide where to focus their efforts.

If limited resources were the only consideration, however, there were other ways that program officials could have optimized their recruitment efforts in their search for the best possible residents, as was their stated priority. Program decision makers, for example, had the option of filtering applications in the Electronic Residency Application Service (ERAS) on the basis of USMLE scores, accomplishments, honor society membership, medical school transcripts, professional experience, publications, letter of recommendation scores, and even felony convictions, which meant officials could have just as easily prioritized high-performing applicants, regardless of pedigree.[19] Stonewood decision makers stressed the importance of recruiting the best residents for their patients but chose to focus their efforts almost exclusively on USMDs rather than carefully assessing the merits of some other cross section of applicants—what some might describe as classic preference-based discrimination.[20] So how did decision makers account for this practice?

Despite the wealth of information about applicants in ERAS, Stonewood officials heavily emphasized the *unknowns* and *risks* associated with non-USMDs, pointing to a lack of tacit information—a gestalt—that they could not necessarily glean from test scores and transcripts. As one attending put it:

> You know, I—we have a sense of what goes on at Tufts, we have a great sense of what goes on at the University of [X]—or at any of the medical schools, really, across the country, and even if we don't, we can call someone who does.

Once you get out of the continental [United States], we really don't have a sense of what goes on in those medical schools, so there's a risk about getting someone who looks great on paper, but you really have no idea. . . . That's the problem. They may have glowing everything, but you don't know if at that school they write that for everybody. Who knows? You have no idea, which is not to say you always know for the US grads either.

So while uncertainty may have existed about USMDs, it was more tolerable than the uncertainty associated with non-USMDs, whose training was more unfamiliar in ways not captured by applicant data. Importantly, nearly everyone at Stonewood admitted they knew very little about osteopathic or international medical training. But unlike at Legacy, this was hardly an impetus to learn more about these schools. Instead, the unknowns associated with non-USMDs, combined with the life-and-death nature of medicine, served as a powerful justification for excluding them from consideration. As this one senior official disclosed, "We are more familiar with the allopathic schools. . . . Because honestly, it's a horrible thing when you have a mismatched or a poorly trained person come in. *It's patients' lives.* And I'm not saying that these folks [non-USMDs] are poorly trained, they may not be but . . . If they come from a US school, we know where they've been; we look at the evaluations they get; we know what those evaluations mean" (emphasis added).

Stonewood officials frequently invoked the high-stakes nature of medical work as a highly convincing justification for excluding non-USMDs from con-sideration—after all, it is hard to argue with wanting to reduce risk in matters of life and death. As one faculty member summarized, "We're not running a shelter for wayward children here. We don't have an obligation to give that person a chance; we have an obligation to our *patients* to make sure that we give them the best possible doctors" (emphasis in original). Another program leader defended their preference for USMDs by saying that non-USMDs come from less familiar schools, so "the level of risk goes up. . . . So now the next question you're going to ask is, How are you ever going to get to know any of these schools if you don't have any students from there? In the end, my responsibility is to the program, not necessarily to the world at large or even to the country at large." This perspective, however, detracts from the possibility that non-USMD applicants might actually have been doctors who are just as good as, or even better than, USMDs.

Stonewood officials therefore both insisted that they provided patients with the best possible doctors (a highly meritocratic approach) *and* justified excluding two-thirds of applicants based purely on pedigree rather than documented performance by emphasizing what they thought was a greater good: mitigating *risk*.[21] When asked to define "the risk," Stonewood officials reasoned that the definition had at least two prongs: (1) the risk of lack of medical knowledge and (2) the risk of unprofessional conduct, both of which could adversely impact patients.

Medical Knowledge Even though they often admitted to knowing little about non-USMDs' training, Stonewood faculty and program officials widely suspected that the clinical acumen of non-USMDs—particularly DOs and USIMGs—was subpar. These suspicions persisted even though applicants had to take the same licensing exams measuring medical knowledge as USMDs, making comparisons between applicants theoretically possible.[22] One faculty member summarized, "Ultimately, the concern is that they wouldn't be able to keep up with the academic rigor that is required in the program that we've set up. Again, patient care first. . . . We can teach them [residency], but we can't teach them med school *and* residency." Similarly, another faculty member who was discussing what it must be like to work at a program with all non-USMDs said, "Your quality of sleep is probably not as good when you are a ward attending [at those hospitals]. Because you just can't be as sure that they [non-USMDs] are going to do the right thing. . . . Certainly we [at Stonewood] like the fact that we keep ourselves *above that level*, if you will, because it does make our lives easier, I think" (emphasis added). Simply put, an all-USMD housestaff gave faculty less to worry about.

In reality, many of these beliefs about USIMGs and DOs being subpar stemmed from widely held assumptions about their inability to gain admission to US allopathic schools in the first place. One faculty member opined, "Here's what I think of those US grads who end up going to Caribbean schools: they are bright kids who fucked around in college and weren't committed. And now they want . . . I mean, some of those Caribbean schools are atrocious." Similarly, regarding DOs, another faculty member told me, "I think again there is a kind of track perpetuation that if you went to a DO school, it's not clear that you are always going there out of choice, and so then that sort of speaks to a lower level of achievement maybe." Thus, it was perhaps not the training per se but rather the presumed personal weaknesses associated with the individuals pursuing that training that prevailed.[23]

These assumptions left little room for alternative explanations: for example, that some DOs or Caribbean graduates might have preferred their training trajectories. This was the case for about half the DOs whose interviews I discussed in chapter 1, and several of the Caribbean graduates, especially those who wanted their previous medical training counted towards a degree—something only offered by offshore schools. Such assumptions also did not account for individual variation within groups. While matched DOs and USIMGs do typically score lower on average on the USMLE than USMDs do,[24] by systematically excluding all non-USMDs from consideration, Stonewood officials precluded the possibility that certain non-USMD applicants might outshine even their USMD peers. Instead, going to a Caribbean or an osteopathic school was invariably associated with having erred somewhere along the way. Medical school trajectories were thus thought to be highly predictive of current abilities at Stonewood, even in the presence of more recent objective measurements of the latter, such as USMLE scores.

Unprofessional Conduct   Far more troublesome than suspected deficits in medical knowledge, however, were concerns about unprofessional conduct. This risk was especially associated with IMGs. Referring to this group, one faculty member explained:

> I'm going to refrain from saying "those people" but . . . they come out of societies oftentimes in cultures that are so hierarchical, that are so male-dominated and oppressive. A lot of the better, higher up [residency] programs view them as just not retrainable. They are very fixed in their ways; a lot of them are incredibly bright but don't speak up; they mumble; their English is crappy; they are not sexist, but they genuinely think that women should be subservient. They don't think about the end of life in the same nuanced way or think patients should make any decisions. . . . Yeah it's crazy the degree to which sometimes those guys are living out the stereotype. . . . They must come over to interview [in the United States], but, boy, sometimes it's just like, *these people are*—there I said it. I didn't want to say it. I didn't want to say "these people" (emphasis added).

Program officials shared similarly unfavorable views of IMGs: "You know, people are from countries where gay people are killed," explained one official. "I don't think I can afford to have someone who is incredibly narrow-minded, so that's one of the risks." It is telling that respondents shared these views so openly. They were simply uncontroversial in a context where USMDs' superiority was taken for granted.

While Stonewood officials may have had valid concerns about cultural differences, it is striking how graduates from virtually any foreign country were often grouped together in the same category without concern for individual variation— or for the possibility that these stereotypes may be wrong. In fact, their perspective had all the hallmarks of "classic racism," where people of color are viewed as undifferentiated.[25] By adopting such prejudiced and xenophobic views, these officials were espousing the very same narrow-mindedness that they were trying to guard against. Interestingly, several of Stonewood's own USMD residents were originally born in Africa, the Middle East, and Asia and were ostensibly raised in contexts similar to those of some IMGs, but this was never raised as a concern by the leadership.

Furthermore, all applicants, including IMGs, are required to pass USMLE Step 2–Clinical Skills (or the equivalent Comprehensive Osteopathic Medical Licensing Examination Level 2–Performance Evaluation for DOs), which is designed to explicitly test patient interaction skills and language proficiency. Passing—or even acing—this test, however, did not seem to allay fears about the "tendency among foreign graduates not to have the fluidity with American patients," as one respondent put it. Some cited patient preferences for "American" doctors as a reason for limiting the consideration of IMG applicants, as though American culture were a single, unified entity. At the same time, there was a paradoxical push to diversify the housestaff at Stonewood, in part because it catered to a large population of refugees. A Diversity Committee was created from the Department of Medicine's Minority Housestaff Association to encourage the recruitment of underrepresented minorities. When asked why diversity was important for the housestaff, a high-ranking member of the program directorship replied, "Because I think that our patient population is diverse [and] our physicians are going to be dealing with diverse populations their entire life. So having a diverse housestaff is important for the patients." But when I asked a member of the Minority Housestaff Association whether they considered IMGs an important source of diversity, they replied, "I don't think that's the diversity they're looking for." IMGs clearly did not represent the kind of minorities being targeted by the program, even though studies find that nationwide internationally trained physicians provide much-needed diversity to training programs and can help reduce social distance between patients and doctors.[26]

Put together, these concerns about non-USMDs lacking clinical knowledge and cultural competency make it clear that decision makers at Stonewood did not *trust* the quality of non-USMDs, even in the presence of objective licensing tests designed to measure both of these skills. These same tests ostensibly made the playing field level for applicants to residency (as I argued in the introduction), but they did little to convince Stonewood decision makers that non-USMDs were comparable to USMDs. Interestingly, physicians in the 1970s and 1980s invoked similar logics to justify hiring male physicians over female ones. Ideal colleagues were "brothers" who could be *trusted* while women were deemed untrustworthy and therefore less desirable candidates.[27] In the same way, Stonewood officials lacked an intangible trust in non-USMDs' training, even in the presence of reliable performance data like licensing exam scores. So instead they relied on pedigree as a surrogate marker for quality they could trust.

These patterns underline the sociological difference between *reputation*, which refers to expected performance based on a previous track record (e.g., licensing exam scores), and *status*, an actor's position in the social order based on ties to other people and institutions (e.g., pedigree).[28] In situations like these, status is a commonly used proxy for quality amidst uncertainty about (or lack of trust in) an applicant's abilities, regardless of past performance (or reputation).[29] Status can become "sticky" in this way. Candidates cannot easily distinguish themselves from the status afforded to them by their medical school—regardless of past performance or reputation—prompting program officials to question whether even top-notch applicants are inferior simply by virtue of being affiliated with a lower-status medical school.[30]

Motivations: Avoiding Threats to the Program's Reputation

Status, however, is a two-way street—it flows and leaks between institutions and individuals, thereby transferring prestige between entities of higher or lower status.[31] Stonewood officials may have relied on applicants' pedigrees to impute quality, but they were also very aware of the effect that applicants had on their own institutional status. To that end, beneath all that talk of wanting to reduce risk, inconsistencies lingered. These inconsistencies shed light on how Stonewood decision makers used risk as a pretext for social closure. When pressed on the issue of patient care, for example, several respondents adopted a more nuanced stance vis-à-vis non-USMDs, suggesting they may have been inflating the dangers associated with hiring them. For example, one program official initially voiced concerns about the quality of non-USMDs by saying "I feel [like] my excellent third- and fourth-year [US] medical students are able to see and verbalize the ambiguity of a situation we're in in a more sophisticated way than some of my [attending] colleagues who are foreign trained." But when asked about the impact on patient care of pooling (ostensibly lower-quality) non-USMDs into community programs, this official espoused a more nuanced perspective: "I have no idea. I don't know. You know maybe, maybe not, because the quality of patient care is so complex. . . . There's a lot of room for US grads to be crappy doctors and for foreign medical grads to be excellent doctors and all in between." Patient care was suddenly more complicated, and there was more room for variability. Studies have consistently shown no appreciable difference in the quality of care provided by fully trained USMDs and non-USMDs, suggesting that any real risk posed to patients by hiring non-USMDs at Stonewood was likely overestimated.[32]

To be sure, concerns about reducing risk and saving resources on problematic workers are part of any organization's efforts to thrive. As one official told me, "Those [residents] who struggle take a hell of a lot of time. Unfortunately, they can create chaos on the teams; they cost a lot to the system from the top to the bottom." Stonewood's risk aversion was not uniform, however. Some risks they *were* willing to take. For example, the program sometimes recruited applicants who failed the USMLE (like Greg from the last chapter), who would most definitely be a risk from a medical knowledge perspective. They also recruited the occasional USMD with disciplinary actions on file, including one with a criminal record, as I will discuss later. So while the same (or even greater) risks may have existed among USMDs compared to non-USMDs, Stonewood officials were more willing to take a chance on the former.

There were also few attempts to correct negative assumptions about non-USMDs at Stonewood. When asked about their opinion of Caribbean medical graduates, for example, one official expressed skepticism about their motivations for going to an offshore school: "I think it's an unknown that *I'm not sure I'm willing to try to find out more about*" (emphasis added). Others were willing to be more open-minded toward non-USMDs only if someone taught them, placing the onus on others to dispel their negative assumptions. As one attending stated, "If someone *teaches* me that people who come from a certain medical school—Caribbean medical school, a DO school, from an international medical school—if I learned that they have what their training entails, if I was better informed on that, I think I would be able to fit them more seamlessly into the way that I would think about all medical schools, but I don't have that exposure" (emphasis added). Thus, in their reluctance to learn more about non-USMDs, Stonewood officials (themselves USMDs) clearly seemed more interested in recruiting residents in their own image than in truly assessing the risks and benefits associated with non-USMDs. Their uncertainty, some might say, was intentional.

Part of this reluctance may have had to do with Stonewood officials' stated commitment to fulfilling their end of the social contract with USMDs, guaranteeing them access to the top residency spots. As one junior faculty member at Stonewood reasoned, "My impression is that the residencies that view themselves or are viewed as higher quality preferentially stick to the US grads . . . out of a commitment to [the fact that] there are more US grads each year and relatively few residency spots. So our first priority is a societal means to train the US grads to be US doctors." Here the faculty member was espousing the widespread myth in the profession of a so-called squeeze in graduate medical education.[33] Despite growing numbers of US allopathic and osteopathic medical graduates, the total number of residency positions has been projected to remain well above the number of these graduates for the next decade.[34] Elite spots, however, *were* limited.[35] So the belief that USMDs were getting squeezed out influenced Stonewood officials' approach to recruitment. As one official pointed out, "I've got a bunch of American schools that I haven't invited applicants from. So is it going to get harder for [a non-USMD] to get an interview here? Yes." Hiring was thus viewed as a zero-sum game at Stonewood: a gain for non-USMDs was seen as a loss for USMDs, which was unacceptable for many Stonewood decision makers, given medicine's implicit social contract with USMDs.

But aside from protecting the elite, these practices and justifications also importantly protected against another, more implicit risk that program leaders wanted to mitigate: threats to Stonewood's reputation. While officials may have emphasized the need to hire the "best" doctors and reduce risk to patients, they were also guided by a desire to maximize prestige, making high-status USMDs (even riskier ones) preferable to non-USMDs. After explaining that Stonewood doesn't consider international graduates because "the training is so different or *may* be so different . . . that we're not willing to take a risk," a senior program official elaborated:

> Whereas there are some programs across the country that rely on interna-
> tional graduates to fill the program, we are not [one of those]. We fill with US
> grads. . . . I think we are in the top half [of all residency programs] because
> there are currently more spots in internal medicine than there are US grads
> to fill them, so *a badge of honor* is filling with US grads. And because we have
> had more US grads applying [than open spots], we don't really have to look at
> the international grads. (emphasis added)

Residency recruitment at Stonewood therefore went beyond simply wanting to hiring the "best" doctors for *patients*—it also involved hiring the best doctors for the *program*: prestigious USMDs.

As a top-of-the-middle-tier/bottom-of-the-top-tier program, Stonewood was acutely aware of its status position and the role that recruitment played in maintaining that position. The consequence was a very low threshold for tolerating even small numbers of non-USMDs. As one official explained, "Historically, international grads have gone to less prestigious programs. I wonder if some folks [current residents] would think, 'Wait, does this mean I'm now in a less prestigious program?' " Indeed, current residents shared these worries. One intern told me, "I think if they accept DOs, it's fine, but if they're *overrun* with DOs, then it also means something about the quality of the program" (emphasis in original). Some were concerned about how it might affect their careers if even 10 percent of the residents Stonewood accepted were non-USMDs. As one intern said, "I would think I invested in the wrong place and wonder what happened to [Stonewood's] standing. . . . I would feel like that decreased my chances of getting into the best fellowship that I could." Thus, even a handful of non-USMDs was perceived as a blight on the program's up-and-coming elite status, with possibly dire consequences for current trainees.

Stonewood officials were also concerned about their chances of recruiting future USMDs if there were non-USMDs on the housestaff—concerns confirmed by the USMDs interviewed in chapter 1 who said they steered clear of programs with non-USMDs. One faculty member reasoned, "I think the greater the number [of non-USMDs], the more of a question you'll get from [prospective] US students who would say, 'Couldn't you get any US students?' So there is that attitude I think that's kept us trying to keep that number low." Stonewood residents showed similar signs of anxiety when I asked what might happen if 10 percent of new recruits next year were non-USMDs. A third-year resident predicted, "They'd come out balls-to-the-wall next year for recruitment. . . . They would recruit the shit out of . . . US grads, to try to overcome that. Because if it's 10 percent, then it's 11 percent, and pretty soon you're at 100 percent." This concern about a slippery slope is evocative of the same sort of moral panic associated with other instances of social "contagion," such as in segregated neighborhoods where whites are willing to tolerate only a certain percentage of black people before deciding they do not want to live there anymore.[36]

Stonewood officials were not always transparent, however, about preferring USMDs because of their higher status. Instead, they often couched their decisions in meritocratic terms that conflated preference with performance. When I asked the senior official why it was a badge of honor to exclusively hire USMDs, they elaborated: "I think, in a way from the US grad perspective that it's badge of honor across the country. I do think it's a national program director perspective. . . . Then I think it's an internal badge as well. You are trying to match with what you perceive as the best students and, again, getting the best US graduates from across the country feels good internally." For this official, USMDs were not just a badge of honor; they were considered the "best" students, when, in fact, their superiority vis-à-vis non-USMDs was assumed rather than systematically assessed. In truth, a more meritocratic approach that evaluated applicants' individual merits, independent of their pedigree, would have likely resulted in an inconvenient outcome for Stonewood, a program seeking to increase its status. The same might not have been as true for a top-tier program. As one intern said, "No one would be like, 'Well, I'm not going to Harvard 'cause there's foreign grads.'" Thus, because of its position as a "trend follower," Stonewood was more likely than other programs to eliminate as many threats as possible to its reputation—including, and perhaps especially, non-USMDs.[37]

Different Rules of the Game

It was not *unheard of*, however, for non-USMDs to be interviewed at Stonewood. Indeed, for a selection process—especially an ostensibly meritocratic one—to be considered legitimate, it has to be at least a little porous.[38] Recall that around

2 percent of interviews were accorded to DOs and IMGs every year at Stonewood. So how did these lucky few make the cut?

To catch the attention of program officials and avoid being simply dismissed as "risky," international and osteopathic applicants had to play by rules of the game that were harder than those for USMDs, thereby ensuring that only a select few would clear the bar. As one respondent put it, non-USMDs "just start lower and have to push themselves up." This approach aligned nicely with Stonewood's emphasis on meritocracy, such that if non-USMDs were excluded, it was because they simply did not measure up to these much higher standards.

Numbers to Numbers   To start, non-USMDs' academic records had to be beyond reproach. Even being at the top of one's class was insufficient because, in the words of one Stonewood official, "maybe they're on top of a heap of not-so-good students." The official went on to add, "We don't automatically reject people. You know if someone's at the top of their class and has done 270s on Step 1 and 2, and . . . we know the people they've done an elective with and they say, 'This kid is better than any American grad I've ever seen,' we'll pay attention to that." In other words, Stonewood would consider interviewing non-USMDs if they scored two standard deviations above the mean on their exams and came with the support of a known faculty member who could vouch for their superiority *over* US trainees.[39] Meanwhile, expectations were not nearly as high for USMDs. As one faculty member said, "There [are] plenty [of] middle-of-the-pack US medical residents that would be preferred. . . . [For non-USMDs] to even get looked at, you have to dot your i's and cross your t's perfectly. Can't have a bad test score."

In this way, non-USMDs were not evaluated "numbers to numbers" against USMDs. As one USIMG resident at Legacy protested, "I mean, theoretically, best case scenario is that your application gets sent without [programs] even knowing where you went [to medical school]. Then it's numbers to numbers, recommendation letters to recommendation letters, and I bet people would be surprised what came out of it." Instead, the very same numbers had very different meanings for non-USMDs versus USMDs. Recall that non-USMDs widely speculated that this was the case in the previous chapter, and now key decision makers at Stonewood confirmed that this was true.[40] These double standards inevitably favored USMDs who perhaps performed less well but whose training was deemed more trustworthy, making them far less risky in terms of the program's social standing.

Electives Grades alone were not enough to catch the eye of busy program directors, however; as one official noted earlier, elective rotations where non-USMDs
outperformed USMDs were also necessary. Advocacy was a key piece of these
electives. Take Farha, for example, an international resident at Legacy who also
applied to Stonewood's residency program. She did several rotations as a medical
student at the various hospitals affiliated with Stonewood University Medical
School and received glowing evaluations from residents and attendings who encouraged her to apply. She even asked the program directorship about their requirements for residency, and they told her the same criteria as on their website.
"I asked them, 'Do you have preference for [Stonewood] students or American
students?' And [they] said, 'No, it is not like that.' " But Farha was never contacted for an interview. "They never take any foreign medical graduates," Farha said
resignedly, with a shrug, "It is not that my scores were low; I had like 98th, 99th
[percentile]. So I don't know why." The reason was that it wasn't enough for Farha
to have had exemplary USMLE scores or even to have rotated at Stonewood. She
needed someone to advocate on her behalf.

But Stonewood made it nearly impossible to secure that kind of support.
Stonewood University Medical School had very clear policies regarding visiting
medical students who wanted to do elective rotations at its affiliated hospitals,
including Stonewood University Hospital. First, it explicitly prohibited all medical students from offshore (Caribbean) schools from rotating at its hospitals on
the grounds that these schools did not have hospitals of their own with which to
reciprocate. For their part, IMGs like Farha, whose school was on an approved
list, could rotate in limited numbers.[41] Remarkably, however, they were forbid-
den from requesting letters of recommendation. Written in bold in several places
on the application form was a statement that, under penalty of dismissal from
the elective, visiting international students were not permitted to ask for reference letters from Stonewood faculty or program officials. The same rules did
not appear anywhere on the application materials for US or Canadian medical
students, however. No faculty member or official ever mentioned this policy to
me during interviews, suggesting they may not have even been aware of it. This
could explain why Farha did not get an interview, despite being encouraged to
apply by her attendings. She could not ask for their support, and they may not
have even known.

The policy regarding DOs was more complicated. Stonewood had a long
history of institutional discrimination toward DOs. One former hospital

administrator "would not even allow [program officials] to put [DOs] on the rank list—plain and simple. Period. Done. End of story," as one official disclosed. In 2010, a medical school official who took a dim view of DOs drafted a policy explicitly prioritizing allopathic students for rotations. It accepted DO students only for "specific clinical rotations," as determined in consultation with the clinical department chairs and only during the less busy months of January through May. To be sure, Stonewood also gave priority to its own students when scheduling clinical electives with visiting USMD students. But this policy meant that DOs could rotate at Stonewood only with special departmental approval, making it harder for osteopathic students to do electives at Stonewood hospitals and eventually match there, regardless of their competence.

In sum, the rotation policies at Stonewood blocked many non-USMDs from gaining clinical experience at the hospital and catching the eye of faculty members, even though that was one of the only ways of getting noticed as a non-USMD. While these restrictions (especially the DO rotation policy) may have been framed as efforts at quality control, they also helped maintain the program's "badge of honor" by ensuring that the Match list was made up almost exclusively of USMDs. They also helped obscure and legitimate the barriers keeping non-USMDs out of Stonewood. As one USMD resident at Stonewood said with a shrug, "The fact that [non-USMD] people do make it through observerships [here] and such, [and] that there's a reasonable process to get in somewhere *if you really want to*, speaks against it being, say, frank discrimination" (emphasis added). This line of thinking led to the widely held belief at Stonewood that if non-USMDs did not match, it was because they did not work hard enough or did not "want" it enough rather than because the deck was stacked against them.

Resident Selection Committee   For the few non-USMDs who did manage to catch the program's eye and get an interview, there was a final hurdle they had to clear before being added to Stonewood's rank list—the penultimate step before getting sent to the National Resident Match Program: surviving the Resident Selection Committee. The committee met five times between November and February to discuss candidates who were flagged during the interview process, either because they were deemed risky or because they might have been over- or underranked by the interviewer.

As a matter of protocol, all international and osteopathic interviewees were automatically discussed at the Resident Selection Committee meetings while only "flagged" USMDs were discussed. One of the rare non-USMDs on the faculty at Stonewood thought this was unfair:

> Frankly, the idea of discussing every IMG at the meeting is a little discriminatory. . . . Why discuss all IMGs? Should we discuss all people that are from Alaska or California? . . . You can discuss everybody that received a [Step] score below 230; you can discuss everybody that has a substellar recommendation letter; you can make that rule. You can discuss everybody [without] publications, but I just don't see the point of having, necessarily, a discussion about everybody that is IMG.

Non-USMDs therefore not only had to impress their interviewers but also had to pass muster with the Resident Selection Committee, a twenty-or-so-member panel of faculty members. They especially had to impress their flag reviewer, a committee member who was assigned to scrutinize their file and lead discussion on their application during the meetings. Unsurprisingly, this practice further helped lower the likelihood of non-USMDs being ranked high enough to match at Stonewood, as there had to be consistently strong support among the faculty at multiple stages to push forward their candidacy.

Aside from being automatically singled out for further discussion, non-USMDs often faced greater scrutiny than USMDs at the Resident Selection Committee meetings, with familiar concerns about risk and the unknown resurfacing. Take, for example, this exchange about a DO candidate:

> "This candidate was interviewed by [Dr. X]. He was really impressed by her real-world understanding of what it's like to practice and had much more of a sense of what it's like out there than most other applicants. She had good questions. He was impressed by her part-time work during undergrad and med school. He was called by [a community attending] who wanted to put [in] an extra special plug for her. And then he noted that the folder wasn't that great," said the committee chair by way of introduction. Someone else pointed out, "She's coming from [a] DO school which I think we're less familiar with." He named the school and asked the flag reviewer if he'd heard of it. The flag reviewer replied, "Yeah, that school has been around for a while." . . . The leader continued, "She was in the top 20 percent of her class. . . . If we're interested in calling someone she rotated with, another one of our graduates is at

[a nearby community hospital where the DO applicant rotated], so it sounds like she could be a good place to go [for more information]." An attending interjected, "It's still going to be tough to compare people doing rotations at [community hospitals]. If [the faculty there] are used to seeing people [students] who aren't that good, they'll be blown away easily by someone. Isn't [a score of] 4.6 reserved for people with publications and stuff?" The leader nodded: "Yeah, it's pretty high." Someone else noted that the community hospital she rotated at is exposed to a wide variety of students, including MDs and DOs. Yet another attending chimed in, "I just saw she did her pediatrics rotation at [a different community hospital]. How many pediatric patients do they have there, *really*?" (emphasis in original)

This discussion about an osteopathic candidate in the top 20 percent of her class nicely captures how the rules of the game were different for non-USMDs. Not only did this candidate need to have an attending "put [in] an extra special plug for her," but also the details of her file were put through extra scrutiny simply because she came from a DO school (a school that has been around for more than thirty-five years). The flag reviewer, who was sympathetic to this applicant, later told me, "Would they have said the same thing if [she had been] an MD that had rotated in a smaller [hospital]? They wouldn't even know it! They wouldn't raise the question!" Indeed, one of Stonewood's most respected attendings (a USMD) had completed their residency at one of the community hospitals in question several decades prior, but that did little to assuage concerns. Instead, the committee challenged the validity of this DO's letters of recommendation by questioning whether the letter writers could really identify excellence among "people who aren't that good." These letter writers were local, however, as was the community hospital in question, which made concerns about the uncertainty—or untrustworthiness—of this DO's training less credible.

In contrast, USMDs were given the benefit of the doubt more often than non-USMDs were, likely because their pedigree posed less of a risk to the program's reputation. In one case, a USMD from a top-tier medical school was flagged for receiving only a "Pass" on their subinternship (sub-I)—a critical rotation in medical school during which students are given responsibilities similar to those of first-year residents. ("Pass" is a relatively low grade for a sub-I clerkship. While different medical schools use different scales, most schools usually award "Honors" and "High Pass" before "Pass" and "Fail.") During discussion about the candidate, one faculty member said, "I worry about the sub-I," and then added snidely, "Granted, [a] pass from [a top medical school] might be better than honors from [the previous candidate's osteopathic school]."

Similar serious red flags on USMDs' applications were not always approached with the same degree of consternation expressed in the case of top-notch non-USMDs. One USMD candidate was flagged because he failed the Step 2–Clinical Skills portion of the USMLE, which is designed to assess physical exam and patient interaction techniques. The interviewer introduced the candidate enthusiastically: "Yes, his résumé is so full of activities and research and presentations and travel history. It's really amazing–I don't know how he slept during medical school! The reason I have him flagged for today is he failed Step 2. He's well rounded so I wanted to see what other people thought." When they expressed concern about his failing Step 2, an attending began to rationalize:

> "[In Step 2], they have like what sounds like a list of no-no's: you forgot to ask for permission to remove a piece of clothing or wash your hands. It looks like an inexact science, and I think if you take twenty physicians, one of them might fail." The flag reviewer interjected, "I was going to comment–it seemed anomalous. . . . Is he worth the risk? And if you read the letters carefully, I was impressed with his personality and now hearing that he failed the interpersonal part of the skills? I don't know what to make that." A discussion ensued; someone said, "I agree that it [Step 2–Clinical Skills] can be very subjective–only it's so hard to know what to do with . . ." Someone else jumped in, "He looks like someone who doesn't respect the tests–[below average on Step 1], fail [on Step 2]. . . . If he's going to come here . . ." The interviewer countered: "He is *so* busy with extracurricular activities," including welding as a pastime. . . . To conclude, the flag reviewer said, "The question is, Is he a risk? I think in terms of what he will bring, he will bring some unique stuff and light up the place." Someone else quipped, "He's going to light up this place because of the welding!" The reviewer laughed, "Yeah, light the place on fire!"

Compared to the previous discussion about the excellent DO student, there was greater effort to contextualize this USMD's poor performance on the USMLE, which was dismissed as a "subjective" evaluation, thereby minimizing concerns about medical knowledge risks. Recall that similar efforts were not invested in DOs and USIMGs; they were just assumed to be risky from a medical knowledge standpoint, even when they scored higher on the same tests.

Program officials also explained away rather serious and concrete risks to professionalism posed by USMD interviewees, although those same theoretical risks were the primary justification used to exclude IMGs from consideration. Consider the following discussion about a USMD with a criminal record:

> The applicant's interviewer, who was in the room, recalled being very excited about meeting the candidate: "He looked absolutely fabulous on paper except for a few indiscretions as a teenager—convictions. So that caught my eye at first, and then he got his act together and worked as a plumber, spent a lot of time [abroad], decided he wanted to be a doctor, then went to medical school where he's been a star—he has two publications—and I was just so excited. And then I interviewed him. And I was disappointed." "Anything missing from your office?" someone deadpanned. The interviewer shrugged: "No, he had a flat affect, just very flat. Difficult to get him engaged. Maybe he was having a bad day." . . . The interviewer concluded, "I think he's someone who almost needs a call [to his letter writers] 'cause he might have just been having a bad day." "Did you look around the office? Did you have everything still?" someone else repeated. The meeting leader said with a nod, "I think his folder is close to a [near perfect score], so it sounds like a phone call is worth it." Someone else agreed: "I don't think his shenanigans as an eighteen-year-old matter. His male prefrontal cortex has developed!"

The levity with which the committee members broached this applicant's criminal record and their willingness to write off a lukewarm interview as the result of a bad day stand in stark contrast to their review of the DO candidate's file discussed earlier.[42] At Stonewood, program directors would regularly make *outgoing* calls to guard against "being unfairly negative" about questionable USMD candidates; for non-USMDs, however, recall that *incoming* calls were necessary to even be considered for an interview. The rules of the game were simply different for non-USMDs, which ensured that only a token number would be interviewed and placed on Stonewood's rank list, thus protecting the program's prestige among its peers.

Stonewood's Match List: Shifting Justifications

Match Day was quite a production at Stonewood. The day began with the program directorship heading to Stonewood University, where champagne flowed and a live jazz band boogied in the lobby, to personally congratulate students who had matched to the Stonewood residency program. Back at the hospital, the excitement continued with the Match list being posted in the residents' lounge. A swarm of residents began to huddle around the list, which, for the first time in recent memory, contained *two* non-USMDs. Reactions were mixed. While most residents hardly noticed the non-USMDs, one PGY-3 pointed to the affiliation of one of the interns and said, "Huh, that's interestingggg . . . ," stretching out the last syllable. She was pointing to one of the non-USMDs. "It's surprising," she added. "Not that there's anything wrong with that," her tone somewhat betraying her words.

From the leadership's perspective, the fact that the Match list contained two non-USMDs was not totally surprising, given that they had ranked those individuals high enough to match. Their explanations for doing so, however, helped shed light on the extent to which officials were preoccupied with the program's prestige. When I asked program leaders to make sense of this outcome, their explanations started sounding an awful lot like the rationales used by Legacy officials: "It's all individualized!" replied one high-ranking program leader, referring to the selection process, even though officials had previously emphasized their use of nonindividualized shortcuts, like pedigree, to justify the wholesale exclusion of non-USMDs:

> These two [non-USMDs] were quite spectacular so we took them. Only a program that has confidence will take [non-USMDs]! . . . So foreign grads and DOs, for many years, when we were building the program, we didn't want to be known as a place that took these second-tier individuals—but that's a pejorative term—that took individuals who were not from allopathic schools in the [United States]. But now that we've been established, it's a badge of honor. . . . [For example], nobody's going to say [Stanford] must be losing it if they took [a guy] from Yugoslavia! They'll say, "Boy, this kid must have been spectacular if they took him." . . . We're not at that level yet, but I don't think people will say, "They must be a crappy program; they can only get DOs and IMGs."

For this official, it was now a badge of honor to hire *non-USMDs*, whereas the leadership had previously stressed the opposite. That they felt the need to neutralize the threat of two spectacular non-USMDs joining the housestaff by emphasizing how "established" the program was speaks to just how vigilant officials were when faced with the effects recruitment might have on Stonewood's standing as an elite institution.[43]

In this way, just like Legacy, Stonewood officials emphasized the importance of a highly meritocratic recruitment process. But they, too, were trying to maximize prestige while minimizing risk, which meant deviating from a purely merit-based approach. Stonewood officials relied on pedigree as a shortcut to cull applicants, which they argued yielded perfectly acceptable doctors, so why branch out further? But it was not a coincidence that those shortcuts also yielded the most prestigious outcome. The almost complete absence of non-USMDs at Stonewood was not due to chance or, in most cases, even a cursory appraisal of their merits. It was "conscious," as one attending put it—an effort intended, at least in part, to fulfill Stonewood's end of the social contract and, perhaps more importantly, to protect its precarious position at the bottom of the top tier of residency programs. Yet, rather than publicizing that preference or outright prohibiting non-USMDs from applying, which would have likely been illegal, Stonewood officials made the rules of the game much harder, making it more difficult for non-USMDs to rise above largely uncorroborated suspicions about their incompetence.[44] As a result, only two non-USMDs (out of thousands of hopefuls) successfully matched to Stonewood's internal medicine program, representing fewer than 5 percent of all new recruits.

CONCLUSION

Residency recruitment decisions do not occur inside a vacuum. Instead, officials at both hospitals selected residents with an eye toward elevating or maintaining program prestige, leading to instances of blatant discrimination and starkly segregated outcomes. To justify these choices, officials from both hospitals emphasized—and likely truly believed—that they made decisions based on merit. But without the immense pressure to stay competitive within the broader field of residency programs, it is unlikely that Stonewood and Legacy officials would have selected such plainly segregated housestaffs. Rather, programs might have pursued different goals, like actively trying to diversify the housestaff, recruiting the "best and the brightest" from around the world, and alleviating obvious inequality. They could have aimed to calibrate their Match lists to reflect the broader composition of residents nationwide, with roughly 42 percent of internal medicine positions being filled by USMDs. Instead, program officials recruited residents that maximized the prestige of their housestaff while minimizing the risks to their reputation, resulting in Stonewood matching exclusively with prestigious (but, in certain cases, lower-performing) USMDs and Legacy matching (fully) with mostly USIMGs.

Unsurprisingly, officials also justified their practices in ways that made their programs look good. Legacy officials specifically underscored the objectivity and rigor of their selection methods—a justification aided by the fact that they mostly matched with high-performing non-USMDs. In so doing, they both distinguished Legacy as less biased than Stonewood and diverted attention away from their own predilection for prestige-boosting USMDs. Incidentally, it was this same predilection that all but guaranteed that even the worst-performing USMDs would secure a residency somewhere—a central promise built into the social contract—because the prestige associated with their pedigree was attractive to lower-tier programs looking to climb the ranks, like Legacy. For their part, Stonewood officials stressed the importance of safely avoiding risk in residency recruitment, thereby justifying their exclusion of lesser-known non-USMDs who could cause harm to patients. But when two non-USMDs matched to their program, their justifications shifted; they now insisted instead that these non-USMDs were chosen using rigorous methods and held them out as evidence of the program's upward trajectory in terms of prestige.

Organizational status and concerns over social position therefore deeply shaped residency recruitment, from the selection processes that led to segregated Match lists to the justifications used to defend those practices. But the sorting of USMDs and non-USMDs into high- and low-status programs like Stonewood and Legacy should not matter much if the training is, in fact, standardized across programs, something the ACGME strives to ensure. Yet, as will become clearer in the next chapter, training differed dramatically between these two settings. The differences in education between the two hospitals only served to reinforce the inequalities evident among residents based on pedigree, thereby further entrenching status separation within internal medicine between USMDs and non-USMDs.

CHAPTER 3

A Day on the Wards

pager went off at Legacy Community Hospital, signaling another admission. It was 7:30 PM, and Blaine (a US graduate of an international medical school [USIMG] in his second postgraduate year [PGY-2]) and Isabel, his intern (an international medical graduate [IMG] in her first postgraduate year [PGY-1]), were on call until 9:00 PM.[1] There were two patients waiting to be admitted in the emergency department: one was a man with chest pain, and the other was a woman with "question-TB" (needing evaluation for possible tuberculosis). With two patients getting admitted at 7:30, the intern-resident team was unlikely to get out by 9:00 PM. They decided to divide and conquer. Blaine followed up with an attending physician on another patient while Isabel went to the emergency department to see the new admissions. They met back on the wards, where Blaine entered orders on the new patients and Isabel updated the team's patient roster. By 9:30 PM, they finished the admissions and went home after a fourteen-hour shift.

The next morning Blaine went to check on the "question-TB" patient and noticed that an ultrasound technician was in the room without the proper infection precautions. (Tuberculosis is airborne, so usual precautions include gowns, gloves, and tight-fitting masks to protect against transmission.) There was a sign on the patient's door signaling the need for these airborne precautions, but it seemed the technician either had ignored it or just did not see it. Blaine and Isabel peered inside the room as the technician hovered mere inches from the patient's face without a gown or mask, administering an ultrasound of the heart—an unnecessary test for potential pulmonary tuberculosis. "Apparently, [the patient's] getting a 2-D echo[cardiogram]!" Blaine announced with a nervous laugh as he quickly shut the patient's door. It was unclear who ordered the echocardiogram, but if the patient did have TB, the technician had undoubtedly been exposed. The patient's nurse, who happened to be nearby, asked, "Does she still need a chest CT [scan]?" Blaine nodded firmly and said with a laugh, "Yeah! *That's* what she needs!" As the nurse's attention shifted toward another patient, Isabel whispered to Blaine, "Did you order a 2-D echo last night [for the TB patient]?" He gave her a half smile and offered, "I don't think so. I was really tired."

A few hours later Blaine bumped into a fellow resident who asked him about the ultrasound: "Did you know the tech went in without a mask?" Blaine gave a small nod. "Does she [the tech] know it was an *accidental* 2-D echo?" his fellow resident pressed on. Blaine replied curtly, "No, and she shouldn't know." He added something about how it wasn't accidental—how he believed everyone should have an echocardiogram at some point in their lives. He was joking, but the expression on his face revealed the gravity of the situation; a staff member may have inadvertently been exposed to tuberculosis, a highly contagious and airborne infectious disease. Isabel clicked through the patient's labs and realized that the ultrasound should have been ordered for the patient admitted with *chest pain*—not for the TB patient. Blaine ordered it by accident, and no one caught the mistake until it was too late.

Meanwhile at Stonewood University Hospital, an attending physician on rounds began asking an intern about a patient who had been admitted for alcohol withdrawal—a potentially life-threatening condition when left untreated. "So he's on CIWA," confirmed the attending, referring to the Clinical Institute Withdrawal Assessment protocol for treating alcohol withdrawal. (The more severe the symptoms, the more medication that should be administered.) However, the intern had forgotten to input medication orders associated with the protocol, so while nurses were monitoring the patient's symptoms, they didn't have orders to treat those potentially deadly symptoms. The attending continued, "How's he been scoring?" The intern paused and then replied, "Uh, not sure." The attending frowned: "So if you put an alcoholic on a CIWA protocol, you have to give them [the nurses] something to do other than look at the numbers. The nurses need to know how to treat him." The attending said he noticed the absence of orders last night, so he put them in for his intern. Thankfully, he caught the error before it had consequences for the patient.

How could such similar scenarios play out so differently at these two teaching hospitals? These examples are not meant to suggest that mistakes always fell through the cracks at Legacy or that they never did at Stonewood. Rather, they raise a different set of questions. How did the residency program training structures explain these two near misses? (It turned out the patient at Legacy did not have active TB, so the technician was fine.) How and why did approaches to resident education differ between these two segregated residency programs? And what were the implications for the residents' training and approaches to patient care?

Sociologists have often conceptualized medical education as being relatively standardized, giving little thought to how it might differ across training contexts.[2] After all, regulatory bodies like the Accreditation Council for Graduate Medical Education (ACGME) issue basic standards to which all residency programs must conform to maintain accreditation, which helps give the impression that graduate medical education is more or less uniform everywhere. But there is good reason to believe that education can vary by setting. Over two-thirds of internal medicine residency programs are currently housed in community hospitals, which tend to have more limited resources, including supervision, than university hospitals.[3] Community programs also tend to be staffed by USIMGs, IMGs, and Doctors of Osteopathic Medicine (DOs) rather than graduates of US allopathic medical schools (USMDs), a situation which lowers their institutional status and may dissuade some attendings from working there.[4] Despite these important structural differences, however, there are few accounts of how medical education can differ between university and community programs.[5]

In this chapter, I follow a typical workday at Legacy and Stonewood Hospitals to highlight the differences in how the two programs approach medical education. At Legacy, the laissez-faire structure of the residency program meant that residents were primarily viewed as *laborers* who were expected to get the job done first and then learn on their own in their considerable spare time. In their clinical work, residents served as surrogates for private attending physicians, who relied on residents to care for their patients in their stead while they primarily worked in outpatient settings. The attendings' absence therefore led trainees to experience what I call *inconsistent autonomy*, whereby Legacy residents were required to both follow their attendings' orders and make independent decisions without support—a pattern that echoed the lack of support typical of the contest mobility track experienced by non-USMDs before residency (see chapter 1). Put together, the conditions at Legacy led to poorer learning outcomes and a more exploitative work environment for the residents, even though they had lower workloads than Stonewood residents did.

In contrast, at Stonewood, residents were first and foremost considered trainees who only secondarily worked for the hospital. The program's structure meant that the residents were strongly supported and supervised, allowing them to gain independence without posing a risk to patients. I call this *supported autonomy* and argue that it is an extension of the professional support experienced by USMDs during medical school, thanks to the social contract. This chapter builds on the previous two by examining the implications of segregation in residency programs for both professional training and patient care. More broadly, it explores the construction and reinforcement of professional (dis)advantage in residency by focusing on the role that formal training plays in exacerbating informal status inequalities.

PREROUNDING

It was 6:30 AM. Lynn, a USMD intern about six months into her residency at Stonewood, shucked off her winter coat in the residents' lounge and immediately received the sign-out from the overnight intern—the handoff of patients between the day and the night teams that occurs at least twice a day. Lynn received two new patients for the day, which maxed out her list of patients at seven. Only months ago Lynn would have been capped at ten, but a new admissions system that assigned interns to specific beds also reduced the cap to six or seven beds per intern. She was one of eight interns covering the teaching wards at Stonewood that month.

Lynn rushed upstairs, where she bumped into Doug, a fellow intern with whom she shared a resident. He, too, was maxed out with six patients, for a total of thirteen for their four-person team of two interns, a resident, and an attending.[6] They exchanged pleasantries but did not waste time. Their notes, complete with vital signs, updated lab results, physical exam findings, and treatment plans, had to be finished by 9 AM, when their resident would come upstairs from morning report. Lynn speed walked from one patient's room to the next, spending about three minutes examining her "old" patients from yesterday and trying to minimize delays from patients who wanted to chat longer. For the new admits who arrived overnight, she spent only a few extra minutes asking about their chief complaint and performing a more thorough exam. Many of Lynn's patients were quite sick, requiring time-consuming, coordinated care between medicine and other subspecialties (which was typical of the patient profile at

Stonewood), but this left Lynn with little time to spare. She quickly scrawled patient information onto a folded bundle of about ten papers stapled together, which contained vital data on each patient. She would eventually transcribe all this information into the electronic health record, where she wrote notes and orders for each of her patients. If she did not finish her notes by 9 AM, the case manager, resident, and attending would not have the information they needed to prepare for rounds. Time was of the essence.

Meanwhile, at Legacy, McKayla (a USMD preliminary intern) started leisurely prerounding over an hour later, at 7:40 AM. Even after having been on call last night until 9 PM, she got only one new admission, bringing her total patient roster to just two. This was not uncommon at Legacy; while the hospital "census" (or patient load) fluctuated considerably, the average number of patients per intern-resident team was only around 3.4 for the days I observed, with a minimum of 0 patients (not uncommon) and a maximum of 12 (rare).[7] There were even times when the housestaff outnumbered the patients. On the rare occasions when a team's patient load would get closer to the six or seven that was standard *per intern* at Stonewood, attendings sometimes quipped that they had better give me, the ethnographer, some patients to handle.

McKayla received the sign-out from the overnight intern and then wandered upstairs to briefly examine her two patients. Because she was on call the night before, she was spared from getting new patients this morning, so she did not join her fellow interns who had congregated around a graying white board behind the nurses' station to get their new assignments. Instead, she busied herself with paperwork after consulting the attending's note in the patient's chart from earlier that morning. As she handwrote her progress notes, she announced, "I'm going to write my note," signing the bottom of the page with a flourish, "and then do nothing for two hours." It was 8:20 AM, and she was done prerounding. She got up to search for her resident.

McKayla's and Lynn's experiences with prerounding foreshadow some important differences between Legacy and Stonewood. Because of the low patient census at Legacy, interns arrived later, prerounded on fewer patients who were generally less sick, read the attending's note in the patients' chart, and waited for their residents to arrive around 8 AM to discuss their patients' status. They did not have an assigned attending who was responsible for their patients and with whom they rounded every morning; this made for a more laid-back workday, but it also meant fewer opportunities to learn. The primary goal, it seemed, was to do the work. At Stonewood, interns would arrive as early as necessary to preround on six or seven usually complicated patients in preparation for 9 AM rounds, when the whole care team would discuss and tweak their treatment plans for every patient. While McKayla had a chance to grab coffee and maybe even breakfast every morning, Lynn barely had time to see all of her patients before 7:30—the time at which she had to begin writing her notes if she wanted to finish by 9:00. As long as McKayla got the job done, she could spend her free time doing whatever she wanted. Lynn, in contrast, had no free time as she prepared for the educational rounds with her superiors that would take up the whole morning and often spill over into the afternoon. Already, their days were beginning to look quite different.

MORNING REPORT

While the interns prerounded and worked on care management (what the housestaff sometimes referred to as "scut" work), residents went to morning report. The purpose of this daily conference was to offer protected time for second- and third-year residents to hone their medical knowledge and sharpen their clinical reasoning skills. Yet the content and format varied importantly from one institution to the other. At Legacy, morning report was formulaic and focused heavily on inculcating medical knowledge. Expectations were modest, and the tone was more informal than at Stonewood, where morning report consisted of a rigorous group exercise in collective problem solving. These dissimilarities exemplified the two programs' fundamentally different approaches to medical education. Legacy was more hands-off and seemingly less invested in pedagogy, which was consistent with its overall approach to residents as *laborers*, while Stonewood was more structured and far more engaged in the residents' learning, emphasizing its commitment to residents as *trainees*.

Morning Report at Legacy

On the first day of every month, the Legacy chief resident cheerfully described the format of morning report to a new group of residents rotating onto the general medical floors. She explained that a different attending physician would come in every day of the week to share their expertise on a given area of internal medicine. "Some of the attendings don't like people coming in and out, so try to arrive on time," she implored, although the housestaff regularly arrived late, sometimes trickling in after grabbing breakfast from the cafeteria, still clutching coffee and hash browns doused in ketchup. She continued, "Now I don't want anyone fighting over reading EKGs [electrocardiograms] or answering questions. Everyone will get a chance." This last comment would usually elicit a round of snickering from the seven general medical ward residents seated at the table, who could hardly imagine fighting over EKGs. As much as the chief resident tried to impose structure on morning report, she was often unsuccessful. The residents' attention would frequently wane, giving way to surfing the internet or exchanging text messages. One day a third-year USIMG resident prepared to give a presentation on Hashimoto's disease at the end of morning report. As he plugged in his computer to project his slides, he announced loudly with a cautionary tone, "I hope I don't get any text messages while I'm presenting," warning his fellow residents not to include him in any of the messages that would regularly bounce back and forth among the housestaff during morning report.

Every session began with the reading of an EKG. The chief resident would pass out copies and ask for volunteers to assess the squiggly lines. Residents were expected to present information in a specific order, beginning with the rate, rhythm, and axis. When they wanted to show off, residents would sometimes skip to the final diagnosis without carefully interpreting every peak or valley. "It's pericarditis!" declared a resident one morning. This was akin to giving away the punch line of a joke prematurely and was frowned upon by superiors, who would urge residents to start from the beginning. When residents struggled, the chief resident or attending would coach them. Their expectation was simply that residents *try*. One day the chief resident brought in an EKG of a heart with a pacemaker. When the chief was met with silence from the housestaff, she jumped in to help them:

> "So there's three letters . . . ," she said, hinting at the electrophysiology lecture from noon conference a few weeks ago where they discussed the North American Society of Pacing and Electrophysiology's codes. "So what are some of the typical letters?" Silence. The chief resident's face dropped. "No? Nothing, guys? I see the blank stares." She explained the three letters (the first was the chamber paced, the second was the chamber sensed, and the third was the response after sensing). "Nothing, guys? Well, I feel sad because it was a really good lecture."

The faculty at Legacy were not in the habit of reviewing concepts covered in previous didactic sessions, so residents had little incentive to retain much from the noon conference on pacemakers. Besides, being a community hospital, Legacy rarely saw patients with pacemakers, rendering this knowledge relatively esoteric for the residents.

After the EKG, the chief would call on different residents to answer practice multiple-choice questions from the American College of Physicians' Medical Knowledge Self-Assessment Program® (MKSAP) in preparation for the American Board of Internal Medicine Certification Examinations (Boards) at the end of residency. One day a resident was answering a practice question about a patient with severe trouble swallowing. Before revealing the answer choices, the chief resident asked him for the diagnosis. "Achalasia," the resident replied. The chief nodded and then continued, "OK, so what are the options to treat achalasia?" The resident began talking through the various treatments (Botox injections, balloon dilation, and surgery), and, unsurprisingly, all three treatments were among the options when the chief revealed the answer choices. The resident began to reason that because the question specifically mentioned that the patient lived far away, the best choice for her might be the surgery (myotomy). "Wanna go with C [myotomy]? Final answer?" asked the chief, and the resident nodded: "Because it's lasts longer." But then the resident began to hesitate and decided to change his mind, opting for the balloon dilation because it was minimally invasive. He ended up getting the question wrong. Myotomy (his first choice) was the correct answer.

Noticeably absent from the discussion was any mention of the scientific evidence for the treatments, even though MKSAP questions/answers reflect the evidence-based standard of care. In stark contrast to superiors at Stonewood, as will become clearer later, those at Legacy more commonly expected the housestaff to know *what* the right interventions were rather than encouraging them to think through *why* those were the right interventions based on the best available evidence. This approach had the potential to stunt the residents' clinical reasoning, as they were not consistently taught how to think critically and empirically about their decisions, including on the wards.

Morning report at Legacy usually ended with a case or topical presentation by a member of the housestaff. The quality of the presentations varied greatly, however, and expectations were generally low. One morning a third-year USIMG resident giving a presentation on pulmonary embolism looked at a pulmonary attending in the room and made a disclaimer before starting—"You're the expert; if you have anything to add, or if there are mistakes, let me know"—immediately releasing herself from ownership over the quality of her talk. As she gave her presentation without enthusiasm, reading directly from her slides, many of the housestaff unsurprisingly tuned her out and began checking their phones for stock prices, text messages—anything to keep them entertained. Meanwhile, the presenting resident consistently mispronounced thrombolysis (saying thromboLYsis instead of thromBOLysis), even though it was a key term in her presentation and English was her native language. She was never corrected, however, and the expert attending did not say anything during or after her presentation. She did not receive feedback, and the other residents were not chastised for failing to pay attention. Educators did little to show that they were invested in the residents' education in this way.

In sum, this low level of engagement by both the housestaff and the faculty was typical at Legacy, where comparatively little was expected of residents other than to simply get by and there were few consequences for failing to meet whatever expectations did exist. Legacy residents were primarily expected to get the job done. Learning, it seemed, was secondary.

Morning Report at Stonewood

In contrast to Legacy's morning report, that at Stonewood was a tightly structured event punctuated with an air of officiality that was markedly absent at Legacy. The conference room was lined with photographs of every previous cohort of residents dating back to the 1950s.[8] On a nearby bulletin board hung seventeen articles published by the housestaff in the past year, with the names of the resident-authors highlighted in yellow. The space itself could comfortably seat approximately fifty people, which it did at the height of interview season when prospective applicants attended morning report. But the table at the center of the room was reserved for residents.

On the first day of every month, the two chief residents leading morning report at Stonewood would spell out the nuts and bolts: "The expectation is that you're here at 8 AM for morning report. . . . I know it's tempting to say, 'Ah, I'll arrive at 8:05, 8:10,' but we also put a lot of work into our morning reports." Indeed, they did; it was not uncommon for the chiefs to be more familiar with the details of a case than the presenting residents themselves, who carried up to thirteen patients on a given day. With few exceptions, residents arrived on time, prepared to discuss. Expectations were clear and enforced: "Know enough about the case to be able to present to us," the chiefs would say. Residents were not to read from their notes. If they wanted to refer to lab values, that was fine, but they were not to read everything from their papers. Residents were also expected to sit at the main conference table. The program director, who attended almost daily, would ask rhetorically, "What about these side seats?" pointing to a semi-circle of chairs surrounding the conference table. In answer to his own question, he would always say, "The correct answer is no," followed by a jovial laugh. The side seats might have been tempting to those residents trying to keep a low pro-file, but they were for the audience. At Stonewood, program officials were quite serious about the residents having a seat at the table—literally and figuratively—as active and alert participants in their own learning.

Instead of following Legacy's formula of EKGs, MKSAP questions, and presentations, morning report at Stonewood almost always consisted of two residents presenting on two different patients and always followed the same classic presentation structure, which mirrored the structure they used upstairs during rounds with attendings: chief complaint, history of present illness, past medical history, past surgical history, social history, complete physical exam, summary, differential diagnosis, labs, and then diagnosis and treatment. Throughout the presentations, the chief residents would emphasize evidence-based medicine, clinical reasoning, feedback, and review of concepts.

Evidence-Based Medicine   Residents at Stonewood were constantly encouraged to use evidence-based medicine (EBM) to support clinical decision-making and guide their clinical practices. For example, presenting residents were routinely asked to come up with a "postcall" question that addressed some puzzling aspect of their case and answer it using evidence from the primary medical literature, thereby informing their approach to patient care. Sometimes the focus on EBM involved reviewing the evidence for the latest clinical guidelines (one chief resi-dent would refer to guidelines as important "vegetables" for the housestaff). Other times the chiefs used EBM to challenge the residents during case discussions. One morning Adam, a chief resident, asked the residents when to give steroids to patients with alcoholic hepatitis. Someone replied, "When the discriminant function is higher than 32."[9] Adam continued, "How do we know that?" Another resident replied, "There are studies!" As the housestaff chuckled, Adam pulled up a forest plot of the studies showing evidence for the use of steroids in alcoholic hepatitis. The studies in question, however, had explicitly excluded patients with infections. So Adam asked whether they should give steroids to alcoholic hepatitis patients *with infections*. When he was met with silence, he replied, "It pervades us up on the floors that we don't give steroids in the context of an infection in alcoholic hepatitis because it's contraindicated.[10] [But] there is *no* evidence to support that statement [because studies excluded patients with infections]. We can 'logic' it any way we want, but until we study it, we don't know the answer." In this way, the chiefs would challenge the residents to think reflexively about the presence or absence of evidence for their practices. At Legacy, in contrast, the discussion would have likely ended with the conclusion that patients with a discriminant function higher than 32 should be given steroids, with minimal discussion of the evidence supporting that practice.

Every so often case presentations at Stonewood would begin with a MKSAP question that was directly tied to a case. This helped reinforce medical knowledge through clinical practice.[11] In one such instance, a chief resident called on someone to read a MKSAP question about the treatment for achalasia (similar to the one that had been discussed at Legacy). However, the chief did not simply ask the housestaff to provide the diagnosis and treatment. Instead, a resident who had just presented a case of achalasia to morning report a few days prior began to review the evidence he had found on various treatment options. He eventually arrived at the correct answer by citing studies that supported the efficacy of one intervention over another. In this way, Stonewood residents were encouraged to learn not only *what* to do but also *why* to do it, which only sharpened their clinical reasoning skills.

Clinical Reasoning Chief residents would also regularly elicit the residents' thought processes during morning report:

> After getting a brief description of the history of present illness, the residents began to ask questions: "Cold intolerance? Heat intolerance?" "Nope," replied the presenting resident. "What are you getting at with those?" inquired Adam, the chief resident. "Thyroid disorders?" replied the resident. "Good," said the chief.... Someone else asked, "Any blurry vision or headaches?" "Why are you asking about that?" Adam inquired again. "I'm thinking of thrombosis from the PCV [polycythemia vera]."

These "why" questions signaled that it was not enough for residents to simply have medical knowledge; they also needed to demonstrate the logic accompanying that knowledge.

By repeatedly asking for the residents' thought processes, the chiefs taught them to be more critical of their practices and reasoning. They also encouraged the residents to be critical of those of others. In one instance, a program director inquired whether a patient with altered mental status had a normal sodium level, but because several people were talking at once, the chief didn't hear the question. Moments later a resident repeated, "Sodium's normal?" having heard the program director just ask the same question. The sodium was indeed normal, but the program director frowned: "Why did you ask [that]?" The resident smiled slyly and said, "Because you asked!" "OK, why did *I* ask?" countered the director. The resident thought for a moment and then eventually replied, "DI [diabetes insipidus]," a condition characterized by high sodium levels, to which the program director nodded, "Right because of the altered mental status." This resident was pushed to offer a reason for asking about sodium other than the fact that the most seasoned doctor in the room had asked about it. He was encouraged to think independently and critically about his request for labs in a way that simply was not done at Legacy.

Precision and Feedback Program directors and faculty members would frequently attend morning report and chime in with teaching points or feedback. In one case, a resident referred to a patient's social history as "significant for male partners," prompting one of the program directors to interject, "Remember, it's risky *behavior*, not orientation [that's relevant]." The resident rephrased more precisely, indicating that the patient had had unprotected sex with a male partner. By being corrected on the spot, residents learned the importance of accuracy. The regular presence of two chief residents, the program directors, and attendings and their frequent interlocutions meant that residents internalized these high expectations and were actively engaged in morning report.

Review A final priority in morning report at Stonewood was the review of important concepts that cemented the residents' newly acquired knowledge. These reviews ranged from ad hoc questions about previous morning reports to week-in-review sessions to a monthly *Jeopardy* game where residents were quizzed on everything they had covered that month. The residents really got into the *Jeopardy* game, playfully competing with one another for the correct answers. These reviews reinforced lessons about what was expected from the residents, as well as what constituted the good practice of medicine at Stonewood. They also showed a level of investment in pedagogy on the part of the chief residents, who created these review sessions, that was not as obvious at Legacy. Residents would then carry their newly acquired knowledge with them on the wards, where they would teach their interns about EBM and clinical reasoning, demanding the same degree of precision and critical thinking from their subordinates.

———————◆———————

While Legacy and Stonewood both set aside an hour per day during morning report to teach their residents, the format, structure, and expectations at the two hospitals were quite different. Consistent with the general nature of both residency programs—as well as with the notable differences resulting from the profession's social contract with USMDs but not with non-USMDs—Legacy's morning report was more informal, laid-back, and hands-off while Stonewood's was more formal, structured, and supportive, with several members of the program leadership and faculty attending regularly. Legacy emphasized medical knowledge through its MKSAP review questions and EKG readings while Stonewood heavily prioritized clinical reasoning and critical thinking. These different priorities reflected the broader conceptualizations of residents as laborers versus trainees; residents at Legacy were expected to have the right answer, whereas residents at Stonewood were expected to show (and grapple with) how they got that answer. Put differently, Legacy residents were taught *what* to think while Stonewood residents were taught *how* to think, which formed the basis for significant bifurcation in their education.

ROUNDS

The bulk of the day at both hospitals was spent on rounds, the ritual of going to see each patient as a team and deciding on a daily plan. This ritual looked very different at Legacy and Stonewood, however. With few exceptions, at Legacy the attending physicians in charge of patients (attendings-of-record) tended to be community primary care practitioners, who admitted patients from private practice, rather than hospital-based doctors (hospitalists). Residents could work with up to ten different attendings per week, many of whom spent only about an hour per day at Legacy, examining patients and updating charts but often without the housestaff in tow. Temporary teaching attendings were hired monthly to spend around three to six hours per week doing "teaching rounds" with the housestaff on the wards, but because they were not attendings-of-record, they could not independently make changes to patient care.[12] They could only offer educational insights while two or three teams of residents (four to eight trainees per attending) presented "interesting" patients to them, often at a conference room table rather than at the bedside.

Stonewood, in contrast, had a large team of dedicated hospital-based teaching attendings who were also attendings-of-record. This meant not only that they were primarily tasked with teaching residents but also that they were ultimately in charge of caring for the patients on the wards. A teaching attending conducted rounds at the bedside with each team of residents every weekday and on weekends, if necessary—thus affording much more structure and support to trainees.

These differences in supervision between the two programs had important impacts on the residents' training, particularly on their autonomy or professional independence. At Legacy, residents would round among themselves, with the intern updating their resident on overnight events, lab results, and new orders requested by attendings for their patient. This meant that interns and residents would often just read the attending's note in a patient's chart to know what the plan of action for the day was rather than formulate their own plan. One morning, for example, an intern announced to their resident, Raoul (IMG, PGY-3), that the attending wanted to send a patient with a skin infection home on Vancomycin, a highly powerful antibiotic. Raoul disagreed, however, with his attending: "I wouldn't do that. I would discharge her on something else." The predicament, while common for the housestaff, was unfamiliar to a medical student who was new to the team. "What do you do in those situations? Would you override that attending?" the student asked. Raoul replied, "No. Because it's *their* patient. Same as you respect the patient's wishes, we respect theirs. They're responsible legally for the patients."

The attendings were indeed legally responsible for patients—as they were in any teaching hospital—but they were present only sporadically to discuss their plans with residents. Aside from impromptu hallway chats when they crossed paths, Legacy residents and attendings primarily communicated through the paper chart and on the phone, with residents often expected to implement attendings' orders in their absence, much like laborers. As one member of the program leadership explained, "A lot of private attendings will come in at 5:00 in the morning, see their patient, write a note which you can't read, and you'll just follow up and call the attending and that's your interaction. . . . So what's the value in that? To me, none. You are becoming a robot responding to something written in a chart." Another official added, "There are some community docs who are awful role models. Take [this one attending]; he comes in, doesn't say anything, [and] writes orders in the middle of the night. I don't know what he does." Many Legacy attendings therefore did not carefully titrate the amount of responsibility they gave to subordinates.[13] Instead, they primarily viewed residents as their substitutes who should implement orders and watch over their patients while the attendings maintained busy clinical practices. The lack of supervision was thus due to limited time and resources more than to a calculated decision to cultivate the residents' independence.

Yet most Legacy residents interpreted their attendings' absence as *autonomy* because they were on their own a lot: "I think the amount of autonomy we have here is pretty impressive. I didn't think I would have this much freedom as an intern or a resident," admitted Harvey, a second-year resident who had trained in the Caribbean. When I asked why that was the case, he replied, "Here we don't round with attendings. We round amongst ourselves, and then we just read the attending's notes and see what he wants."

Legacy residents therefore viewed themselves as autonomous insofar as they worked separately from their superiors. But absentee attendings meant that the residents' clinical independence was often curtailed, especially when they were simply implementing orders. At the same time, residents were regularly expected to make important clinical decisions by themselves, without supervision. Some attendings even expected them to take the lead and just keep them informed. As mentioned earlier, I call this arrangement *inconsistent autonomy*—an experience of autonomy that varied by attending, swinging between nonexistent and maximal in the same day or even the same hour, and that was characterized by a common defining thread, being alone. It was further evidence of how Legacy offered a more exploitative training environment for the residents, who were primarily treated like laborers for the hospital rather than trainees.

In contrast, consider the following example from the first day of rounds at Stonewood: Dr. Katz, an attending, addressed his new team, composed of two interns, one resident, and a medical student. He looked at Nick, the third-year resident (USMD), and told the group, "I would never hope or dream of getting in Nick's way—he'll be leading things—but I like to be kept informed. . . . In terms of specific expectations, specific expectation #1: I expect to be made aware of a deterioration in a patient's status—no matter what time it is. I don't think I've gotten a call after 7 PM that hasn't started with 'Sorry to bother you!' But you're not bothering me. I'd rather find out about it at 2 AM than the next morning."

Compared with Legacy, rounds at Stonewood were highly structured with clearly articulated expectations. Interns would present pertinent clinical findings while the residents and attending asked probing questions, tweaked the interns' plans, and taught on the fly. Rounds therefore were a team effort, as well as an exercise in group problem solving, as the team would confront management issues and diagnostic puzzles together, under the expert guidance of the attending. Thus, despite having more supervision, in practice Stonewood residents consistently had more autonomy than Legacy residents. As also noted earlier, I call this arrangement *supported autonomy*, in that subordinates could make their own decisions but always felt reliably buttressed by superiors. This made the housestaff much more like trainees than laborers, offering them a better training environment.

Next I detail how these different kinds of autonomy affected the residents' training, particularly with respect to clinical reasoning, ownership and accountability over patient care, patient communication, and approaches to patient care.

Clinical Reasoning

Because attendings were often absent from Legacy, residents were not privy to much of their supervisors' clinical thinking. In fact, the housestaff sometimes described how they had to guess their attendings' rationales for decisions. As Todd, a USMD intern, explained, "Basically, you learn what the private attendings want, and you try to understand why they're requesting certain tests and why they're doing certain things. It doesn't always make sense." This lack of interaction with attendings sometimes hampered the development of the residents' clinical reasoning. One morning, for example, an intern updated his third-year resident on an anemic patient's hemoglobin level, which was low at 8.5 g/dl (a normal level for males is 12.4–14.9 g/dl). The intern asked whether they could discharge the patient, as his condition had improved. The resident shook his head no: "[The attending] is going to go for the number, so let's [get] him above a 9. Let's give him another unit of blood." Rather than rely on his clinical judgment to decide whether this patient was symptomatic and thus in need of a blood transfusion (which has added risks), this senior resident made a decision that would please his attending. Without seeing the patient for themselves, the Legacy attending understandably might have felt more comfortable "go[ing] for the number," but this did little to advance the resident's education or reinforce evidence-based practice.[14]

By way of comparison, the attendings at Stonewood always told their residents to "transfuse symptoms, not a number," and if a resident elected to transfuse, they were often asked by superiors for scientific evidence to support that decision. Interestingly, some sociologists have pointed to EBM as a potential threat to physicians' autonomy, but at Stonewood, EBM was a common language used by trainees to demonstrate progress toward becoming an autonomous clinician.[15] As one chief resident (who often played to my identity as an ethnographer) explained, "That's the dance you do when you are in this tribe . . . that's how you show that you fit in [by citing evidence]." In contrast, at Legacy EBM came up less frequently in conversations with attendings, in part because they were mostly absent.

In fact, Legacy residents were sometimes actively discouraged from disagreeing with their attendings. One morning, during a one-hour teaching session, an intern and a resident told Dr. Black, a teaching attending, that a patient's attending-of-record had ordered a colonoscopy but that they felt this would not yield relevant results. (Recall that as a teaching attending, Dr. Black was not in charge of this patient's care.) "What are we even looking for?" the resident complained. "Stalagmites and stalactites," his intern replied sarcastically. Dr. Black replied, "Piece of advice? Try not to be feisty. Because at the end of the day, you're the lowest of the totem pole. . . . Even though you don't agree with some of the attendings, this is how we practice. Everyone has their own way. You can practice however you want when you're an attending. So don't ruffle any feathers." This comment would have been highly out of place at Stonewood, where the faculty frequently encouraged residents to imagine how they might practice as attendings in order to develop their independence. However, because the attendings-of-record was often absent at Legacy, the residents could not engage with them—whether to convince them that the residents were right or to learn from them why the residents may have been wrong.

To be sure, Legacy residents would sometimes find ways to push back against their attendings when they felt something was necessary for a patient, like once when a resident instructed his intern to call the attending: "Don't ask for permission; *tell* him we'll prep [the patient] for a colonoscopy." Furthermore, not all attendings had the same expectations. As one intern put it, "Every patient has a different attending and a different style, and you have to chase them down every day, and you're not sure what to do. . . . So you come up with your plan and you present it and then you see what happens." Another resident added, "We basically call [attendings] up and tell them, 'This is what I am going to be doing. Are you okay with that? I just want to let you know,'" which highlighted that some attendings allowed residents to make most of the decisions on their own as long as the attendings were kept in the loop. This was especially true with late-night admissions, when residents were usually expected to put in their own orders and these were then adjusted in the morning, as needed, by the attending. Still other attendings, however, would get furious when the housestaff made decisions without consulting them. Marco, an IMG intern, explained:

> You have to play it by ear. . . . One of [our patient's] medications was causing renal dysfunction, and it was stopped. Then it was restarted again [by a specialist]. And the attending was *livid* that we restarted it without telling him. So what do you do? I'm just the intern! People tell me what to do and I do it . . . I don't feel I make a lot of decisions now on my own. I could, but I don't.

Being caught between two attendings, Marco was too busy implementing orders to form a clinical impression of his own.

Perhaps unsurprisingly then, Legacy residents rarely took the initiative to come up with independent plans of their own, preferring to wait instead for their attendings' orders. Faisal, an IMG and PGY-3 resident who completed residency training in his home country prior to coming to Legacy, complained about a perceived lack of trust in the residents:

> If you are training your residents to be primary care [doctors], then why are you not trusting those residents? You don't trust them and by the end of

third year, how will you make those decisions if you've never been trained to make those decisions? . . . I remember [my first] day here [as an intern], we started on call. I had a patient come with dehydration, hypernatremia [elevated blood sodium levels], and pneumonia. So, sitting with the resident, I said, "I think that I need to do one, two, three, four [*enumerating action items on his fingers*]. Are you OK with this plan?" [And my resident responded], "Oh, I don't know; just call the attending." . . . That doesn't make sense to me at all. . . . Why is there a resident carrying the patient with me if he can't make a single decision?

In Faisal's experience, the attending structure at Legacy impinged on the residents' development as future attendings because it discouraged them from developing their own clinical reasoning.

In contrast, because of Stonewood's team structure, its housestaff were fully expected to make independent decisions for their patients in consultation with, rather than under the thumb of, their attendings. For example, one morning an intern was discussing the management of one of her patients with uncontrolled high blood pressure and asked her attending, "Want to change his blood pressure meds? We have a lot of room to grow in a lot of medications. So you tell me what you want." This sort of deference to the attending's wishes, which was common at Legacy, was unacceptable at Stonewood. The attending replied, "Excuse me? Tell me what *you* want. We're your training wheels," referring to himself and the resident. Stonewood interns were thus expected to make independent decisions— which could be corrected or debated but were independent nonetheless—rather than simply wait for attendings to issue orders.

While interns and medical students wrote notes and presented on patients, residents at Stonewood watched over them carefully as team coleaders in conjunction with the attending physicians. As one Stonewood attending explained, this arrangement helped prepare residents as future attendings: "I'm happy to run the team, but I think the reason you have a senior resident is for the senior resident to get an opportunity to do that. I mean, ultimately, they're going to be attendings; at some point, they need to feel comfortable making some of the major and initial decisions. . . . I want [them] to have a junior attending type of role." In this way, residents shared the decision-making alongside their attending physicians and were often asked to weigh in on a given intern's plan or assessment depending on their level of experience. Unlike the didactic questions directed at interns or medical students (where superiors were testing their subordinates), the questions aimed at residents were usually more consultative in nature, evidence of the more horizontal nature of the relationship between attendings and residents.

The supported autonomy experienced by the Stonewood housestaff also came with a safe space for testing out one's independence as a clinician. As Blake (USMD, PGY-1) explained, "They [the attendings] give you the chance to really think on your feet rather than tell you what to do. . . . I don't like to be outspoken unless I absolutely have to, and I think they really are doing a great job of creating a very safe environment for someone who's more introverted to really express their thinking process." This supportive space thus made it possible for Stonewood residents to gain more confidence in their abilities than was the case for Legacy residents, who sometimes doubted themselves without that support.

Ownership and Accountability for Patient Care

Being bound to their attendings' orders, Legacy residents often lacked a sense of ownership over their work, which sometimes alienated them from their patients. This was especially evident when attendings ordered residents to frequently consult specialty services like nephrology and cardiology. Because attendings-of-record were not in-house, many of them consulted more liberally with specialists, who *were* in-house and could therefore keep a closer eye on patients. Notably, Legacy relied on advanced practice providers (like nurse practitioners and physician assistants) to staff several specialties, which meant that while residents learned a lot from these non-physicians, they were not necessarily trained to educate physicians. Attendings also frequently consulted specialists without a specific question in mind, which further gave the residents the impression that they were just pushing paperwork around rather than serving as primary caregivers for patients. One attending was so notorious for overconsulting that one day, after getting a new admission, an intern joked, "Guess the attending: she wants a cards [cardiology] consult, urology consult, pulm[onology] consult. . . . It's unreal, like think for yourself!" Even the housestaff made fun of this attending for outsourcing her clinical thinking.

The teaching arrangement at Legacy, which involved residents sitting down for an hour or two per day with a temporary teaching attending and discussing cases, did little to bolster their sense of ownership over patients. This was partly because the teaching attendings were not usually in charge of their patients' care. One day during teaching rounds, a team was discussing a patient who had a foreign body in her foot and also complained of severe headache, suggestive of possible meningitis. After examining the patient, the teaching attending turned to the resident and asked, "What do you think about getting an LP [lumbar puncture], given the headache? Who's the attending? Check that she doesn't want the LP." Here the teaching attending advised the housestaff to ask their attending about this important diagnostic test, rather than ordering it herself, because it was not her patient.

Unsurprisingly, teaching attendings lacked the motivation to invest much effort in these rounds because they were not in charge of the patients' care. As one teaching attending put it, "If I was listening to [the residents] present [on *my* patients] . . . I unfortunately would have a lot more interest in what [they] have to say, right down to the nitty gritty. . . . When I'm covering [teaching], I know that the other attending [the attending-of-record] has their own ideas, so I just kind of let the [residents] talk about it. [I ask them,] 'What are the academic points?' But it's not down to the nitty gritty." In other words, this teaching attendant admitted that aside from touching on the main learning points from each case, she invested little in rounds because she had little say in the patients' care. Even the residents didn't see much point in teaching rounds, given the way they were structured. As Marco, the IMG intern, told me, "[Teaching] rounds don't do an awful lot because that attending doesn't have any responsibility. . . . Now if *our* attending was there, wouldn't that have been better? Then [we could have] heard her think out loud and then think about what she's going to do; we could have talked about it, discussed it."

Teams at Stonewood benefited from exactly that kind of pedagogical support. As one resident told me, "I feel like here that the bigger asset is not only do you have smart people [as attendings] but you have smart people who want to model their being physicians and are invested in people, they're invested in their hospital, they're invested in the residents and the medical students, and they're dedicated." This degree of investment further meant that Stonewood residents exhibited greater ownership over patient care. Teams consulted specialists only when they had reached the limits of their own expertise (including that of the attending), and even then, they only took the specialists' recommendations under advisement. As one attending told his team, "If you feel uncomfortable [with the consultants' recommendations], call them. It's *their* job to sell you on their rec's [recommendations]. It's what we do as primary doctors; we ask for opinions." This instilled in Stonewood residents a degree of ownership of and often protectiveness toward their patients. For example, one day an intern informed her attending that she was refusing a recommendation from the pulmonary medicine team. In response, her attending nodded approvingly and replied, "I'm empowering you to feel like you're not just a scribe. You have patients' lives in your hands, and your job is to make them feel better." Stonewood residents were therefore more engaged in their work and felt less alienated than Legacy residents did.

One result of the teaching infrastructure at Stonewood was that attendings had high expectations for their housestaff. With teams regularly maxed out at thirteen patients (six to seven per intern), time was scarce, making rounds a perpetual exercise in efficiency and parsimony. Precision was key. One morning an intern had just finished presenting on a patient with a history of drug abuse when his attending interjected, "Let's work on our vocabulary words. . . . This patient has a past medical history of drug dependency; we know this. Can we be more precise? Is it misuse? Full-blown addiction?" These types of interruptions taught residents to report physical exam findings in fine detail. Instead of simply referring to a heart murmur, for example, the housestaff were trained to say "He had a 2 out of 6 systolic ejection murmur with a click, best heard at the right upper sternal border." This expectation of precision encouraged the housestaff to be all the more diligent in their encounters with patients, knowing they could be asked any detail at any time.

At Legacy, however, the teaching attendings did not expect as much from the housestaff. As one teaching attending disclosed, "I struggle with, How much do I try [to enforce expectations]? I don't want to be nasty, but how much do you try to hold people up to a standard as well that they're going to have to perform at [after residency]?" This meant that attendings generally intervened very little in the housestaff's case presentations. It was common for Legacy residents, for example, to refer to patients as simply being in heart failure, without specifying whether it was left-sided or right-sided, diastolic or systolic, or acute or chronic—including in patients' charts, where such detail is important for clinical, billing, and legal purposes. One day during teaching rounds, an attending sheepishly told the housestaff, "One thing I've been bad about [is that] you have to [specify] diastolic or systolic, acute or chronic heart failure." She sounded apologetic, as though expecting precision from the residents was too much to ask. Legacy's attending structure, with off-site attendings-of-record and disengaged substitute teachers, meant that there simply were not the same expectations of precision and diligence from the housestaff as there were at Stonewood.

Patient Communication

While it is beyond the scope of this book to assess how these two approaches to medical education impacted patient outcomes, several aspects stood out as having had an influence on residents' interactions with patients. For one, the lack of regular supervision and role modeling at Legacy meant that sometimes residents excelled at patient communication and at other times they struggled. One morning, for example, Terry, a third-year USIMG resident, went to talk to a patient about her diagnosis: "So you did bleed, obviously, because of your coffee ground emesis," he said. The patient, who did not understand Terry's jargon, just responded with a blank stare. Terry continued, "But your hemoglobin is normal." Another blank stare. Terry was trying to say that the patient had vomited blood but that her blood levels appeared normal, suggesting that the bleeding in her digestive tract had stopped. If an attending had been present at the bedside, they could have clarified the diagnosis for the patient and reminded the resident to avoid using such technical jargon.

Intern-resident pairs at Legacy also had a tendency to talk *over*, rather than *with*, their patients, as they chatted with one another while flanking both sides of the hospital bed. These conversations would involve patient care but often ignored the presence of the patient—or, worse, referred to the patient in the third person. In one example, two residents were examining a patient's abdomen. The first resident asked his colleague, "So what's the plan for her? Should we give her more blood?" The other resident responded, "Yeah, we have another unit for her." Meanwhile, the patient between them followed the conversation with her eyes, looking from one resident to the other without a word. Patients at Legacy were generally low-socioeconomic-status and elderly individuals, many of whom had grown up in an era when it was considered impolite to ask a doctor for clarifications, so patients rarely asked questions in these cases.[16]

At Stonewood, by comparison, residents would regularly benefit from observing their attending talking with (rather than over) patients during rounds, so they tended to be much better communicators. Patients were routinely included in discussions, with attendings often asking questions like "Do you know what we're treating you for?" to make sure they fully understood what was happening.

This kind of modeling rubbed off on the residents, who made it a priority to include patients in conversations and use lay terms whenever possible. And when they did use jargon, the attendings were there to step in and take over the patient encounter if necessary.

In one example, Blake, a USMD intern, and Louise, an attending, went to see a patient whose heart symptoms were so severe they were concerned she would not survive. There was talk of sending her to the coronary care unit (CCU), an intensive care unit for heart patients. Blake told the patient and her daughter, "We may send you to the step-down unit or CCU." What he meant was that she may be sent to either the intermediate coronary care unit, which provided a more intensive level of care than the general wards did, or the full CCU, which offered the highest level of care, but he did not explain what these acronyms stood for or how they differed. Sensing that he was having some difficulty, Louise stepped forward and gently took over the conversation from her intern. She started from the beginning and explained in layman's terms that the sac around the patient's heart seemed to be enlarged, and then she went on to describe the treatment plan in plain English.

The examples from Blake at Stonewood and Terry at Legacy highlight the fact that trainees of all kinds can struggle with patient communication. The difference was that at Stonewood, an attending was there to correct the resident and make sure that patient care was not compromised when they struggled. One could argue that because Legacy residents were predominantly non-USMDs, they might have been unfamiliar with American cultural standards for patient communication. But Stonewood hospital residents used jargon too, and Terry, from the previous example, was a USIMG nearing the end of his three-year residency at an American hospital. Thus, the biggest difference between these two examples was not cultural but rather structural, the result of the supervisory structures in place.

Approaches to Patient Care

Finally, inconsistent autonomy at Legacy also meant that residents were regularly left on their own to make clinical decisions—from the mundane to the emergent— without much support. As the ACGME has noted, insufficient supervision can compromise patient safety and quality of care, in addition to hampering trainees' opportunities to receive formative feedback and assessment.[17] This was one of the problems caused by Legacy treating residents primarily as laborers rather than trainees; compared to the program at Stonewood, the program at Legacy neglected the residents' learning, leaving its housestaff ill equipped to deal with the various impromptu clinical situations that are inherent to hospital medicine.

To be sure, some residents at Legacy liked having this much freedom; they felt it made them better doctors. One chief resident said, "You grow to get comfortable with it, you are not scared, you can make your own decisions." Another noted, "I think there are advantages to not having great supervision; . . . you [get] to make decisions on your own." In the opinion of these seasoned residents, the attendings' absence made for more confident residents. But others, like Simon (a DO intern), expressed concern: "I don't want it so structured that I'm suffocating or just blindly writing an order because somebody tells me to write orders. That's not the way you learn, but I also don't want to be alone in making the decisions that I might fear." Legacy's structure, however, ensured that both extremes (too little and too much autonomy) were happening simultaneously.

As a result of such inconsistent autonomy at Legacy, sometimes residents got to know their patients better than their attendings did and were able to offer better care than if they had simply waited for instructions from their superiors. Other times, however, patients were not upgraded to higher levels of care when they should have been.[18] Occasionally, important diagnostic tests were overlooked, as was the case with a patient who had a heart infection and also happened to have classic indicators of colon cancer.[19] An intern presented this patient during a didactic conference, and after citing a few lab values, a cardiologist interjected, "Where's the colonoscopy [to rule out colon cancer]?" The intern replied meekly that none was ordered. This omission was not caught by the patient's attending, who should have ordered a colonoscopy or documented why one was unnecessary.

Sometimes serious diagnoses were also missed, like one morning when Toby (IMG, PGY-2), the overnight resident, signed out a patient to Farha (another IMG, PGY-2). The patient had presented to the emergency department the night before with chest pain, and Toby's diagnosis was acute coronary syndrome (ACS). All Farha had to do, he said, was follow up on his labs and send him home. As Farha scanned through the patient's lab findings, she stopped at a value that was highlighted in red, meaning it was critical: the patient's creatine phosphokinase was in the 800s (the normal level is 10–120 mcg/L) while his troponin (heart enzyme) levels were normal.[20] This meant that instead of having

ACS—as Toby had diagnosed—the patient was likely experiencing rhabdomyolysis, a breakdown of muscle tissue that can cause serious kidney damage. Edward (DO), Farha's intern, erupted angrily at Toby, who had already gone home, for failing to mention anything about rhabdomyolysis during his handoff. He began mimicking Toby: "Ohhh, 'Straightforward ACS. Straightforward! Just discharge [the patient] and send out!'" spat Edward, adding "Then I'm sitting, looking at the chart and he's in *rhabdo*! And no fluids!" referring to the standard treatment for rhabdomyolysis to protect the kidneys from damage. "I'm so pissed!" As Edward and Farha tried to figure out why the patient was in rhabdomyolysis, Farha suddenly realized that Toby had also forgotten to order a second set of cardiac enzymes last night to rule out a heart attack—standard procedure for a patient presenting with chest pain. "Oh my God, Toby! I just assumed he would put in troponins! I didn't even check!" At this point, a pharmacy student on the team asked the obvious question: "How does [Toby] not get in trouble?" Toby was known among the housestaff for these kinds of oversights; the residents actually got in the habit of ordering costly STAT (urgent) morning labs because Toby would forget to order routine bloodwork overnight. Edward answered bitterly, "'Cause we save everyone," referring to a professional "code of silence" that is common throughout the profession.[21] He continued, "But this could be really bad! This could be serious; the patient could go into kidney failure!" Neither he nor Farha reported Toby for the incident. The attending never found out, in part because at Legacy, attendings did not round with the residents every morning to monitor precisely these kinds of decisions. Had Farha been a less astute resident, however, and simply discharged the patient as Toby suggested, the patient could have suffered severe consequences. Stronger oversight by attendings might therefore have been beneficial not only to the housestaff but to patients as well.

In contrast, the hospital structure at Stonewood meant that attending physicians were much more involved in patient care, acting like safety nets for the residents. As one attending explained, "I think my role . . . first and foremost is to the patient, making sure I really see those patients as my patients, just as much as the residents' patients, and making sure that the care that they receive is excellent and centered around them." This meant that the attendings were much more able to catch errors and turn them into teachable moments before they had consequences for patient care.

Two highly emblematic examples can be found at the beginning of this chapter. Recall that Blaine, a second-year resident at Legacy, mistakenly ordered a heart ultrasound for his patient with possible tuberculosis, which could have exposed the ultrasound technician to TB. The attending never picked up on the error, and, luckily, the patient tested negative for TB, so the ultrasound technician was not accidentally infected. In a comparable near miss at Stonewood, an intern forgot to order life-saving medications for a patient in alcohol withdrawal, but unlike at Legacy, his attending caught the mistake during a routine review of the housestaff's work.

These two examples share several similarities: a trainee gave a mistaken order, and the penalty could have been death. The key difference, however, was the hospital structures. Trainees are always prone to making mistakes, but at Stonewood, there were layers of supervision in place to help make sure these mistakes did not have disastrous consequences. To be sure, the CIWA incident at Stonewood took place just after a new cohort of interns had begun their training, so it is possible that the supervisors were reviewing the interns' work with exceptional vigilance. But even later in the year, when interns and residents were more seasoned, attendings still viewed themselves as the housestaff's "training wheels," ready to spring into action whenever they were needed. At Legacy, in contrast, the interns and residents were comparatively on their own in a program that exploited their labor but lacked the resources to supervise them more closely.

CLINIC

> *Clinic—everyone hates it.*
>
> Paul (USIMG, PGY-2, Legacy)

> *Oh, I love clinic!*
>
> Lynn (USMD, PGY-1, Stonewood)

While rounds dominated the morning at both hospitals, the residents at Stonewood and Legacy would spend at least one afternoon a week working in an outpatient clinic setting, learning to treat ambulatory patients.[22] As of their second year, Stonewood residents also spent an additional half day per week at a specialized clinic (or "second site") of their choosing. As the preceding quotes suggest, however, the residents' outpatient experiences were quite different. At Legacy, clinic was a huge source of vexation for the residents, as it took time away from their main job—caring for patients on Legacy's inpatient service. At Stonewood, it was a welcome opportunity for outpatient practice and additional subspecialty training.

Despite the fact that nearly 40 percent of Legacy residents took positions as primary care practitioners after graduation (see chapter 5), the program did not place much emphasis on outpatient (i.e., nonhospital) medicine. As one senior Legacy official admitted, "It really is the case that medical education is too concentrated in the hospital. These people [residents] are going to go out and be outpatient doctors, and you learn a lot in a hospital and all that, but, really, some of the stuff is not going to be useful for them. Some of it they're doing . . . because *the hospital needs them to do it*" (emphasis added). While residents in all specialties nationwide complain that there is too much emphasis on inpatient training during residency,[23] the attending structure at Legacy only exacerbated this complaint, with residents providing twenty-four-hour inpatient coverage for medical (and occasionally even surgical) patients.[24] The program openly prioritized inpatient over outpatient medicine because it *needed* that coverage, but in so doing, Legacy may have potentially neglected important aspects of the residents' training.

Legacy's deemphasis of outpatient medicine manifested itself in different ways. For example, the housestaff were expected to complete all their ward work in the hospital before going to clinic in the afternoon—if they did not, they would have to come back to the wards after clinic to finish it. This lent a sort of primacy to inpatient work, making it seem more important than outpatient work. In contrast, Stonewood interns would hand over their pagers to their residents on clinic half days, along with any remaining tasks. Once they left for clinic, the focus was to be exclusively on outpatients. Similarly, when residents attended a full day of clinic per week in their second and third years at Stonewood, they were replaced on the wards by "day float" residents, allowing the residents in clinic to focus exclusively on their outpatient duties for the day. There was no such system in place at Legacy, however, such that when team members were at clinic, the remaining housestaff had to improvise. One month an intern and a resident with the same clinic day were inadvertently assigned to work together, leaving no one to care for their patients or accept new admissions for one afternoon per week while they were both at clinic. Instead of alerting the chief resident, however, the intern-resident pair made an informal arrangement with the on-call resident to surreptitiously divert their admissions to other teams.

During the hours that this intern and resident were in clinic, however, no one was looking after their patients—an issue that took the on-call resident by surprise one day when a patient of theirs experienced a precipitous drop in blood pressure. If Legacy had provided systematic coverage to the housestaff during their clinic hours, they may have been more able to focus on their outpatient duties without compromising patient care.

Given this arrangement, the Legacy housestaff viewed clinic as a "corvée," according to one IMG resident—a burdensome obligation rather than a valuable learning opportunity. Many Legacy residents dreaded clinic for a variety of reasons, not the least of which was its location. Housed in a rundown office building across the parking lot from the hospital, the residents' clinic constituted a depressing work environment by all accounts. The walls emanated the stale stench of cigarette smoke, the examination rooms were crammed five wide into a corridor that could comfortably accommodate three, and the work area in the back was cramped, with two round tables and a row of computers competing with the residents for space. The clinic had a distinctly claustrophobic feel. Between seven and ten residents were assigned to the clinic per half day, but with only five exam rooms, they had to take turns. The setting communicated to the residents that the program did not prioritize outpatient training. Every year the program promised to renovate the residents' clinic, and every year there was little progress in this regard. One day a program official announced gleefully, without a hint of irony, "The money was approved last fall and we're just waiting for construction to start in the basement of the morgue"—an even less appealing location than the current clinic. Two years later, however, the new clinic still had not been built. Consequently, and over time, the housestaff grew distrustful of the leadership's promises, which only added to their cynicism about clinic.

By comparison, outpatient medicine was a stated program priority at Stonewood. Outpatient care came up often, even in the inpatient setting, as chief residents and attendings would frequently encourage the housestaff to think about what they might do "on the outside." This kept outpatient medicine relevant, even while on the wards.

Like those at Legacy, Stonewood interns and residents spent half a day per week in clinic where they followed a small census of outpatients. About three months after I began observations at Stonewood, a brand-new residents' clinic opened its doors, boasting twenty-six exam rooms, portable computers, and shiny new medical equipment. In contrast to the Legacy clinic, where limited resources constrained the leadership's responsiveness to the residents' needs, this new Stonewood clinic was designed with the residents in mind. After a third-year resident gushed about the new clinic, an attending replied, "Oh, yeah, it's great! The advent of the new space has pushed us to rethink what the clinic is, what we want it to be. 'Cause we got to design that space based on our goals." Third-year residents could now use more than one exam room at a time, and there were even rooms with two-way mirrors to allow preceptors to observe unobtrusively while residents interacted with patients. While the new space clearly reflected Stonewood's considerably larger pool of resources, it also communicated the program's commitment to improving the residents' outpatient education.

Beginning in their second year, Stonewood residents also spent an additional half day per week working at a subspecialty clinic of their choosing (on top of their usual half day in regular clinic). These second sites ranged from outpatient offices in traditional medical subspecialties like nephrology and gastroenterology to disease-specific clinics dealing with HIV and substance abuse. Toward the middle of the interns' first year, the program sent them a list of approximately eighty-five biographies of potential second site clinicians, asking them to rank-order their top five choices. The program also gave interns the option of proposing their own clinic mentor. Over 95 percent of residents were paired with either their first or their second choice. These second sites offered residents not only supplemental outpatient education (with Stonewood residents spending 60 percent more time in clinic than Legacy residents) but also ample opportunities for mentorship (see chapter 4).

Given the newly renovated clinic and the large selection of second sites, Stonewood's relative emphasis on outpatient medicine was clear and comprehensive. Compared to Legacy, it had the resources, networks, and workforce to free up residents from work in the hospital so that they could train more extensively in outpatient settings. While Stonewood residents, like Legacy residents, sometimes complained that too little of their education focused on the outpatient setting, their experiences were still markedly different. Stonewood viewed clinic time as yet another opportunity to learn, whereas Legacy viewed it as a requirement for maintaining accreditation. Stonewood's approach made clinic more enjoyable for its residents, while Legacy's approach left its residents believing it was an annoying detractor from their primary task: working on the wards.

FREE TIME

After rounds, didactic conferences, and clinic, the residents at both hospitals had very different amounts of free time. Tellingly, after spending a month on an elective rotation at Stonewood, Farha (IMG, PGY-2, Legacy) exclaimed, "It was like being on call every day! I would stay until at least 7:30 every night!"[25] She said she missed Legacy's "good old" general medical floors, where "even when you're on call, you're not working *all* the time." The low census and laissez-faire approach of the program at Legacy meant that residents had a lot of free time. On some days, rounds would be over at 8 AM (especially when teaching rounds were canceled, as they often were), leaving the housestaff with a full two hours before morning report. Interns would work on patient management and discharges in the afternoons while second- and third-year residents would spend hours in the residents' lounge until they signed out for the day at 4:30 PM. Teams were on "long" call until 9 PM and "short" call until 6 PM only once a week ("Q7" days) and usually admitted no more than two or three new patients per night. As Harvey (USIMG, PGY-2) told me, "It's pretty laid-back compared to other programs. There's less stress here [because of] the amount of patients we carry. . . . We won't get as much experience. But we get to balance our social life and our work life."

The program actually advertised itself as laid-back, touting free time as an opportunity to do research, study, and learn. This was an integral part of Legacy's approach to medical education: get the job done first, and then learn in your considerable spare time. As Todd, a USMD intern, explained, "There's supposed to be a larger emphasis on learning by yourself. . . . If you have a lower patient census, you have more time to read and study on your own. [But] that's only the assumption—that you *do* read and study on your own." In practice, however, residents spent most of their free time on leisure activities. The housestaff even set up social rituals like the much-anticipated *cafecito* hour after lunch, when Latin American and Middle Eastern residents would prepare strong, syrupy coffee from their homelands. There were innumerable hours spent playing video games or watching TV in the lounge. A smaller proportion of time was spent studying or doing research (a situation that I'll elaborate on in chapter 4).

In contrast, Stonewood residents had something of the opposite problem. Because of the large patient loads and the complex nature of those patients, the housestaff hardly had a moment to themselves on most days. I learned early on in my fieldwork at Stonewood to use the bathroom before morning report at 8 AM because I knew I probably would not have another break until noon conference. Thirteen patients per team meant that residents had to keep their attendings and interns on track if they wanted to finish rounds before noon.[26] Sometimes morning rounds ended in the afternoon. Chief residents actually had to make sure that the housestaff took *at least* four days off per month, as required by the ACGME. Overwork was a known problem at Stonewood; while I never heard of a single Legacy resident exceeding the eighty-hour workweek limit set by the ACGME, it was a monthly occurrence at Stonewood, especially in specialized units like the CCU and the intensive care unit. The hospital's Graduate Medical Education Department eventually took notice and decided to conduct an internal review to make sure the program was respecting duty hour limits.

Partly in response to concerns about duty hours, Stonewood changed the way it allocated new admissions. Instead of receiving a large number of new patients once every four ("Q4") days (known as a "bolus" approach), Stonewood teams would now receive a smaller number of new admissions on a "drip" basis every day. At first, the new system was not well received by the housestaff. As Ken, a PGY-3 resident, put it, "There is the perception that you are doing more work. In the old system, you [could] get your mind around the fact that one day out of four [was] awful. . . . You [were] going to be in the hospital for sixteen, eighteen hours, but then the other three days [weren't] so bad." With the new system, however, interns were getting new patients almost daily. This created a perverse incentive to *keep* patients, rather than discharge them, because every discharge meant a free bed and every free bed meant a new admission, which created more work. When patients were discharged, it was usually toward the end of the day, so new admissions came only later in the evening or at night (once the beds became available). This meant that a nighttime resident would often handle new admissions instead of one of the daytime interns.

Many residents expressed concern that their interns were not admitting their own patients under the new system and were instead relying on the notes, orders, and initial diagnoses of a more experienced nighttime resident. One focus group with PGY-2s summarized this concern:

RESIDENT 1: The worst about that is all those admissions are coming in to residents, not the interns who need to be getting [them].

RESIDENT 2: That's the big issue.

RESIDENT 1: I mean interns need to become efficient, they need to become competent, and that doesn't happen if you don't admit patients fresh. Because when they come after I've already written an H&P [history and physical], which gets copied and pasted, and then putting in the orders, they basically just . . .

RESIDENT 3: They don't know how to admit.

The worry was that interns were not learning to be independent clinicians because they were not admitting their own patients; they were simply implementing the orders already input by the admitting resident. There is a remarkable parallel to Legacy here, where residents regularly implemented orders from their superiors. But unlike at Legacy, this was a cause for concern among the residents at Stonewood rather than an acceptable status quo.

Despite the problems with the new system, Stonewood residents seldom complained about their work hours. If anything, many of them said that they viewed residency as a unique training opportunity and would not prefer a residency with a lighter patient load if it meant they worked less. In this way, free time was anathema to the Stonewood housestaff. As one PGY-2 resident said, "You learn by working hard and seeing patients, and if you're not working hard and not seeing patients, there's no learning to be had." In fact, "working hard" was one of the ways Stonewood residents distinguished themselves and their elite program from lower-tier residents and residencies (as I'll explain further in chapter 6). At Legacy, in contrast, free time was one of the program's prime selling points. Time therefore helped delineate the contours of status within residency, with free time being associated with lower-status, almost lethargic training and overwork being associated with a more rigorous, robust education.

LABORERS VERSUS TRAINEES

The dual nature of residency as a form of both employment and training can raise a tricky issue of balance, as programs must decide how much education to give to their residents versus how much labor to take from them. At Legacy, the program decidedly prioritized the latter—getting labor from the residents. This was evident in how the program invested comparatively little in didactics and outpatient medicine and in how the residents were used as stand-ins for their attendings on the wards, although they were given inconsistent amounts of autonomy. When I asked the residents what they would change about their program, they overwhelmingly replied that they would make education more of a priority. To emphasize this point, Yasmin (IMG, PGY-2, Legacy) contrasted her experience with that of the residents at Stonewood: "Everything [there] is set up for someone to teach them and for them just to be learning." She went on to compare the situation at Legacy: "Our hospital, even though it is a teaching hospital, [it's] not really teaching, because if it was teaching, *residents [would] come first.* . . . We are the most important part of this hospital because if we weren't here, this hospital [and] the attendings would be screwed because who is doing the work here? We are. But they don't give us the credit we need" (emphasis added). As noted earlier, even the leadership admitted that Legacy residents do much of what they do because "the hospital needs them to do it." Internal medicine residents were therefore primarily used to fill important gaps in human resources at Legacy.

This effectively made them cheap labor. As one Legacy resident (IMG, PGY-3) put it, "We make their [attendings'] life so much easier." Stonewood residents agreed. During focus groups, the Stonewood housestaff openly criticized community programs like Legacy for being exploitative, citing their lack of focus on education as a major drawback. One resident explained, "[Lower-tier programs] are the ones that are exclusively community based. . . . [They're] where the residents don't have a presence; they're just the manual labor that's doing the work."

To be sure, Stonewood residents also performed work for the hospital—even exceeding their mandated eighty-hour workweek limit, as noted earlier—but the hospital had the resources to make education more of a priority than at Legacy. For example, on the general medical floors, residents collectively cared for approximately fifty patients, and after that point, the hospital relied on the nonteaching hospitalist group (NTHG) of attendings to pick up the rest of the work. As one teaching attending explained, "NTHG are a working group. They work. They're hired to work. We [teaching attendings] are hired to educate." A faculty member echoed the program's commitment to learning: "Our whole goal is that at the end of the day, we take good care of patients, number 1. But number 2 [is] that we learn something through that experience of taking care of patients." In this way, the residents at Stonewood were learning to work; at Legacy, they were working to learn.

CONCLUSION

Approaches to medical education looked very different in these two hospitals. Legacy's highly decentralized structure with off-site attendings meant that the program was far more hands-off than that at Stonewood. One consequence of that structure was that attendings' expectations were low and generally emphasized knowing *what* to do, rather than *why* to do it, because there were few opportunities to model and hone evidence-based reasoning. The attending structure also meant that residents experienced *inconsistent autonomy*—inconsistent in the sense that residents were unaccompanied and unsupported most of the time, variously implementing their attendings' orders and making in-the-moment decisions without guidance or supervision. This made it easier for omissions in care to take place and did little to nip bad habits in the bud.

Spotty supervision at Legacy was not the result of a deliberate pedagogical logic carefully tailored to meet the learners' or the patients' needs; instead, it was mostly the product of constrained time and resources. It made Legacy residents more like workers than trainees, serving as twenty-four-hour stand-ins for superiors who offered variable support, thus prolonging the familiar pattern of disadvantage that had faced non-USMDs in the profession since early in life. Legacy residents may have marveled at the autonomy they experienced, but, paradoxically, they often had less of it than Stonewood trainees, who worked *with*, rather than *for*, attendings. Instead, what Legacy residents misidentified as autonomy was actually simultaneous abandonment by and subservience to attending physicians—an exploitative arrangement that hindered the development and refinement of the residents' skills, resulting in poorer learning outcomes. In exchange, residents were given the promise of free time and a work-life balance made possible by the low patient census and relatively low expectations of the program. It was a continuation of the lack of support they experienced on their way to residency, as described in chapter 1.

Stonewood, in contrast, offered a far more centralized program with a stronger hierarchy and greater structure, which was reflected in its more dedicated approach to education. This approach was consistent with medicine's broader social contract with USMDs (introduced in chapter 1), whereby trainees are shepherded through their training, making it nearly impossible for them to fail. Residents at Stonewood experienced *supported autonomy*, where the interns were buttressed by layers of training and supervision from the residents and attendings, who served as training wheels supporting the interns' autonomous thinking and action. The structure of supported autonomy therefore reflected an approach where the residents were treated primarily as trainees and where the program's main priority was to train excellent physicians rather than staff the hospital. In this context, the housestaff came prepared to learn. Free time was considered antithetical to a good education, and many residents explicitly preferred to be exposed to more patients rather than fewer. Ironically, in the end, this may have made them better "laborers" (who worked longer and harder for their patients) than the residents at Legacy (who prioritized their free time).

In this chapter, I have made the case that program structures are responsible for such stark differences in training between the two hospitals. Some might counter that Legacy residents may have been weaker doctors from the outset, which could explain the observed differences. The evidence, however, strongly indicated that structural inequalities, rather than differences in competency, were behind these results. Residents from both programs made errors and struggled with communication; the key difference was between Stonewood's and Legacy's approaches to their education. Stonewood residents were afforded fundamentally different opportunities to learn than Legacy residents were, thereby further helping separate the two in status.

These findings on the effects of the *formal* medical curriculum indicate the need for a closer examination of the *informal* or hidden curricula at Stonewood and Legacy. In the next chapter, I examine how the programs' approaches to socialization and professional development affected the residents' ability to prepare for life after residency, further driving them apart in terms of status.

CHAPTER 4

Grooming

O ne October afternoon during a quiet shift in the intensive care unit (ICU), I sat down with Laurie, an American graduate of an international medical school (USIMG) in her second postgraduate year (PGY-2) at Legacy Community Hospital. The unit had no patients on that particular day, so we had some time to chat. We began chatting about the residency program, which she immediately described as "laid-back." Laurie elaborated:

> The hospital doesn't really [care] as long as the work's getting done. . . . It's more about what you want to do in this program, what you want to gain, rather than . . . [*she trails off*]. You can totally get by, you know, slip by under the radar and be not as great of a physician, or you can, you know, take whatever you have here and really work with it and better yourself. So some people, for example, for fellowship, will match at a really good place. But then there's some that just won't match at all. So it's very based person-to-person.

Laurie felt that the program didn't invest much energy in the housestaff's professional development or long-term success—all of this was incumbent upon the residents themselves. She was not alone in thinking this way. It was widely accepted at Legacy that the residents' success was left mostly up to them and was by no means guaranteed. As one senior member of the Legacy leadership even confessed, "I don't stay in touch with them [residents] a lot but every now and then I do hear and . . . I'm surprised at how well they've done sometimes. *I have doubts about whether they'll succeed or not* and they have and that's no small thing" (emphasis added).

The culture at Stonewood University Hospital was almost diametrically opposed to Legacy's. After being asked to describe their duties as a program leader, one member of Stonewood's top brass replied, "I think the overarching mission is to enable the residents under me to thrive and professionally develop so that they can ultimately achieve their goals." Another put it even more concretely: "Our job is to take you, work with you, be facilitators, guides, *enzymes to catalyze you going to the next step*" (emphasis added).

In the previous chapter, I focused on the residents' clinical education. But there is more to succeeding as a physician than just mastering clinical knowledge. In this chapter, I explore how the two programs groomed their residents differently for the future. First, I compare their approaches to professional development by examining the residents' training beyond the wards, including those nonclinical skills, like research competency and professionalism, that are necessary to play the game after residency and succeed in the profession. What did Legacy's "laid-back" approach look like, and how did Stonewood "catalyze" their residents to get to the next step? As will become clearer, the hospitals' different approaches echoed broader patterns of sponsorship and isolation that were present on the wards (chapter 3), that date back to early life (chapter 1), and that have consistently advantaged US-trained medical graduates (USMDs) and disadvantaged non-USMDs. If there ever was a metaphor to capture the essence of the profession's consideration (or promise) in the social contract with USMDs, it was providing the "enzyme" to "catalyze" their success.[1]

Second, I make the case that these different approaches instilled very different *values* in the housestaff, thereby leading to important differences in professionalism between Stonewood and Legacy residents. Sociologists have long been fascinated by doctors' socialization into the profession, but most studies focus on a single setting, or type of setting, which obscures how different learning environments can effectively produce different kinds of trainees and reinforce status hierarchies.[2] But professional norms and values do not emerge in a social vacuum; they are influenced by the structure of the training programs and by the social location of those programs within the broader field of medical education.[3] A residency program's resources, organization, and priorities all shape residents' socialization and professionalism—the set of standards and values that trainees internalize about how to succeed in medicine—affecting not only the residents' attitudes but also their behavior.[4] In turn, those attitudes and behaviors can go on to shape, and often reify, the program's status position within the broader field of medical education, thereby reproducing the current social order. This kind of relational perspective therefore allows us to see how structure affects agents and how agents, in turn, affect structure, reproducing broader structural inequalities.[5]

The hidden curriculum is a useful concept for analyzing how structural differences between the programs' professional development strategies can produce different values and behaviors among residents. In the late 1990s, Hafferty urged scholars to consider the latent messages being transmitted to trainees in medical education by asking "What are the fundamental values and messages being created and transmitted within each or all of these activities?"[6] He maintained that there is an important distinction between what is taught and what students learn, pointing to "a set of influences that function at the level of organizational structure and culture," which he called the hidden curriculum.[7] Hafferty notably urged researchers to pay special attention to the allocation of resources as a way of distinguishing what is considered important and unimportant in a given setting. In this chapter, by reflecting on the "larger structural picture," as Hafferty urges scholars to do, I explore how the programs prioritized professional development differently and groomed their residents based on these different priorities.

This chapter is divided into two parts. First, I begin by describing the different structures of professional development at both programs and making explicit the tacit, latent messages being communicated to the housestaff. I define these structures as programmatic efforts, arrangements, resources, and leadership that shaped individual trainees' development into full-fledged members of the profession. In the second part, I trace the impact of these messages on the residents' professionalism. I define *professionalism* as "those behaviors by which [physicians] . . . demonstrate that [they] are worthy of the trust bestowed upon [them] by [their] patients and the public, because [they] are working for the patients' and the public's good."[8] I find that Legacy's more passive and "laid-back" approach, as described by Laurie, produced residents who were self-starters in some respects but more complacent in others, sometimes encouraging them to act unprofessionally. Stonewood's approach, by comparison, was more active and supportive and even bordered on coddling. As such, Stonewood's efforts again reflect a continuation of the social contract with USMDs, helping ensure that they reach fulfilling careers after getting admitted to US allopathic medical schools. Thanks to its relative abundance of resources, Stonewood prioritized its residents' success, thereby producing residents who were more motivated but also more smug. Professional development in these two hospitals therefore helped consolidate and exacerbate status separation between USMDs and non-USMDs, helping USMDs accrue advantages over non-USMDs and providing the former with the support necessary to outperform the latter.

THE STRUCTURES OF PROFESSIONAL DEVELOPMENT AT LEGACY AND STONEWOOD

Adjusting to Residency

Quite literally from day one, Legacy and Stonewood approached their new interns' transition to residency very differently, communicating dissimilar degrees of investment in their professional development. At Legacy, orientation consisted of a single two-day event held prior to the beginning of internship, where the chief resident and a parade of hospital personnel would cover the basics like note writing, dictation procedures, infection control, parking policies, and employee health. Long periods of downtime punctuated the two-day session, however, with some speakers arriving late and others leaving early to go back to other pressing tasks. The chief resident was mostly absent during these intervals, leaving the new interns to chat awkwardly among themselves while they anxiously awaited the next speaker. The program leadership made an appearance, but didn't stay long. Recall that Legacy program leaders spent three to five half days per week in private practice and on their other duties, effectively running the program on a part-time basis. This made it difficult for them to attend much of the orientation with the new housestaff. It was emblematic of the program's relatively weak structure and hands-off approach, already communicating to the new residents that they would be competing for the attention of busy attendings and program officials. After the initial two-day orientation, there were no further formal attempts to help ease the transition into residency for Legacy trainees. Their success, it seemed, was not going to be "ensured" the way Stonewood residents' success was, reflecting a fundamentally different social bargain with the profession. They were on their own.

Perhaps unsurprisingly, some Legacy interns struggled to adjust to life as a house officer. Many of them were foreign nationals who had to contend with learning a new language, culture, and health care system, in addition to all the medicine interns had to learn. Raoul, an international medical graduate (IMG) and a third-year resident, remembered how difficult it was to write notes in English for the first time: "Just to write a progress note in a different language, it's a big thing," he recalled. Others had difficulty adjusting to the US health care system. For example, one Middle Eastern resident (IMG, PGY-3) said, "I was trained the British way and the British usually don't use the lab. [In the] British way, you need to diagnose before the labs. . . . Here people ordered all these tests . . ." A few noted differences in the doctor-patient relationship, as they were used to more paternalistic models where doctors' orders went unquestioned. Another subset struggled with the realities of returning to internship after having already practiced autonomously abroad as fully trained clinicians.

These struggles are not uncommon among internationally trained residents. IMGs often face dual learning curves as immigrants and new interns[9] and may need to find ways to overcome important cultural differences.[10] Research also shows that these obstacles are surmountable with targeted orientation programs, which Legacy notably lacked.[11] While the transition may still have been challenging, additional orientation could have benefited the roughly 35 percent of Legacy's categorical housestaff who were IMGs. Instead, they were left to fend for themselves, with the impression, as Laurie put it, that "the hospital doesn't really [care]."

Meanwhile, new intern orientation at Stonewood lasted nine full days.[12] In mid-June, dozens of interns would gather for five days of internal medicine orientation and four more days of housestaff training by the Graduate Medical Education Department. In between barbeques and baseball games—all of which were paid for by Stonewood's comparatively larger budget—the internal medicine program offered sessions covering resuscitation, wellness, the resident clinic, and general wards. The program also offered a daylong clinical skills workshop that was specifically designed to transmit Stonewood's culture and expectations to the new interns—the program leadership preferred not to leave such things to chance. It helped that program directors and chief residents had few competing responsibilities besides running the program. They could be present at each of these events and carefully begin cultivating the interns' perceptions and priorities through targeted socialization efforts, unlike at Legacy, where the interns didn't know what to make of Legacy's disorganization.

Orientation at Stonewood did not end there, however. In addition to regular orientations at the beginning of every wards month and a mandatory half-day retreat at the end of the intern year, interns benefited from a weekly intern conference designed just for them by the program directors to help ease them through the first year. Intern conferences were considered protected time for the interns, who would relinquish their pagers to their residents for forty-five minutes each week while they attended these didactic sessions. There were thus structures in place to prioritize interns' socialization as future residents, which communicated to the interns how important their success was to the program.

Some interns complained that these supportive structures verged on hand-holding, however. At the end of each month, for example, the intern conference would often culminate in a friendly competition; the interns were split into two teams, and one team would provide a "one-liner" description of an interesting case (e.g., "sixty-eight-year-old female presents with altered mental status") while the other team had to correctly guess the diagnosis. Like most things at Stonewood, the tone of the competition was friendly, and the approach was supportive—perhaps too supportive for some interns, who sometimes criticized the program for "coddling" them, as one put it. One day, for example, a program official reminded the interns, "I told you, the pressure's really low. We always try to end with a tie." As the teams traded one-liners and diagnoses, one program leader leaned to the other and said, "Maybe next time, we'll have them stump the other team. Oh, but we don't want them to stump each other! We want them to work on their presentation [skills]." After six rounds, however, the score was 5-6, so the program leader interjected, "One more! We have to have 6-6. We have to! I don't like to leave Fridays without a tie!" The losing team guessed the next diagnosis correctly, and the competition ended with a tie, even though the seventh round was only half over. This example is emblematic of the highly encouraging but sometimes patronizing approach adopted by Stonewood, where virtually everything was done to protect the residents from failure—the very essence of medicine's part of the bargain with USMDs.

Mentorship

Mentorship was another key difference between the two programs that signaled divergent levels of investment in the residents and their futures. At Legacy, there were few formal mentorship opportunities available to the housestaff beyond biannual meetings with an assigned advisor who would review their evaluations and offer career advice. These advisors, however, did not necessarily align with the residents' career goals, partly due to the limited range of clinicians at Legacy. Instead, it was often up to the housestaff to find suitable role models in their area of interest. One Legacy official, when asked about the benefits of training in a small residency program, replied:

> If you recognize it early enough in your training and you take advantage of it . . . you have easy access to physicians that . . . can be mentors for you on a one-on-one basis and they get to know you very well. So if you know what your identified area of interest is and if you, I don't want to say latch on, but you *find yourself a mentor that is willing to work with you* one-on-one, they can provide new contacts, they can provide you with research opportunities. (emphasis added)

The program was not in a position to systematically facilitate mentorship ties, so the onus was largely on the residents to find themselves a mentor. Some were successful—especially those interested in pulmonary/critical care, thanks to a particular ICU attending at Legacy who enjoyed mentoring residents. Those attendings, however, were rare. Instead, mentorship at Legacy was very much contingent on the residents taking initiative. This taught the residents self-reliance, but it also communicated to them that the program did not, or could not, prioritize their professional development and future success.

In contrast, mentorship was a stated priority at Stonewood. While describing the program's features to a group of overwhelmed-looking applicants one day during interview season, a program director said, "Our philosophy is that we really like you and we really like to be part of your nurturing and training and *getting you where you want to go*. So we have three to five mentoring programs" (emphasis added), and she began listing them:

> Firstly, you are assigned to a chief resident who is at least one person . . . in a nonevaluative role. They can help you with medical and nonmedical things. Need a dentist? Second, you're assigned to one of us [a program director]. You'll meet with us at least two times a year, but often more than that, to discuss evaluations, research interests, when are you taking Step 3. That sort of thing. And third, . . . you're assigned a mentor, who is also in a nonevaluative role, and you're matched usually because of something in your history that brings you together—you're from the same place, you have overlapping research interests, you both like kiteboarding, whatever. So those are three initial mentorship relationships right away.

In addition to providing these initial mentors, program directors helped residents set up relationships with other faculty members in their desired areas of specialty through the second site clinics (introduced in the previous chapter). Second sites often served as a major source of mentors, in addition to providing residents with extra clinical exposure to their field of interest. As a program director explained to prospective applicants, "That preceptor you work with once a week for two years, so they're a very formative mentor for you personally and professionally for things like letters of recommendation, research, jobs, and future planning." Larry (USMD, PGY-3, Stonewood), for example, wanted to pursue a fellowship in nephrology, so he set up a second site in a kidney clinic. He explained, "Second site is a big help because it really puts you in the world of the people you are trying to be like essentially and that's how I met two of my letter writers . . . I think that is excellent for getting fellowships."

Stonewood residents therefore benefited from wraparound career guidance, support, and encouragement from a wide variety of mentors provided by the residency program. In the words of one program director, "You have a research mentor, you have a program director, you have a big buddy, you have a chief resident. We say that people are *mentored to death*. There are too many people looking out for your well-being" (emphasis added), which communicated to residents that their success *mattered* to the program. It was also consistent yet again with the social contract between USMDs and the medical profession—i.e., once they got into medical school or residency, the profession would help them succeed. While it was up to Legacy residents to find themselves a mentor, the structure at Stonewood and its status as an elite hospital enabled it to provide residents with a ready-made network of rich ties they could later draw on in the labor market.[13] The message was clear: at Legacy, the residents' professional development seemed incidental to their work; at Stonewood, it was central.

Research

There were also important differences in the ways both programs approached research, which conveyed different programmatic priorities. These priorities, however, had direct implications for the residents' future career paths. While the national guidelines of the Accreditation Council for Graduate Medical Education (ACGME) required only modest amounts of research for graduation, involvement in scholarly activity was especially crucial for those residents interested in subspecialty fellowship training, particularly in more competitive fields.[14] This made research an important determinant of residents' mobility after graduation (as I'll explain further in chapter 5).

Making Opportunities at Legacy Research was hard to come by at Legacy, a community hospital with few clinician-scientists. Earlier, when the hospital had been affiliated with Stonewood University, there was more research being done, but when the university dropped Legacy as an affiliate, most of the research left along with the faculty. Basic science projects in areas such as stem cell research remained, but clinical research was scarce,[15] which meant residents had few opportunities to get involved and even fewer role models to mentor them if they wanted to start their own projects.[16] The program's more recent affiliation to Carter Medical College, a medical school located in a nearby state, did little to help build the research curriculum, as the medical school's core faculty rarely spent time at Legacy except to give an occasional talk.[17] The affiliation was so loose that Legacy residents did not even have access to Carter Medical College's library resources, including electronic access to medical journals. Instead, residents had to rely on Legacy's more modest holdings, and this lack of access sometimes dissuaded the housestaff from searching for articles. This is a prime example of how institutional resources can influence behavior—in this case, discouraging the search for primary sources. The hospital's limited access to scholarly resources also communicated to residents that evidence-based scholarship was not an institutional priority at Legacy and thus not an integral part of a physician's professional development.

To be sure, many Legacy residents still found a way to get involved in some sort of research, usually because scholarship was a must for fellowship. About half of the housestaff presented posters at the local American College of Physicians (ACP) conference every year, for example, while one or two presented talks. But even when encouraging the housestaff to do research, Legacy officials conveyed mixed messages. One day at noon conference, a program official halfheartedly tried to encourage the housestaff to prepare a poster for the ACP: "If you have a project that has some data, those make nice posters. Give it to the attending so they can review it. Sometimes when residents do stuff on their own, it turns out fine; other times it doesn't. . . . Just have someone else read it and fix it up a bit. And if no one else will help you, I'm happy to help you." The tone of voice exuded little confidence in the residents' abilities and acknowledged the broader problem with getting help from attendings. On the whole, the program leadership did little to explicitly encourage research at Legacy.

One thing that did make research a bit easier at Legacy was the program's much-touted flexibility. Legacy residents had comparatively more elective months than residents at Stonewood did, and according to the Housestaff Manual, they were encouraged to use these electives to " 'flavor' their training."[18] The residents could choose the topics of their electives as long as these were authorized by the program, and they often had to make connections with subspecialists with whom they could write case reports or collaborate on other forms of clinical research.

This flexibility was at least partly designed to make up for Legacy's lack of clinical and research offerings. In practice, however, what it actually meant was that Legacy would not *get in the way* of residents wanting to set up outside rotations. As Aaron (USIMG, PGY-3, Legacy) explained, "We don't have a cath lab that's interventional," referring to a catheterization laboratory used for interventional, as opposed to diagnostic, heart procedures like angioplasty during heart attacks. "But if you are really involved, if you are really interested, you can always go to an outside cath lab. *They don't really stop us from doing that*" (emphasis added). Thus, what Legacy touted as flexibility was really an arrangement whereby it was incumbent upon the residents, rather than the program, to identify and address deficiencies in their education. They had to be self-starters.

This arrangement was especially disadvantageous for residents wanting to eventually subspecialize in highly competitive areas like gastroenterology and cardiology—areas in which Legacy did not have a fellowship program—as they sometimes had to travel considerable distances to other hospitals to find suitable electives or research opportunities. Here again they encountered barriers. Even though Legacy was affiliated (on paper) with the out-of-state Carter Medical College, "It's not like we have an open door to rotate in their hospital," said Trevor (USIMG, PGY-2), referring to the lukewarm relationship between the two hospitals. Another obstacle was medical licensing; to rotate at Carter Medical College, Legacy residents had to secure out-of-state licenses. Rodney (USIMG, PGY-3) told me he tried to arrange a cardiology elective at Carter Medical College Hospital, but it took two to three months just to secure the license before starting the approvals process at the hospital, so he gave up: "I mean, people still do make it out there, but it takes advanced planning and patience," he said.

Cody (USIMG, PGY-2) was a case in point. He was determined to pursue a fellowship in allergy and immunology—a highly competitive subspecialty in which

Legacy lacked a fellowship program. So he got licensed and went to Carter Medical College several times to arrange what were called "away" electives. His colleagues marveled at his determination: "Your passion for allergy is crazy," a third-year resident told him one day. But Cody *had* to be crazy about allergy, given the absence of opportunities at Legacy. As he put it, "At a place like this where they don't do a lot of research, they are not going to look for you. *You have to go look for them*, and if you are adamant about it, if you want something, the attendings will help you find it" (emphasis added). He contrasted his experience to those of residents at Stonewood who wanted to pursue a similarly competitive fellowship in cardiology: "It makes it much [easier] because they have a cardiology fellowship. You have the program director, you have the attendings, you have everything right there, and because there's a fellowship there, guess what they have there: research." Cody was highlighting a fundamental dissimilarity between Legacy and Stonewood; while opportunities were made easily available to Stonewood residents by the program, they were self-made at Legacy and thus much harder to come by. At the same time, this paucity of opportunities engendered a degree of initiative and determination in residents like Cody. His story illustrates how the program's structure and its broader location in the field of medical education—as a smaller community hospital without many fellowships in competitive specialties—influenced the residents' attitudes and behaviors, discouraging some from pursuing research but galvanizing others into making opportunities happen for themselves.

"Having Everything Right There" Unsurprisingly, compared to Legacy, research abounded at Stonewood, thanks in large part to the institution's considerable resources. In 2012, Stonewood University Medical School boasted about having tens of millions of dollars in research funds, more than three-quarters of which it funneled directly into Stonewood University Hospital, where residents could work alongside clinician-scientists. The case mix at Stonewood also helped; as a tertiary care center with transplant services, Stonewood attracted far more publishable cases than Legacy did. One day, for example, Lucy (USMD, PGY-3, Stonewood) spoke to an attending about an intriguing patient with a rare kidney condition: "Only, like, thirteen other cases [have been] reported!" she blurted out excitedly. The attending urged Lucy to publish the case: "With thirteen cases, this is something—however it evolves—that should be written up [and published] 'cause there's a lot to learn here." Cases like these, which were much rarer at Legacy, were low-hanging fruit for Stonewood residents looking to establish a record of scholarship.

These hospital characteristics made it easy for the Stonewood program to create opportunities for the housestaff and ultimately make good on its promise to ensure USMDs' success. There were also monthly noon conferences focusing on research, which helped clue residents into research opportunities and underscored the value of scholarly projects. The hour-long sessions would begin with the program director circulating a twenty-four-page booklet entitled *Research Overview* that listed nearly one hundred ongoing research projects categorized by medical subspecialty, from cardiology to rheumatology, along with the principal investigators, their projects, and their contact information. For the residents, having an actual catalog full of people willing to work with them took the guesswork out of cold-calling researchers.

Importantly, research was also a pedagogical requirement at Stonewood. In addition to Senior Research Day, during which the PGY-3s were required to present some kind of scholarly work, the program mandated that second-year residents complete a quality improvement project. All of these curricular requirements signaled to the housestaff that research was a fundamental part of their training as future physicians. Not all residents at Stonewood wanted to pursue fellowship after graduation, but if they changed their minds (as some did—see chapter 5), they at least had a scholarly foundation on which to draw, thanks to the program's curricular emphasis on research. Research opportunities were thus planned, packaged, and promoted for Stonewood residents in a way that simply did not exist at Legacy—yet another example of the many structural advantages enjoyed by Stonewood residents and of the social contract in action.

Despite the relative abundance of opportunity and support, some Stonewood residents still felt that research projects were hard to find. Several reported having to fight to get access to mentors and projects, despite the research-focused noon conferences. Some even struggled to find basic projects for Senior Research Day. As Logan, a USMD and PGY-2 interested in gastroenterology, explained, "I wanna get this project going, but I'm having a hard time getting people to . . . [*he trails off*]. My hand needs to be held a little bit, at least at the beginning. . . . I can't just generate this thing out of thin air." Thus, some Stonewood residents struggled with finding research, but there was a big difference between them and Legacy residents; while the former may have mainly struggled to get their *own* research projects off the ground, the latter often had to go to other hospitals—even travel out of state—just to get involved in *others'* research projects.

Conferences

Perhaps one of the best ways to appreciate the differences in grooming between the two hospitals is to compare their approaches to didactic conferences. Per ACGME requirements, both programs held a regular assortment of noon conferences, journal clubs, grand rounds, and morbidity and mortality conferences (M&Ms)—rituals designed to help socialize residents into the profession.[19] The tone and content of these didactic sessions varied dramatically between the two hospitals, however, communicating very different messages to the housestaff. While Legacy's informality seemed to signal indifference (or, at the very least, inattention) to the residents' professional development, Stonewood's formality confirmed its importance and signaled that it held its residents and faculty to a high standard. Following are examples from noon conferences and M&Ms.

Noon Conferences Noon conference was a daily lecture at both hospitals where the residents would listen to a faculty member give a talk while they ate lunch. At Legacy, it was held in the bowels of the community hospital in a dank conference room with grey industrial carpeting and plastic stackable chairs. The chief resident would occasionally take attendance, an uncharacteristic attempt by the Legacy leadership to keep tabs on its residents, who sometimes took liberties with the program's laissez-faire approach. Still, residents would arrive late, leave early, or occasionally skip noon conference altogether in favor of spending lunchtime in the residents' lounge.

At Stonewood, attendance was not recorded, but internalized norms about professionalism meant that if residents did not go to conference, it was usually because they were tied up with patient care. In fact, the orientation packets distributed to ward interns each month admonished the housestaff to "attend all conferences as if you stood a good chance of winning $1,000 just for showing up. The acute care of a patient always comes first but many of our clinical care activities can wait until after attending rounds or noon conference or Grand Rounds. Attend these conferences, be on time, and reflect on what you have learned." Directives like these, which were regularly reinforced by the chief residents and program directors, helped Stonewood residents internalize early on in their training the importance of showing up to conferences.

Noon conferences also often differed in quality between the two settings. Stonewood attendings were skilled teachers who consistently supported their talks with evidence-based medicine, carefully listing works cited on their slides and thereby modeling proper citation practices for the residents. They sometimes even referred to research that took place at Stonewood itself. For their part, Legacy fellows and attendings were generally less skilled presenters, and their slides were sometimes poorly organized, peppered with spelling mistakes, and rarely supported with references. One day I entered the conference room only to be momentarily confused because the title slide projected on the screen listed an unknown female author affiliated with a different hospital. The male attending stood in front of the housestaff and announced with a wolfish grin that he had decided to give a talk prepared by someone at Georgia Medical College four years ago. "If ever you need to give a talk, I would recommend you just Google whatever the title of your presentation is, and someone has probably shared it generously," he advised. "Why would you make your own slides when they're already made online?" He went on: "Notice, I gave her credit? I didn't change her name to mine. I left Medical College of Georgia and everything!" The degree of effort exhibited by the attendings communicated to the housestaff that they were not a priority—to say nothing about the importance of research, knowledge translation, and the associated professional behaviors that should accompany those endeavors. Consequently, residents' attention would often wane during such talks, giving way to cell phone surfing and text messaging. The attendings and the housestaff at Legacy did not take noon conference as seriously as their counterparts at Stonewood did. It was yet another example of how program structures communicated hidden messages to the housestaff about professional development.

Morbidity and Mortality (M&M) Conferences   Monthly M&Ms were another key difference between the two programs. At Legacy, M&Ms replaced noon conferences and, with a few exceptions, were mostly run by the residents—even though, according to ACGME guidelines, they should have consistently involved faculty.[20] Every PGY-3 was expected to present a case involving errors in medical care that resulted in the patient getting sicker (morbidity) or dying (mortality). After going through the case details, the resident would elaborate on the relevant learning points. The aim was not to point fingers but to learn from mistakes in order to avoid them in the future.

In one example, Rodney (USIMG, PGY-3) presented on a patient who was suspected of having tuberculosis upon admission in the emergency department and was therefore given a mask to prevent possible disease transmission. The mask fell off, however, during transport, and no one realized it in time. The admitting residents did not document their suspicion of TB or the fact that the patient was put on infectious precautions, so by the time the CT scan came back, showing raging active TB, the patient had already exposed several hospital workers. The moral of the story (like that of so many M&Ms) was to "document, document, document," in Rodney's words. In this case, however, despite the involvement of the emergency department, radiology, infectious diseases, and the patient's attending-of-record, there were no attendings present during the M&M to help unpack what happened. Two nurses from infection control were the only unfamiliar faces in the room, even though hospital policy regarding isolation procedures changed after that incident.[21]

Thus, once again, Legacy residents had little commitment from the program to help them improve as physicians. Rituals like M&Ms at Legacy were more about going through the motions—perhaps to maintain accreditation—than about improving the residents' professionalization.

M&Ms at Stonewood, by comparison, were much more elaborate. They were held in lieu of morning report in Stonewood's flagship mahogany-paneled auditorium with upholstered seats, were attended en masse not only by the housestaff but also by fellows and faculty from every division in the Department of Medicine, and were simulcast to two other hospitals. Attendance could easily approach one hundred, if not more. Many of the audience members were faculty who earned continuing medical education credits for attending, thereby incentivizing their continued professional development. The monthly event, organized by the chief residents, consisted of an evidence-based, interactive case discussion with a panel of three or four experts—usually fellows and attendings who were directly involved in the patient's care. While the housestaff regularly attended, they seldom participated in M&Ms, unlike at Legacy, unless they were asked to present the case or weigh in on their specific roles. Attendings mostly ran the show.

The event had a distinctly performative air, a public mea culpa of sorts, complete with microphones, video cameras, a stage, and a panel.[22] The serious tone of Stonewood M&Ms echoed the seriousness with which the program approached professional development. Consider the following excerpt from my fieldnotes:

> The program director began by introducing the panel by name, preceded by the ubiquitous "Doctor" prefix, which added to the formality of the session. The panel was composed of attendings from the emergency department (ED),

radiology, neuro-critical care, and endocrinology. A PGY-3 resident involved in the case began describing the patient's symptoms before presenting to the ED. Periodically, the program director who was moderating would interrupt and address the panel: "So, at this point, we'll stop. Dr. [ED attending] was involved in the emergency room. What was going through your mind?" The emergency attending took the microphone and began to describe the patient's course in the ED. He walked in through triage, and she saw him about fifteen minutes after his arrival. The young patient apparently sustained a severe stroke.

What is remarkable is how involved the attendings were compared to those at Legacy; unlike in the previous example with Rodney, attendings from no fewer than four different departments were on hand to explain their thought process and reflect on the incident. At the same time, because M&Ms mostly featured attendings, the residents at Stonewood were more removed from the process than those at Legacy, giving them less hands-on experience with this sort of accountability. Still, the formality associated with Stonewood M&Ms and the wide attendance of faculty, fellows, and the program leadership reinforced in the residents the importance of critical reflection at all career stages.

Evaluation and Remediation

Finally, evaluation is an important aspect of any training program and offers key opportunities to reinforce, and correct, professional development with trainees, particularly those who are struggling. Aside from regular feedback from attendings (which was spottier at Legacy due to the attending structure—see chapter 3), both programs relied on clinical competency committees to discuss residents' overall progress and identify those with clinical knowledge or professionalism deficits as potential candidates for remediation. But in what has become a now familiar pattern, Legacy officials were often more passive—even in the face of egregious lapses—while Stonewood officials intervened as often as necessary to usher even the weakest residents through residency, thereby fulfilling their implicit social contract with their trainees.

Despite strict language in Legacy's Housestaff Manual ("Any incidence of unprofessional conduct will be included in the overall evaluation of clinical competency"), disciplinary action was rare. For example, one time a resident secretly attended an out-of-state wedding, leaving his intern unsupervised for a whole weekend. When program officials found out, they "sent a dramatic email say-ing this *might just* get written up" (emphasis added), as one resident put it, but aside from the threat, it's not clear whether there were any actual consequences. Certainly, with more-minor infractions, like getting behind on discharge summa-ries or signing (absent) friends' names on the occasional noon conference atten-dance sheet, Legacy officials rarely did much more than gently scold the residents.

To the best of my knowledge, fewer than 3 percent of residents were officially put on probation during my time at Legacy.[23] One example was a resident with an eccentric personality. They[24] would go off topic during rounds, say outlandish things, and inevitably end up in conflict with the housestaff, the administration, and even patients. One official explained, "People kept trying to help [them] and failing. . . . We met with [them] and we tried to do stuff, [but they] just kept get-ting into conflicts." The individual was eventually informed toward the end of the year that they had three months to improve; otherwise, they would be put on probation, and their graduation would be delayed. After the three months, the resident was indeed held back for a few more months. The program also imposed more structure on this resident, as described by a senior official:

> We sat [them] down, and we said, "This is how you are to act: you may not yell, you may not raise your voice, you cannot have any fights." . . . We wrote all this down, a checklist you know, show up on time, leave on time, don't do this, do that. . . . So, yeah, that took hours and hours of time. You can just imagine time, effort, you know worrying about [them] at night, losing sleep, writing reports, keeping track of all [the] meetings.

Eventually, the program's efforts paid off; the resident's behavior improved, and they were able to graduate. Tellingly, however, what this resident needed was more defined rules and structure to keep them on task, something that the pro-gram did not offer much of to its residents.

To the best of my knowledge, this resident's probation was a somewhat rare instance of Legacy actively tailoring an intervention to a single trainee; usually, officials opted instead for a more passive, one-size-fits-all approach that put the onus on the residents to succeed. For example, Legacy was very lenient about the yearly In-Training Examination (ITE), a practice test taken by all residents in ACGME-accredited programs to prepare for the American Board of Inter-nal Medicine Certification Examination (Boards) administered at the end of residency. In the Housestaff Manual, Legacy promised to use the ITE scores to "focus on areas where a majority of Housestaff were deficient." In practice, however, the program did little to intervene, despite substandard performance among some of the housestaff. Take Raoul, who did poorly on his ITE: "I was expecting someone to come in and yell at me, to say something, and then when I [went] to my advisor, he said, 'Well, you know, maybe you're a poor test-taker.' No, not really! . . . That's probably one of the reasons why people do so badly on the Boards, because [faculty] don't put pressure on you."

The program was well aware of its residents' substandard performance on the ITE, but as Raoul noted, it seemed ill equipped or unmotivated to do much about it. As one program official observed, "I go down to the auditorium [during noon conference] and say—you've heard me say this—there are people in this room who took the In-Training Exam and scored in the 90th percentile, so that means it can be done; the content is here. . . . But I've got people also who scored in the first percentile, and either they're not listening or they don't know how to take tests or whatever it is. *I don't think we have to do all these things to try to improve that performance*" (emphasis added). The implication was clear: it was not the program's responsibility to remediate residents who scored poorly on the ITE; instead, it was up to the residents to ensure their own success. Extra help with passing the Boards was yet another area that the program simply could not, or would not, prioritize.

Stonewood, however, was explicitly devoted to shepherding its residents through residency—very much in line with the social contract between USMDs and the profession. As one program official boasted, "We have a commitment to ensur[ing] their success and it's unusual that we can't get that." Stonewood adopted a systematic approach to identifying and resolving individual residents' problems, whether they involved medical knowledge or professionalism. Among individuals at risk of failing the Boards, for example, mentors would usually suggest minor remediation; for those struggling with interpersonal issues, they would often recommend counseling. If, despite all efforts, problems remained, residents were put on formal remediation. Those residents had six months to improve before being put on probation.

In one case, a resident struggled with synthesizing medical knowledge into a plan of action and working efficiently. The program put together a plan of nearly ten action items for the resident to accomplish before being taken off remediation, including things like asking for help when necessary. The plan involved meeting with chief residents for an hour or two per week to go over case presentation skills. The program also arranged for the resident to meet with a cardiology fellow once or twice a week to discuss high-yield topics to help brush up on their cardiology knowledge. Program officials took an interest in individuals' performance and offered interventions tailored to their needs, thereby ensuring success to everyone, just as they promised.

At the same time, the program may have had a deeper motivation beyond the residents' self-actualization for so steadfastly upholding its end of the social contract in this way. If the housestaff failed their Boards after graduation or if, heaven forbid, a resident had to be dismissed after failing probation, this situation would represent a considerable blemish on Stonewood's carefully maintained reputation as a rising elite program (see chapter 2). The residency's social location as a top-of-the-middle-tier/bottom-of-the-top-tier program therefore likely encouraged Stonewood to do everything possible to avoid such an outcome—as much for its benefit as for the residents'. To be sure, Legacy's reputation would have probably also taken a hit if it lost a resident, but the immediate concern would have likely been staffing rather than standing. At Stonewood, in contrast, officials regularly experienced anxieties about prestige. During one noontime discussion about Board pass rates, for example, one official was concerned that Stonewood had scored only around the national mean that year: "I would bet that some of the [programs] we're in competition with are probably [above the mean]. . . . I don't think we think of ourselves as an *average* program!" (emphasis in original).[25] In this way, Stonewood had not only the means but also the motivation to ensure its residents' success on the Boards.

Some worried that Stonewood's efforts went too far, however. One group of graduating Stonewood residents criticized the program for coddling the housestaff too much:

RESIDENT 1: [Stonewood is] very responsive to the residents; if there's a problem, they are more than willing to help, but I think . . . they tolerate more than [other programs]. . . . They tolerate it almost to a fault at times. Like problems where people are having difficulty with things, like catching up or keeping up, they will do whatever they can to help you, but at the same time, it might be to a fault sometimes.

RESIDENT 2: They don't let a lot of people fall down.

RESIDENT 3: They do not.

RESIDENT 2: Maybe people need to [fall down]. It's hard to know.

An attending echoed similar sentiments with respect to Stonewood—and the profession more generally—giving people too many chances:

> I think that we are also a field that has become more like take all comers rather than a field that says, "We've given you every chance under the sun here; you might not be good enough; medicine just might not be the calling for you. We understand that you have gone through four years of medical school and an additional year and a half of training, but there are issues that we've identified that are beyond repair, and without repairing those issues, you should not be practicing medicine."

He went on to give an example of a Stonewood resident who would arrive late, was not on top of patient care, and lacked medical knowledge:

> At some point, we have to sort of say, "Look, you got this far; you obviously are able to make a career out of something. You're bright; you should be able to do something, but it is clear that medicine is not the field for you because you can't, when it matters, put something else ahead of yourself." *And we don't do a good enough job of telling that to people.* . . . I think there is something to be said for a program that wants to give the residents every bit of support possible. I think it's great. But I think there has to be a line somewhere. (emphasis added)

Given how rare it is for USMDs to leave or be dismissed from medical school or residency, these findings from Stonewood raise questions about whether and how substandard physicians get filtered out as programs strive to protect their reputations.[26] Clearly, Stonewood invested countless hours ensuring its residents every success, even when some were not always up to par. This made it nearly impossible for the USMDs at Stonewood to fail. In fact, protecting "insiders" is a classic feature of sponsored mobility,[27] and in this case, it clearly distinguished a selected elite group from those, like the residents at Legacy, who were competing on their own to make it to the top.

———

To summarize, as a result of Legacy's overworked program officials and limited resources, its residency program adopted a far more detached approach to professional development than Stonewood did. Comments by Legacy officials like

"You *find yourself* a mentor that is willing to work with you one-on-one" and "I don't think we have to do all these things to try to improve that performance [on the ITE]" were in stark contrast to comments made by Stonewood officials, such as "We say that people are *mentored to death*" and "Our philosophy is that we really like you and we really like to be part of your nurturing and training and *getting you where you want to go*." In this light, it is remarkable that Legacy residents did, in fact, succeed, as the senior Legacy official confessed at the beginning of the chapter: "I'm surprised at how well they've done sometimes." Legacy residents had to sink or swim mostly on their own—just as they had prior to residency. In contrast, compared to Legacy, Stonewood seemed to spoon-feed opportunities to its residents, who were already more advantaged on the aggregate compared to non-USMDs. These efforts represented a continuation of the sponsorship inherent in the social contract with USMDs, designed to ensure that they reached fulfilling careers after getting admitted to US allopathic medical schools (see chapter 1).

IMPLICATIONS FOR PROFESSIONALISM

Now that it's clear that these two programs groomed their housestaff differently, what type of professionals did they produce? How did these different structures of professional development, and their latent messages, influence the residents' professionalism—those behaviors and values that make physicians worthy of public trust?[28] I argue that Legacy, being more laissez-faire, and Stonewood, being more engaged, activated different attitudes among the housestaff, with outlooks being transmitted from superiors to subordinates and effectively reproducing themselves, leading to very different understandings about what it meant to be a "good" physician in both places.

"Laid-Back" Professionals at Legacy

It was no secret that Legacy prided itself on being a "laid-back" program. As a senior member of the program leadership told me, "[This is a place where you can] take an internship, where you can learn something, have a baby and not get killed. So we're happy to offer that." Legacy's website advertised the program as offering a "balanced approach" to residency training that assures a "humane" experience, in sharp contrast to so-called malignant programs known for violating duty hour limits and humiliating residents during rounds.[29] The program leadership, for the most part, was aware that residents were becoming complacent. One even called them "spoiled": "They're a little bit spoiled and I have always told them. . . . One thing doesn't go [their] way and people throw temper tantrums: 'I want to do this!' You [would] not get away with this anywhere else. They get away with it because they can." A different leader, however, was unconcerned about the type of residents being produced by the program: "Now do I think the laid-back approach leads to complacency? Absolutely. Do I think it's a good thing that we try and make this program 'trainee-happy'? Yeah. People have family. . . . So laid-back goes a long way." This official recognized that having more spare time could lead to complacency but believed that it was more important for Legacy residents, many of whom were older and had families, to have time to spend with their loved ones—an approach that also probably benefited the residents' mental well-being.[30]

The problem arose when that complacency impacted their work. One afternoon I was sitting in the residents' lounge during the downtime after lunch that was common at Legacy. Four residents were playing a video game. A pager belonging to one of the players went off. The beeping ran its full course—perhaps ten beeps—and then went silent. The resident eventually paused the game to return the page. A patient's blood work had come back with a critical lactate level of 55 mg/dL (a normal level is 4.5-19.8 mg/dL).[31] Elevated lactate can be a sign that organs are failing and/or that the body is not getting enough oxygen, so it can be an important lab test. The resident hesitated for a while about what to do: finish the game or go see the patient. The other players egged the resident on, telling them to finish the game first.[32] Someone joked that the patient should be upgraded to the ICU (to "turf" the patient to another service). Another resident asked with forced seriousness, "In your medical opinion, is she stable, yes or no?" The resident shrugged and admitted that, yes, the patient was stable. "So let's finish the game!" replied another resident with a laugh. And they did. After a few minutes, however, the resident put down the video controller and went to check on the patient, perhaps feeling guilty for having ignored the page.

To be sure, most of the time residents at Legacy were responsible clinicians who consistently made patient care a priority, even without the constant supervision of their superiors. One resident, for example, told me he would regularly check his patients' lab values and vital signs from home before going to bed every night. But the conditions at Legacy made it such that the incident with the resident playing video games was not as isolated as it should have been. Implicit in Legacy's general approach to the residents was the sense that the leadership was too busy, or too resource-poor, to seriously invest in the residents' education, so the residents, in turn, did not always take their education and work as seriously. Here was a critical lab value that needed immediate attention from a resident, and that resident elected to keep playing a video game before going to see the patient. In the absence of higher expectations at Legacy, where the level of supervision was low and complacency predominated, this resident was able to do what would have been unfathomable at Stonewood—put themselves before patient care. Stonewood chief residents even prepared monthly orientation packets for residents on the wards, urging them to "answer pages, listen to nurses, learn their names, say thank you, be polite, and discuss your plans with them and case managers. Although you may be the conductor of this patient care symphony, they are your orchestra and actually make the music." Clearly, differences like these in the programs' hidden *and* explicit curricula had the potential to produce very different kinds of residents.

It didn't help that Legacy's temporary teaching attendings would sometimes model unprofessional behaviors themselves, thereby teaching the housestaff that such behavior was, in fact, acceptable within the profession. One day an attending accidentally spilled an entire cup of coffee on the floor in the emergency department and left without even attempting to clean it up. Another time, during a discussion about how obese Americans were, an attending joked, "They have a gland problem. Salivary gland!" Given this sort of modeling, it was unsurprising that, when residents were discussing gastric bypass surgery during rounds on another day, a senior resident exclaimed, "What these people need is not a gastric bypass—it's a brain transplant!" Similarly, given how often the faculty would give uninspired lectures during noon conference or grand rounds, it is perhaps to be expected that the residents' own presentations during didactic conferences, such as morning report, would also be of low quality. Indeed, studies find that individuals are more motivated when they are surrounded by positive role models.[33] Legacy residents watched their superiors put in minimal effort and establish low standards, so they learned to do the same.

Consequently, senior residents at Legacy, just like their own attendings, were quite hands-off with their interns and medical students—often preferring to spend leisure time in the residents' lounge rather than helping their subordinates—which taught interns to look forward to the days when they could do the same. By leaving early or prioritizing leisure time over education, residents left an impression on junior trainees about what was acceptable behavior. Consider one medical student's description of her first day at Legacy:

> I ended up sitting by myself for about an hour and a half because they [the program officials] were like, "Oh, follow the intern." And when I came back after lunch, they [the residents] were all playing video games, and that was my first day, so I was just kinda sitting there against the wall, so awkward. . . . I didn't know if I should stay or I should leave. I stayed till 4:30 with nobody talking to me; then I just left.

She went on to describe another instance when a patient's kidney function deteriorated to the point that he needed emergency dialysis, but the housestaff realized it only when it was too late. She attributed it to the general culture at the hospital:

> It just seems like everybody is on this different wavelength, and then I think it translates to the staff. . . . Nobody is worrying about, OK, why did this guy's creatinine level need to get 10 [a normal level is 0.6–1.2 mg/dl] before he urgently needs to be dialyzed because we didn't have a PICC [peripherally inserted central catheter] line? . . . I feel like everybody is like, they wanna clock in and they wanna clock out and they just wanna do what they have to do. . . . But when you're in the medical [field], . . . it doesn't matter what you have to do today.

By picking up on subtle cues and observing her superiors, this medical student learned that it was acceptable to simply put in the bare minimum and get away with it at Legacy.

More Engaged (and More Smug) Professionals at Stonewood

In sharp contrast, Stonewood attendings and program officials made a concerted effort to inspire engagement and enthusiasm in their trainees. This enthusiasm rubbed off on the Stonewood housestaff, who were often more excited about their work than the residents at Legacy were and, consequently, were perhaps more diligent. One day, for example, a medical student was reporting on a patient who had received an ultrasound of the heart (echocardiogram): "We heard it [a murmur] on the echo and then went back and listened [to the patient's heart]," she told her attending. In response, the attending complained lightheartedly, "Why didn't you come get me? I love murmurs, and we don't get to hear them very often!" Remarkably, this medical student and her intern went back to listen to the patient's heart murmur after recognizing it on the echocardiogram, even though that was not clinically necessary—a manifestation of both their curiosity and their thoroughness. That curiosity was further stoked by their attending, who exhibited similar excitement at the prospect of hearing a murmur. At Stonewood, curiosity and diligence were integral to being a good doctor.

Of course, it helped that the case mix at Stonewood was more interesting than that at Legacy, but this same level of engagement extended to more mundane tasks as well, such as regular attendance and participation at noon conference. Some residents even exceeded expectations, like the time a patient's cell phone battery died and an intern rounded up several types of chargers so that the patient could call home to make travel arrangements for his discharge. When the intern's attending found out, he shook his head with a smile and said, "It's amazing, residents who go above and beyond." Then he told another story about a resident who went to the pharmacy to buy a glucometer for a patient who needed to check their blood sugar regularly but could not afford to buy one.

This level of engagement was facilitated by the fact that Stonewood laid out clear expectations of its residents, supervised them closely, and rewarded good behavior—all of which communicated Stonewood's deep investment in the residents. For example, the housestaff's handbook reminded residents as follows: "When in doubt about a course of action, do what's best for the patient. Responsibility to one's patients is the cornerstone of professionalism in medicine." While similar instructions appeared in Legacy's Housestaff Manual, Stonewood residents better internalized these professional norms because superiors were constantly monitoring them and modeling these same behaviors. Peers also monitored and encouraged each other. As Lynn, a Stonewood intern, told me, "Your peer group dictates your level of motivation. I'm surrounded by people who really care, who want excellent patient outcomes. They worry about these people [patients], and I would say I worry about my people, I want them to do very well, and I take it very personally when they don't. And I think that kind of camaraderie and that shared morale is critical." In other words, environment and context matter to the way residents behave and learn, just as Hafferty asserts.

At the same time, while Stonewood residents were more motivated than Legacy residents, they were also more smug. They considered this sense of diligence to be a point of pride and used it to distinguish themselves as (morally) superior to community hospital trainees. Recall that Stonewood residents rotated at three clinical sites. At one of those sites—let's call it Tri-Hospital—Stonewood residents would interact with the housestaff from nearby Solomon Hospital, another community hospital affiliated with Stonewood University that was staffed mostly with IMGs. Stonewood residents would frequently criticize Solomon residents for their lack of diligence. Several residents, including a third-year USMD resident, told me about a similar, possibly apocryphal, story:

> We work with the Solomon residents at Tri-Hospital, and sometimes we're like, "Oh, patient's crashing; it's three o'clock. Oh, the Solomon team signed out [left] early; oh, it's a Solomon patient that's crashing." I don't know if that's just like a coincidence but sometimes it seems like they don't wrap things up as well. . . . Here [at Stonewood], I feel like people stay until like nine o'clock following up like a CT scan and not have signed out, you know?

According to this third-year resident, a Stonewood resident would stay late to follow up on the results of CT scan, whereas Solomon residents would sign out when their shift ended. As will become clearer in chapter 6, these limited interactions with Solomon residents would often form the basis for widespread judgments about the competence of community hospital residents *in general*, without taking into account structural factors (like the ones described in the first part of this chapter) that may have impacted their training and professionalism.

At this point, it may be germane to ask whether it was truly the *structure* of the programs, rather than the *agency* of the residents, that was responsible for these differences in professionalism between Stonewood and Legacy. Were Stonewood residents perhaps simply more professional clinicians at baseline than Legacy residents were? An especially illuminating example from morning report helps counter this proposition and sheds light on the extent to which structural differences helped produce the kind of outcomes described in this chapter. Recall from chapter 3 that Legacy residents would frequently tune out during morning report in favor of surfing the internet on their cell phones. In contrast, electronic devices were used almost exclusively at Stonewood to look up relevant data, such as the latest clinical guidelines on the case in question. One notable exception occurred one morning at Stonewood when the program directors and attendings were delayed by inclement weather; only one chief resident had arrived on time for morning report. The absence of more senior officials seemed to have prompted the residents to act more casually than usual because one resident began browsing Facebook on her cell phone during a resident's presentation while another had his feet up on the table, shoes and all. When the chief resident left the room briefly, the housestaff were even more relaxed. The PGY-3 resident presenting a slide on data analysis freely admitted, "I don't know what any of this means now that [the chief] has left the room." His comments were met by a round of laughter. He continued, "And I included this table which goes all the way to the third floor just because [the chief] wanted me to."

This example suggests that without the close supervision and clear expectations of superiors, the residents at Stonewood may not have been that different from Legacy residents in terms of their professionalism. What is certain is that the two programs were vastly different in terms of the support and presence of multiple chief residents, faculty members, and program officials at Stonewood who demanded more from their residents, likely prompting them to act more professionally than the residents at Legacy, where less was expected from the housestaff.

CONCLUSION

In sum, I found that very different program structures produced very different kinds of residents. Legacy's approach to professional development was more passive and laissez-faire—largely the result of the program's limited resources—leaving the residents to make their own opportunities rather than having the program structure opportunities for them. As Laurie said at the beginning of the chapter, "You can take whatever you have here and really work with it," the onus being on the residents to make the best of what little was given to them. I argue that this hands-off approach encouraged Legacy residents to be self-starters in some respects but to be more complacent in others, which sometimes affected their professionalism. Stonewood, by comparison, was more active and supportive, thanks to its abundant resources and strong desire to remain elite, enabling it to shepherd the housestaff toward success by offering them structured opportunities for enrichment. This instilled greater motivation in Stonewood residents, as well as a corresponding sense of moral superiority over community hospital residents.

These broader patterns of isolation and support in professional development echo the same patterns elucidated in chapters 1 and 3 and served to further entrench status differences along educational pedigree lines. I showed previously that non-USMDs had fewer supports in place from early life to guide them into and through medical school. This isolation followed them into residency at Legacy, where research, mentorship, and learning were explicitly the trainees' responsibility. Legacy offered little structural support to ease its residents through the process but was quick to lay responsibility on the housestaff for their professional success. These medical graduates, who had to fight from the beginning to make opportunities happen, continued to have to do so during residency at a place like Legacy. Indeed, if they succeeded, it was largely *in spite* of their training programs.

Most USMDs, in contrast, had all the family and scholarly support they needed from early in life to make it into medical school and through residency, thanks in part to medicine's social contract with its trainees. Stonewood's supportive approach to the residents' education and professional development was a continuation of that support. Just as the social contract promises, once these USMDs joined the ranks of the profession in medical school, it was the profession's responsibility to help them succeed. Stonewood consistently assisted its residents along the way—providing everything from three to five different mentors on the first day of residency to a twenty-four-page booklet cataloging nearly one hundred research projects they could join. All these efforts communicated to the housestaff how to be successful and made it easier for them to thrive. The program's dedication to their success represents the profession holding up its end of the social contract. It also likely reflected Stonewood's desire to zealously maintain its status as an elite program, as the residents' success was intimately linked to the program's success. It is hardly surprising, then, that Stonewood residents had more career options upon graduation than those at Legacy did, as I'll explain in the next chapter. Stonewood's residents succeeded largely thanks to the tailwinds of support provided to them by their residency program.

CHAPTER 5

Graduation

I don't know anyone [at Stonewood] who's not going to match [to fellowship]—in any field.

Ted, a US-trained medical graduate in his third postgraduate year
at Stonewood University Hospital

For them [graduates of US allopathic medical schools], it's more a question of if I want to do it or not, and sometimes for us [international and osteopathic graduates], it's more a question [of] can I do it or not?

Trevor, a US citizen and international medical graduate in his
second postgraduate year at Legacy Community Hospital

After three years of residency training, internal medicine graduates can embark on one of two career paths: they can either (1) remain generalists and practice as internists in hospitals (as hospitalists) or in outpatient settings (as primary care practitioners) or (2) pursue more specialized training, known as a fellowship, in one of ten internal medicine subspecialties.[1] This decision needs to be made long before the end of residency, however. Two weeks into their third year, on July 15, fellowship applicants submit their materials to the Medical Specialties Matching Program run by the National Resident Matching Program. Interviews are scheduled through November, when residents must finalize their rank list. As with residency, applicants rank-order their preferred programs while programs rank-order the applicants, and the Match algorithm determines an optimized outcome. Match Day is in late November, allowing successful applicants about seven months to complete residency before transitioning to fellowship.

This timeline really gives residents only two years to prepare for fellowship if they want to start right after residency, as most do. Prior to 2012, residents had even less time, with fellowship applications due in November of the *second* year and Match Day held in October of the third year. The timeline was delayed in order to give residents sufficient experience to make fellowship decisions and to allow program directors more time to get to know their residents better before writing letters of recommendation.[2] The new timeline reduced the pressure on residents to make career decisions early in their residency, but it also increased the stakes of the game. Just as with getting into medical school and residency (see chapter 1), residents understood that there was a series of boxes to check off—a game to play—to make it into fellowship. The longer timeline meant that there were now more boxes to check off because residents had more time to accumulate accomplishments.

In this chapter, I examine Legacy and Stonewood residents' trajectories out of residency and demonstrate how status and training inequalities during residency can have lasting impacts on physicians' professional mobility. Graduation from residency is a critical turning point because it represents the juncture at which the formal elite and rank-and-file emerges. At the end of residency, some residents become part of the formal knowledge elite (by pursuing fellowships to become subspecialists) and the formal administrative elite (by becoming chief residents who may go on to become program or hospital administrators) while others form the formal rank and file (by remaining generalists). Perhaps unsurprisingly, a greater proportion of Legacy graduates than Stonewood graduates ended up as generalists (50 percent versus 33 percent). This outcome did not occur randomly, however. I argued in previous chapters that the informal distinctions between the elite and the rank and file begin long before this point—even before medical school—forming informal horizontal status distinctions among supposed equals (internal medicine residents). It is at graduation from residency, however, that we can observe how the mechanisms elucidated in the previous chapters translate into formal, *vertical* status hierarchies between specialists and generalists.

Importantly, the goal here is not to suggest that because a greater proportion of Legacy residents ended up as generalists, they were somehow less accomplished than Stonewood residents who mostly subspecialized. Becoming a generalist is hardly a failure, especially given the current critical need for more primary care providers than any kind of specialist.[3] Instead, I intend to shed light on the structural conditions that sometimes pushed residents toward careers they may not have otherwise chosen for themselves. I highlight how unequal residency training can give way to different opportunity structures after graduation. I argue that these differences in opportunity were due in part to the fact that international and osteopathic medical graduates (non-USMDs) (1) had less help playing the fellowship game, (2) faced harder rules of the game, and (3) had to combat stigma associated with being a non-USMD resident at a community hospital. They were also partly due to (4) concrete differences in merit and achievement between Legacy and Stonewood graduates arising out of the unequal training structures I described in the two previous chapters. It is here that we begin to see the game as a kind of self-fulfilling prophecy, whereby US-trained medical graduates (USMDs), who received the most support before and during residency because they were deemed more worthy from the outset, unsurprisingly outperform (at least on some key measures) those who got the least amount of support, effectively blurring the lines among structural advantage, merit, and achievement in medicine.

MAKING SENSE OF POSTRESIDENCY OPPORTUNITIES: STRUCTURE VERSUS AGENCY

The Emphasis on Self-Determination

Many residents at Legacy felt that little was out of reach for them when it came to postresidency opportunities. They did not deny that significant obstacles existed. Rather, they insisted that those obstacles were surmountable with enough will and dedication. For example, when I asked Reed, an international medical graduate (IMG) in his first postgraduate year (PGY-1) at Legacy, whether he felt certain fellowships were off-limits to him, he replied, "Honestly I don't think so. I guess it depends on who you are and what you are willing to do to get it." Another PGY-1, Rashad, acknowledged that being an IMG would make it more difficult for him to match into fellowship, but he felt strongly that by "working hard enough, you'll get the research and you'll get lucky. Nice CV. You'll get accepted eventually." Throughout their careers, Legacy residents had internalized that it was incumbent upon them to make their own success; fellowship, it seemed, was no different.

Cody's story is one that I will return to periodically throughout this chapter. He was the Legacy resident I introduced in the previous chapter who had aspirations of subspecializing in allergy and immunology—one of the most competitive fellowships. Residents at Legacy knew that allergy/immunology was going to be tough for Cody, both because he was a US citizen who trained at an international medical school (USIMG) and because Legacy did not have a fellowship program in allergy. Yet they constantly referred to him as proof that anything was possible. They spoke as though he had already matched before he even applied: as one second-year USIMG resident said, "Cody is doing . . . a lot of extracurricular work to get himself a spot in allergy. Allergy is one of those things that are very competitive. He'll get it. He might not even have to go do a chief residency or a year of research; he might get it right out [of residency]. But *he has done the work.* He used what was available to him, and he is probably going to get it" (emphasis added). While Cody was still a PGY-2, the chief resident would even advertise to prospective applicants that Cody was likely to match into allergy/immunology as evidence that such an accomplishment was *possible* from a place like Legacy. There was thus a strong collective belief that with his hard work, he could beat the odds.

Cody himself acknowledged the importance of effort and dedication in achieving his ambitions. When I asked whether certain opportunities were more difficult to achieve than others, he replied with a shrug, "Nothing is off-limits, and I say that to applicants for internship all the time." When I asked Cody whether cardiology, another highly competitive specialty, would be achievable for someone coming from Legacy, where residents had little exposure to complex cardiac patients because the hospital lacked a catheterization lab to perform angioplasty, he admitted, "Just like with allergy/immunology, it's difficult. . . . But could you do it? Yeah. I think you can. . . . The question is, *Do you want to work hard enough to get it?*" (emphasis added).[4] Cody thus attributed professional success to the individual's willingness to work hard: "If you want something, you just have to work hard to get it. Nobody is going to hand you a fellowship in allergy or cardiology just because you're nice . . . and everybody likes you in the hospital. It just doesn't work like that. You have to—because there are people in other places doing the work—so you better do the work, too, to make yourself a good applicant, you know?"

This emphasis on hard work placed the onus on the individual for their own success and suggested that effort (or agency) prevailed over structural constraints when it came to trajectories out of residency. To be sure, competitive fellowships *did require* hard work, and some residents consciously chose not to invest their time and energy into pursuing them. As Reed (IMG, PGY-1, Legacy) explained, "You know you can do a lot of work here and you can get a lot of publications in research if you *want* to, but most people don't do that and so most people don't do prestigious fellowships from here" (emphasis added). The implication, however, seemed to be that it was *only* a matter of effort—that if Legacy residents simply chose to work harder and do more research, prestigious fellowships would be within reach.

The Legacy leadership was instrumental in helping perpetuate these beliefs. When asked whether residents from Legacy matched into highly competitive fellowships, an official replied enthusiastically, "Yes! We do rank in some of the highest, best fellowship programs, including in pulmonary/critical care and GI [gastroenterology]!" At the time of the interview, however, no Legacy resident had matched directly (i.e., without taking time off between residency and fellowship) into gastroenterology or cardiology in recent institutional memory. Yet when referring to cardiology fellowships, this same official exclaimed, "Yes, they did [match]! At the University of Miami, I believe, but [the resident] turned it down. He realized he didn't want to go into cardiology." His account was improbable, however, given that offers made through The Match involve a firm commitment on the part of both the applicant and the program that cannot be waived except in cases of "serious and extreme hardship."[5] Furthermore, the official's reply sounded suspiciously similar to the story of one Legacy resident who was interested in cardiology and even did out-of-state rotations in Florida but who ultimately decided not to apply for fellowship, given the odds against him.

Still, Legacy program leaders remained optimistic that nothing was out of reach for their residents. While admitting that the hospital could not provide exposure to residents in all fields—namely, in cardiology—a different official insisted that the lack of a catheterization lab at Legacy did not affect residents' chances of matching into a cardiology fellowship: "[The impact is] zero as far as I know. Someone correct me if I'm wrong, but if you want to be a cardiology fellow, you can learn how to do caths [catheterizations] [during fellowship]."[6] Yet this same official told me that he would advise applicants *against* choosing Legacy for residency if they were interested in careers in cardiology. When I pressed him on whether the absence of a catheterization lab foreclosed residents' opportunities to become cardiologists, he replied, "Not at all." He then proceeded to tell me about a resident who graduated two years prior and had matched at Stonewood.

"He was one of ours; he trained here. It can be done." When I pointed out that this resident had actually matched into pulmonary/critical care—not cardiology—he shrugged and said, "Yeah, well, I'm just saying, you know?"

Like the residents, Legacy officials also emphasized the role of hard work in achieving fellowship success. After noting that she would discourage prospective applicants from applying to Legacy if they wanted to pursue cardiology, one official still demurred when asked whether cardiology was off-limits to Legacy graduates: "They work hard. No, they can still go to cardiology. I think like maybe five, six years ago one of our chiefs went into doing cardiology, but that was part of the homework he had to do. . . . So it's not like you can't; there is no can't; *it's just how much work you have to put into it. Do you really want it?*" (emphasis added). Once again, she invoked hard work and dedication as the keys to unlocking virtually any career path.

It is possible that by virtue of being program leaders, these respondents may have wanted to paint their residency program in a more positive light by aggrandizing their residents' potential for matching into prestigious or highly competitive fellowships. All of them alluded to (perhaps apocryphal) examples of individuals who had "made it" as proof that competitive fellowships were possible rather than as evidence of their rarity. In actuality, I was unable to find any evidence of anyone matching directly from Legacy into cardiology, gastroenterology, or allergy/immunology—three of the most competitive subspecialties. Still, there remained a kind of lore among Legacy residents and officials about phantom residents who had indeed succeeded in these desirable fields, which fed the belief that with enough work and dedication, anything was possible.

For their part, Stonewood residents—who were more advantaged competitors in the hierarchical social system—shared similar beliefs in individual self-determination, often emphasizing how much of their futures was a function of their own choosing: "It's a rare person who doesn't get into fellowship *who wants to go* in the field" (emphasis added), said one resident, noting how little was out of reach for them. The program leadership echoed similar emphases on choice. As one senior program official at Stonewood remarked one day, "You know, eight of our residents went into cardiology last year. I'm thrilled, and my job, my joy is getting them where they want to go," before going on to question, as an aside, whether the health care system really needs more cardiologists. His residents, however, had the choice to pursue that subspecialty in a way that most Legacy residents did not. Gunther (USMD, PGY-3), who matched into cardiology from Stonewood, explained that in contrast to community residency programs, "it's not as much a question of *whether* someone from [Stonewood is] going to do it [match to cardiology]; it's really a question of *Where* are you going to match? Are you going to match big time, or are you going to match little time? Not *if* you're going to match" (emphasis in original). Stonewood residents therefore not only chose their future career paths but also were often successful in reaching their goals.

To account for these successes, Stonewood residents would often emphasize individual attributes over institutional ones. One Stonewood resident noted, for example, "I would say that if you look at our prior [fellowship] match list for the past few years . . . we have not had a very strong match list [in terms of where residents matched]. I think that's probably because of the quality of the residents that were applying rather than a reflection upon this institution. If you look at this year, we have a very strong class . . . it's more a product of *who you are* and what you bring to the table" (emphasis added). This perspective emphasized individual accomplishments over structural advantages, and just like Legacy residents, those at Stonewood identified hard work and dedication as the keys to future success.

Importantly, Stonewood residents believed these views also extended to non-USMDs. As one Stonewood resident noted, "If you're putting out good stuff from community hospitals, you're putting out good stuff. And that's what they care about. And if you're sitting on your ass at Johns Hopkins Hospital, people stop caring that you're from Johns Hopkins, and they just see that you're sitting on your ass." This view, of course, overlooks the fact that opportunities for producing good research were significantly higher at institutions like Johns Hopkins. Stonewood residents also cited examples of people who had "made it." During one focus group, a resident talked about a rare attending at Stonewood who went to medical school abroad: "He was [South American]; he grew up there and went to med school there. . . . I think he did his residency [in the southern United States], in a decent community program. Probably had to work really hard there and got a lot of publications there and was able to jump up to the fellowship he did here . . . then stayed as faculty here until he got enough publications and then you know now he is a kind of a premier . . . about as high up as you can go if that's your goal." Another resident immediately interjected, "And look how many times [the other resident] said publications."

So indeed it seemed possible for an IMG to jump from being a resident in a community program to being a fellow in a prestigious hospital. But as one Stonewood intern put it, it required being a "pioneer." As will become clearer, sheer will and hard work, while important, were not always enough to surmount the considerable structural obstacles facing Legacy residents. Cody is a case in point; recall that he situated responsibility for fellowship success in the individual: "Don't complain that you don't get the fellowship if you're not going to put the work in." But despite having put in the work—getting involved in research early on, doing external electives, and presenting at conferences—Cody did not match into an allergy/immunology fellowship directly after residency. It seems there were limits to the agency so fervently championed at both hospitals.

As I will argue, for all their belief in hard work and dedication, Legacy residents still had a harder time playing the game of getting into fellowship, a game that often starts long before residency. It's not that hard work didn't matter—it arguably mattered *more* at Legacy than at Stonewood because of the Legacy program's training deficits, as described in chapters 3 and 4. Those same educational deficits meant that Legacy residents were less well prepared for fellowship than Stonewood residents—in other words, they were less meritorious than Stonewood residents were—which limited their prospects after graduation. In addition, Legacy trainees faced now familiar processes of exclusion—stigma—based on their educational (including postgraduate) pedigree, resulting in different, and often harder, rules of the game for them compared to Stonewood residents. In this way, while merit was part of what determined Legacy residents' futures, it was by no means the whole story.

For their part, while Stonewood residents could pursue any subspecialty of their choice, the acceptable range of options was constrained both by the residents' need to satisfy internalized definitions of "success"—themselves a product of the profession's norms and structures—*and* by their financial creditors.[7] Many USMDs at Stonewood faced severe debt burdens and expected great returns on their investment in a medical education, particularly from fellowship training, which carried more lucrative salaries after graduation. These factors—many of which predated residency—importantly influenced Stonewood residents' decisions to pursue a subspecialty or remain a generalist. In this way, the past had a way of shaping the future for residents at both hospitals. Next I detail how structural forces influenced their trajectories out of residency, thereby moderating their individual agency.

STRUCTURAL CONSTRAINTS SHAPING TRAJECTORIES
OUT OF RESIDENCY

Starting to Play the (Fellowship) Game Early

The game for getting into fellowship, like those for getting into medical school and residency, began early in life as applicants strived to keep doors open for the future. However, as I explained in chapter 1, USMDs enjoyed more early support, which better prepared them to plan accordingly (known as planful competence) and thus to play more strategically.[8]

Most Stonewood residents interested in fellowship began thinking about it back in medical school, or even earlier, as some of them pursued electives or research opportunities to position themselves for those postresidency trajectories. At the end of medical school, as I mentioned in chapter 1, most USMDs were advised to apply to residency programs in university hospitals so as not be limited when it came to fellowship. Part of the calculus at every stage for USMDs was ensuring that doors remained open—a mentality that may have ironically constrained them, as I will argue later in "Definitions of Success").[9] Cassandra, a Stonewood intern, explained, "Really it's just [having] control over what choices you have each step along the way." Importantly, Cassandra's use of the words *control* and *choices* highlight the role of agency in the process. USMDs likely overemphasized their choices in playing the fellowship game because they benefited from having structures that, for example, provided guidance during medical school and from having the right pedigree, which made those choices *possible*.

In contrast, as I illustrated in chapters 1 and 2, Legacy residents were much more constrained in their range of options for residency, in part because they faced stigma and other barriers to entry that did not apply to USMDs. This made it harder to keep doors open for fellowship in the same way. Joe, an IMG from Legacy, for example, applied to and interviewed at several university-based programs that he did not match to in the end. He explained, "If we [could] choose between this program and [those programs], you don't have to ask which one everyone would choose. I would choose [a university program] first . . . because you have a better chance [of] getting a better fellowship later." So clearly Legacy residents knew that going to a university program would help them play the game, but they had to keep their career plans flexible to account for their lack of choice in the process. Thus, when USMDs were unsure about what they wanted to do, they fought to keep as many doors open as possible. Non-USMDs, for their part, would often fight simply to keep one door open at a time, like matching into *a* residency program rather than *the* residency program that would offer them the best opportunities.

Interestingly, for all that they emphasized agency, residents from both hospitals—including Joe and Cassandra—alluded to a kind of path dependence for matching into fellowship. This path dependence challenges the idea touted by the profession (see the introduction) that fellowship—and medical training more broadly—is both standardized and meritocratic, for if it was, applicants would ostensibly be assessed on their current merits, independent of institutional context. Instead, structural (dis)advantage and status muddy the meritocratic waters, making prospects for fellowship more complicated than just a matter of hard work and dedication. One USIMG, for example, strongly suspected that decisions he made before medical school could be limiting him now that he was applying for fellowship, as these decisions shaped where he went to medical school (the Caribbean), which in turn shaped where he went to residency (Legacy). Contrasting himself to USMDs, he explained, "They got started on an earlier path and that made the rest of the path maybe a little easier, but they didn't have to work less. They still had to put in work, but the path was easier." This resident's views speak to the lasting effects of how well one plays the game, as well as to the "stickiness" of disadvantage. If he had played the game more strategically earlier on, this USIMG reasoned, he would not be in this position, although this particular USIMG was a first-generation college graduate who struggled to play the game as well as USMDs did. In this way, the path-dependent game had a way of reproducing (dis)advantage, making it a structure unto itself.

Ted (USMD, PGY-3, Stonewood) echoed similar views about the kind of inertia that can result when USMDs successfully get started early, a phenomenon he likened to "cruise control":

I think people always think that it's money and prestige [that drives us to medicine], but I think it's literally *the easiest path* for most people. Meaning that people are always very driven and very smart and in the top of their class and in science, and it becomes like, "Oh, okay, what will I do? Oh, look, here's something [medicine] that like only really smart people do." . . . It's just like the next step; this is easy ... I feel like fellowship, it's the same way. They don't even have to tell us anything because we've done this step four times now, so it's literally *so easy*—you fill out the ERAS [an electronic application system], you go do some interviews, you walk in. You've done this for med school, residency; it's the exact same process, like it's just the next easy step. ... It [is] like cruise control. (emphasis added)

Here Ted was referring to the path set out for USMDs that leads them naturally to the next step—in this case, fellowship. It also harks back to the notion of a "runaway freight train," which some Stonewood residents used to describe medical training in chapter 1. This train emerged as a result of playing the game wisely from the beginning and accumulating advantages at each stage of training, such that getting into fellowship became a matter of just maintaining that momentum.

The trouble was that non-USMDs had a harder time creating such momentum, and even when they were able to play the game strategically, they were not always successful. Cody is one such example; between medical school in the Caribbean and residency at Legacy, he took a year off to work (unpaid) on cardiology research and increase his chances for fellowship. As he explained:

You have to play the game for residency and you have to play the game for fellowship ... it wasn't so much that I wanted to do cardiology, but this was a great opportunity for me. ... I knew that I wanted to do a fellowship; I didn't know if it was cardiology or if it was going to be allergy/immunology or anything, but I knew that I needed my name on research. I knew that I needed to have manuscripts; I knew I needed to have abstracts in order to even have a shot at getting a [fellowship] spot.

Despite accumulating important research experience early on—and therefore starting the game for fellowship even before residency—Cody was unable to match into his desired subspecialty right away. As will become clearer, starting the game early wasn't enough for Legacy residents. Non-USMDs in community hospitals, like Cody, faced several disadvantages when applying for fellowship during residency, including a lack of program support, stigma, and different rules of the game (i.e., higher expectations than those for USMDs). I deal with these in turn.

Program Support

If Stonewood residents had an easier time getting fellowships, it was at least partly thanks to numerous advantages they enjoyed over Legacy residents. First, it helped that Stonewood University Hospital housed fellowships in almost every medical subspecialty, providing built-in support for fellowship applications. As one program director told prospective applicants to Stonewood, "The culture here is that fellowship directors are also very much your mentors. If you're applying for fellowship, you'll meet with the fellowship directors here; they'll advise you, make calls for you." The presence of fellowship directors was thus a huge advantage for Stonewood residents, who benefited from their guidance and networks. Because it was also common for residents to stay on at Stonewood for fellowship, they also benefited from building relationships with program directors, who generally preferred to hire locally.

Second, Stonewood carefully shepherded its residents through the fellowship application process. For example, program officials organized an evening information session with a panel of fellowship program directors to help demystify the process. Topics covered included not only how to apply for fellowships but also what to emphasize in the application, how to strategize ahead of time, and whom to talk to. In lieu of simply giving them the application deadline, a program official further encouraged them to apply by the date the application system *opened*—July 15: "There's a phenomenon," he explained, "in highly competitive programs where some program directors say, 'I'm only going into ERAS [the electronic application system] once, on July 15,' and if they go in only once but you only have one [recommendation] letter uploaded . . ." He trailed off, implying that their application would be disregarded if all their recommendation letters were not in the system by that time. He then said with emphasis, "I want your applications to be entirely completed by July 15. That to me is a hard deadline." He also shared other bits of insider information: "At least one letter should be from people you've done research with. . . . If you're applying to ID [infectious disease], become a junior member of that division—go to their conferences, go to their retreats, . . . get known by the division director. Their emails and phone calls should reflect your participation in the division while here." Those emails and phone calls, of course, were all informal efforts by the faculty to set up back channels on behalf of the residents and were needed along with the (required) formal letters of recommendation they would submit. The program official concluded by reminding the residents that "the culture here is that if you apply to fellowship, the fellowship directors really take you on as advisees. [They] really work with you to advise and add places to your list [of applications]."

In essence, the Stonewood housestaff were taught the unofficial formula for applying to fellowship and offered assistance with its execution. It is unsurprising, then, that the housestaff felt well prepared for fellowship applications. When I asked a focus group of residents about applying for fellowships, one of them replied, "They [the program] tell you what to do. . . . Like they'll set you up with someone, an attending, who acts as your mentor in the subspecialty that you're thinking about." Strong guidance toward fellowships was a point of pride for the program. As one official told me, "Kids do well getting fellowships. We work with [them]. You know it's not an accident; we tell them that they do well. *We make sure of it*" (emphasis added). With that kind of informal sponsorship—a hallmark of the profession's social contract with USMDs—it is little wonder that Stonewood residents felt that virtually any subspecialty was within reach. But by emphasizing their agency in achieving it, they overlooked the substantial structural supports that helped them along the way. They mistook the collective social contract for individual merit.

By comparison, Legacy residents received considerably less guidance about the timing and strategy of the game and had fewer in-house fellowship programs on which to rely for support. This left them feeling a bit lost. As Adrian (USIMG, PGY-2) explained rather poignantly, "[At a university program], you do this, you follow this guideline, this algorithm. You publish this paper about this, you do a little research in this lab that we already have set up for you, you do this rotation. . . . It's a well-worn path. There are signs pointing that way. [If] you want to walk the distance, you'll go. Here [at a place like Legacy], it's having that location but not having the map in your hand, kind of just finding your way." Thus, while Stonewood residents had all the support they needed to get to where they needed to go, Legacy residents were on their own yet again, making it more difficult for them to exercise that agency they so strongly emphasized.

Stigma and Merit

Aside from having less help with the game, Legacy residents also had to contend with the disadvantages—both nominal and substantive—associated with their pedigree. For non-USMDs, there was a sense that the stigma related to their medical school pedigree never fully disappeared. It carried on into fellowship, even after they had completed their residency at a US allopathic institution. As Ivy (USIMG, PGY-1) explained, "The fact that you might be a foreign grad could still come back to haunt you when you're trying to get a fellowship . . . because they think at some point you weren't as qualified to be a medical student in the [United States], so there must be something about you that makes you not as good."[10] Not everyone saw it this way, however. A few respondents from both Legacy and Stonewood felt that medical schooling no longer carried any weight after residency. One Stonewood chief resident said, "Ten years out, it does not really matter [where you went to medical school]."

Yet some attendings, who were further along in their careers, disagreed. In an interview, an attending who was one of the few non-USMDs on the faculty at Stonewood (let's call them Dr. Taylor)[11] recounted how it was an uphill battle to overcome the stigma associated with their medical degree, from hiring to promotion and beyond: "Someone tried to, I'm told by a good source at the time, stack the deck against me because they were very upset about my being a [non-USMD] at Stonewood," referring to their promotion process. "Obviously this individual, I think he had abject prejudice [against non-USMDs] and it's interesting again, [with] academic freedom being so important for me." Dr. Taylor went on to recount how their family had experienced extreme oppression overseas. "I mean, here, this kind of prejudice is *nothing* like that. But growing up, with the coming to America, the stories from my father because of the freedom, and being able to earn a living no matter who you are, and then living something like that!" (emphasis in original). As an attending at Stonewood, the discrimination persisted. Dr. Taylor felt so strongly that they drafted a letter to the Stonewood president about their experiences: "Here I am at a place like [Stonewood] which has fought prejudice and here this is how [non-USMDs] as minorities are being treated in all places at [Stonewood]." But Dr. Taylor never sent the letter. "I think I had fear of profound retribution from a powerful person, a group of people figuring out a way to squash me. And who would protect me? So . . . really, what I was fearing was my livelihood." Here was a promoted and accomplished attending physician who feared enough for their livelihood that they would not speak out against the injustices they sustained because of their pedigree. No amount of research or accolades or clinical experience—in other words, individual effort—could change the fact that Dr. Taylor was a non-USMD at an institution like Stonewood, which did not highly value non-USMDs. Even the residents, when referring to this physician,

TABLE 5.1 Fellowship Match Rates by Medical Specialty and Applicant Type (2015)

Specialty	% USMD Applicants Matched (Odds Ratio)	% Non-USMD Applicants Matched
Allergy and immunology	85.7 (5.11)***	54.0
Cardiovascular disease	91.3 (7.41)***	58.7
Endocrinology, diabetes, and metabolism	93.4 (6.01)***	70.2
Gastroenterology	83.5 (6.39)***	44.2
Geriatric medicine	95.6 (1.20)	94.7
Hematology	16.1 (1.64)	10.5
Hematology and oncology	84.3 (3.87)***	58.1
Infectious disease	94.1 (2.62)*	85.9
Nephrology	98.8 (9.48)**	89.3
Oncology	14.7 (0.68)	20.3
Pulmonary disease and critical care medicine	85.1 (5.04)***	53.1
Rheumatology	86.3 (2.28)*	73.3

$^*p < 0.05$

$^{**}p < 0.005$

$^{***}p < 0.001$

Source: Data from National Resident Matching Program (2015d), *Results and Data: Specialties Matching Service® 2015 Appointment Year.* Washington, DC: National Resident Matching Program.

would almost always use a qualifier, like Dr. Taylor is "brilliant" or "one of the smartest doctors," as if to offset the blemish of their medical pedigree.

Statistics nationwide suggest that medical school of origin is strongly correlated with fellowship outcomes (see table 5.1). A chi-square test reveals that in 2015, the odds of a USMD matching to gastroenterology were 6.39 times that of a non-USMD; in cardiology, those odds rose to 7.41 times. In fact, there was a statistically significant difference in the odds of USMDs matching to fellowship compared to non-USMDs in nearly every specialty except the least populated ones.[12] Furthermore, while the likelihood of matching was still higher for USMD applicants, the specialties in which the largest numbers of USIMGs and IMGs matched were nephrology, endocrinology, and rheumatology—which are among the least competitive (and least prestigious) fellowships for USMDs.[13]

These numbers reveal that medical pedigree is at least correlated with subspecialty outcomes. It is telling, for example, that fellowship data at a national level are still reported by *medical school graduate type* when the applicants are in residency.[14] What remains less clear is whether this correlation is a function of the stigma or prestige associated with certain medical school types or whether it is due to the implications of that training—namely, that it impacts where one goes to residency, which more directly impacts fellowship—or whether it is the result of both.

Regarding program prestige, one Stonewood attending explained, "The top tier, [if] you go to residency there, it doesn't matter if you graduate last in your residency class. You want a fellowship? You are going to get a fellowship, because it's name recognition and so much of what we do is *who you know* and what you know" (emphasis added). In this way, program status could be just as important as, if not more important than, medical knowledge for fellowship, according to this attending. A fellowship program director admitted as much during the fellowship information session held at Stonewood: "I look at where they did their residency. We get three hundred applications for four positions. If the person came from a residency program I've never heard of, unfortunately, that's probably the end of their application." He added with a shrug, "It's sad because of the track—sometimes they have a hard time in med school, and they could be a star resident, but . . ." Even a star resident from an unknown residency would have little chance of matching in his fellowship, which speaks to the relative power of structure (or the "track," as he calls it) over agency. There is little this star resident could do to change their fate, once again reflecting the stickiness of status.

But the name of a residency program does a lot more than signal prestige; it is also a proxy for the quality of training its residents receive.[15] The training at university hospitals was widely assumed to be superior to that at community programs, an assumption supported by the findings in chapters 3 and 4. Even Legacy residents recognized that their training was less rigorous than that at Stonewood, and they felt this put them at a disadvantage for fellowship. Consider the perspective expressed by Laurie (USIMG, PGY-3, Legacy): "It's harder [at Legacy] because when you come from a place like [Stonewood Hospital], your patient load is a lot more, it's more structured, so overall, you're going to be a better resident—not necessarily smarter, but you're just trained better, so that's an advantage." Laurie was right; not only was the training more structured at Stonewood, but also the patient exposure was simply not comparable between university and community programs. For example, Gunther (USMD, PGY-3, Stonewood) relayed a conversation he had with residents from Solomon Community Hospital, which was affiliated with Stonewood University and had a program similar to that at Legacy. One Solomon resident was complaining that his chances of matching into a competitive fellowship were lower than Gunther's. Another Solomon resident interjected, "Have you ever been to the ICU [intensive care unit] at [Stonewood]? It would make the ICU at our hospital look like a nursing home, with the acuity of patients. . . . You need to understand that these two places are not the same, and even if you're better than this person and you don't train in that environment, how are you going to react to those patients?" He raised a valid point: Without being exposed to a certain level of acuity, how could one respond effectively as a fellow at a high-acuity university hospital, where most fellowships are housed? Clinical exposure therefore was understood to be a critical aspect of how residency affected fellowships. Once again, however, this speaks to the path-dependent nature of medical training; by virtue of training at a community program with less case variety, residents found it much harder to move up to a competitive fellowship program, despite widespread beliefs in the power of hard work and dedication.

It didn't help that in the aggregate, Legacy graduates typically did significantly worse on their American Board of Internal Medicine Certification Examinations (Boards) than Stonewood residents did—perhaps unsurprisingly, given the lack of programmatic emphasis on the In-Training Examinations at Legacy, described in chapter 4. In 2012–2014, the percentage of Legacy residents passing their Boards was more than one standard deviation less than the percentage of those passing at Stonewood—a statistically significant difference.[16] While residents take their Boards only after residency (and thus after applying for fellowship), fellowship program directors still have access to previous years' pass rates, making it possible for them to form opinions about prospective applicants on the basis of their programs' previous results—before applicants even take the exam.

Legacy residents therefore had to contend with the stigma associated with their pedigree, as well as the disadvantages of completing their residency at a community program with less-structured training and more-limited patient exposure. This meant that matching into fellowship required going above and beyond to overcome those handicaps—with less help—effectively making the rules of the game harder for Legacy residents than for Stonewood residents.

Different Rules of the Game

Indeed, just as when they applied for residency, non-USMDs generally faced higher expectations than USMDs did when applying to fellowship. For example, after stating that IMGs had to be exceptional when applying for fellowship, a fellowship director at Stonewood explained, "Yes, well, it's expected. . . . Some degree of extra achievement is understandable to make it worthwhile for people to take the small or big additional risk for giving them an opportunity to thrive." Thus, the same beliefs about merit and risk described in chapter 2 regarding residency recruitment carried forward into fellowship, thereby making the bar higher for non-USMDs. Just as before, non-USMDs had to go beyond what might be expected from a USMD at a university hospital by engaging in more research, cultivating stronger mentorship ties, and better presenting themselves. Yet they also were the least well equipped to meet these additional expectations precisely because they trained at a community hospital like Legacy.

Research projects, for example, were scarce at Legacy, as I mentioned in chapter 4, and even when they found one, residents were not always confident that it would be enough for fellowship. When I asked Cody what he thought his chances were of matching into allergy, he replied, "50/50—maybe. . . . I'm just very insecure about it because I know that you need a lot of research. What does a lot mean? Does it mean two manuscripts? Does it mean five? Ten? Abstracts? Two? Ten? Twelve? What does that mean? . . . So until I get it, I am going to continue to work hard and when they tell me to stop is when I'll stop."

In contrast, Stonewood residents received lots of support with research endeavors, with virtually 100 percent of the housestaff involved in some kind of scholarly project throughout their three years. For example, Ken, a PGY-3 who matched to cardiology, described doing a few poster presentations and a small internal study on heart failure: "It's a homegrown grassroots sort of project, but it's something to talk about, and that's all you need. You just need something. . . . It doesn't matter if it gets published because all it is is you are generating a topic during your interview so that you can sound enthusiastic and interested and knowledgeable. So it's a game. It's a *game!*" (emphasis in original). Compared to Cody at Legacy, who obsessed over the quantity and quality of publications he would need to be competitive for fellowship, Ken viewed research more pragmatically—as a box to tick off in the fellowship game. As Ken put it, he just needed *something* (even if it was unpublished) rather than the *many* (published) things Cody needed. In this way, Stonewood residents may have had greater access to research, but they may have needed it less than Legacy residents, who had to work harder to prove themselves.

Perhaps even more important than research, however, were social networks. As one Stonewood attending put it, "The fellowship process really becomes about having connections." Legacy residents understood this; as one resident said to an intern one day, "It's not what you know but who you know," referring to his upcoming fellowship applications. But it was more difficult to forge valuable networks at Legacy, given the limited access to academic faculty.

Importantly, not all connections were equal. Because the subspecialty community is so small, connections were more valuable if they were with well-established academic faculty, like the attendings at Stonewood, not the community practitioners who predominated at Legacy. To be sure, Legacy officials advocated the best they could for their residents, with the chief of medicine serving as one of the most vocal advocates. In 2013, when a resident failed to match to a fellowship, it took only one phone call from the chief to help the resident scramble into a position. Still, without the clout of renowned subspecialists like the ones at Stonewood, Legacy residents were at a comparative disadvantage.

This was especially true for highly competitive fellowships, where superlative research records and strong personal connections were even more necessary than usual for Legacy residents. Cardiology, gastroenterology (GI), and allergy/immunology were widely understood to be among the most competitive specialties, even for USMDs, which made them nearly unattainable for Legacy residents right after residency. One Legacy intern, Rashad (IMG), joked that short of marrying the GI chief's daughter and spending six to seven years doing research, his odds of matching into GI were very low. This was in sharp contrast to the confidence exuded by Stonewood residents, who did not feel bound by the same restrictions. Dale (USMD, PGY-3), who matched into a prestigious cardiology program, said, "I was confident that I would match. . . . I think my CV was competitive enough to compete with residents from the best programs in the country." As residents from Stonewood, with all the structural advantages that this entailed, Dale and his colleagues did not have to worry about the feasibility of matching into any specialty. Aside from highly research-intensive fellowships (which were more difficult to get because of Stonewood's heavy clinical focus), virtually everything was possible for Stonewood graduates.

In light of these constraints, some Legacy residents initially talked about being interested in sought-after specialties but then switched to less competitive fields because they were more within reach. These fields included rheumatology, endocrinology, and nephrology. Roughly 50 percent of categorical residents at Legacy pursued fellowships, but most of these fellowships tended to be in less competitive specialties, and even these successful matches were hard-won.

One resident who eventually matched into a prestigious nephrology (renal) fellowship applied to thirty-five programs after completing outside electives in neighboring states. (Recall from chapter 4 that Legacy residents had to get out-of-state licenses to rotate in neighboring states.) A renal fellowship was within reach for Legacy residents but by no means easy to attain. In contrast, a PGY-3 at Stonewood described having his pick of renal programs: "I'm doing nephrology, so I basically decide where I want to go. . . . It's not the most competitive subspecialty in the world." Another resident chimed in, "Not a lot of American grads want to go into [nephrology], so when there's an American grad that goes into it, they love them." In 2014, ninety out of ninety-one USMDs applying to and ranking nephrology fellowships successfully matched.[17] So while this Stonewood PGY-3 still had to play the game (he was involved in research and networking at Stonewood), he applied to only five nephrology programs and got into his top choice.

Legacy residents faced numerous structural *constraints* on their trajectories out of residency, some even dating back to the assumptions and perceptions surrounding their medical school of origin. For their part, Stonewood residents mostly enjoyed structural *supports*, helping propel them toward the careers of their choice. Those choices were not entirely unconstrained, however. While on the surface Stonewood residents may have had more options for the future than Legacy residents, the range of acceptable choices was limited by two primary considerations: debt and internalized definitions of success.

Debt

Debt was a major concern for Stonewood graduates, many of whom graduated several hundreds of thousands of dollars in the red. The issue weighed so heavily on the residents' minds that it often made its way into everyday conversation. One morning, for example, a resident was frustrated because the computer asked her to change her password. "Just put a dollar sign at the end," suggested her intern, with a laugh. "It's all that matters in the end, after all!" The team's fourth-year medical student looked disgusted and said, "Oh my God, that's terrible," but the intern shot back, "Says the person who's six months away from a quarter million dollars in debt!"

He was not exaggerating. The median four-year cost of medical school attendance in 2014–2015 was $226,447 for public schools and $298,538 for private schools, with interest rates for state and federal loans ranging between 6 to 7 percent.[18] That means that over 84 percent of US medical students graduate with some form of educational debt.

Decisions about whether to generalize or subspecialize therefore often centered on future earning potential. As one Stonewood PGY-2 resident explained, "I think that guides most of our decisions, you know, what salaries are going to be." Another agreed: "It is certainly an incentive." A third chimed in, "I think the people that do the subspecialty services *are* interested . . . in that specialty. [Money] does certainly guide the decision, [but] it's not the only thing." Monica, for example, a Stonewood PGY-3, was debating between remaining a generalist and subspecializing. Her partner had matched into a subspecialty and would thus continue earning a trainee salary for the next three years:

> Between me and [my partner], we have half a million dollars in medical school loans and debt. . . . By the time we make an attending's salary, it's going to be more than our mortgage payment [going] to loans every month and so it's just a burden. . . . You know, this is the time when we want to get married, we want to buy a house, and we don't have any funds because we're just so in the red that . . . We're going to be in our thirties, and we have nothing in our 401K because for four years we earned negative dollars and now we're earning not a lot for how much we work. . . . We're kind of behind, and all the stats say that we'll catch up, and that's fine, but it doesn't make it any less stressful right now, thinking of that burden of debt.

Monica's anxiety was palpable. And just when she was trying to plan a future—get married, buy a house, start a nest egg—she also needed to make important decisions about subspecialty. She debated whether to start working as a hospitalist now (and start earning an attending's salary to help support her family) or to pursue subspecialty training and defer gratification even longer, although she would make more money in the long run: "And so . . . that still plays into my mind, should I apply [to a subspecialty] so that we can be more comfortable?" As a result, some USMDs deferred their dreams, like one resident who put off working in Africa until she paid off her loans, while others modified them to make ends meet. As one intern put it, "The cost of our education I think ends up dictating what you do. If you have $500,000 of debt, waking up every morning and facing that is awful. . . . It's do or die."

This was the unsavory underbelly to the American medical profession's social contract: work hard, sacrifice years of life, and pay exorbitant amounts of money in exchange for a lifetime of job security, prestige, professional autonomy, and a considerable living wage. However, this agreement, which was made implicitly with all USMDs upon admission to medical school, works only if both sides get the promised benefits. As Dale (USMD, PGY-3) noted, "It's a big financial commitment to become a physician in this country," and in exchange for that commitment, USMDs expected to earn enough to make it worth it. Another resident explained, "[IMGs] are not coming out of medical school $400,000 in debt, and yet they're coming here and they're making the same salaries as we are. We're kind of paying our dues to get these spots in some sense. I don't know how other countries pay for the medical schools, but I can guarantee the majority of them are not carrying as much [debt] as ours are." This indebtedness—both financial and professional in the sense that USMDs felt *owed* for their sacrifice—is absolutely fundamental to the social contract. USMDs had put in the money, and they were driven to subspecialties to receive enough in return to make their investment worthwhile.

The result of feeling like one put in more than they got out is often disillusionment—a common sentiment among physicians, particularly USMDs.[19] Some residents at Stonewood referred to medical school as the "$1 Million Mistake," quoting an article by that title circulating on social media.[20] A group of second-years gossiped one day about someone who had left medical school to become a physician assistant and was now working in anesthesiology and making $120,000 per year. "He's probably made the best financial decision ever," someone quipped. The residents actually applauded the decision to leave the profession to become a physician assistant and even warned against going to medical school in the first place, given the million-dollar mistake of investing in a career that they felt returned so little in exchange for so much. Debt was one of the rare constraints facing USMDs, but it was an exceedingly important one.

Residents at Legacy were not immune to financial concerns. The majority of IMGs graduated debt-free from medical school in their home countries. USIMGs and graduates of osteopathic medical schools (DOs), on the other hand, often had *more* debt, and some of them, by virtue of attending medical school abroad, were unable to secure federal loans, which meant they paid even higher interest than USMDs did.[21] Toward the end of my fieldwork, Legacy merged with a holdings company, becoming a for-profit hospital, which had implications for federal loan forgiveness and gave residents plenty of reasons to be concerned about money.[22]

Yet, remarkably, debt came up far less at Legacy than it did at Stonewood. Compared to all the other constraints facing Legacy residents, finances did not seem to be at the forefront. They had entered into a fundamentally different bargain with the profession than USMDs had, one whereby they expected less in return, making debt less salient for them. When I asked one Legacy PGY-3 who went to medical school after having trained as a paramedical professional whether he was considering a fellowship in cardiology, he mentioned his loans only in passing, focusing more on the difficulties associated with matching to fellowship from a place like Legacy. Referring to lower reimbursements in primary care, Trevor, a USIMG who managed to train debt-free in Southeast Asia, noted, "If you don't feel like you're adequately reimbursed, then people don't want to go into it." But he added, "I'm not one to complain; I mean you're going to be able to support your family with a doctor's salary. It would be kind of arrogant for me to say we're not being paid enough . . . you're putting food on the table; you can take care of your family. You're fortunate enough to be able to say so compared to other people." As someone without debt, it was perhaps easier for Trevor to feel satisfied with his earnings. Yet even among those who were heavily indebted, the issue rarely came up. Kamal, an IMG who trained debt-free, told me about at least four residents he knew at Legacy who were in debt: "I feel sorry for them. They will never be able to excel and get out of that debt." None of the residents he named mentioned money to me, however, when I asked them about their career decision-making. Of course, they may well have been more comfortable confiding in this resident than me, especially given the sensitive nature of personal finances. By comparison, however, Stonewood residents were very open about such sensitive matters, suggesting that debt may have been a more pressing concern for them.

A Legacy program official who trained at Legacy shed some light on why debt and money may have been less pressing for Legacy residents. She began by explaining that USMDs were subspecializing en masse and that "we need primary care everywhere because everyone is subspecializing. Because the guy from Harvard is not going to be a PCP [primary care practitioner], he is going to be running his cystic fibrosis clinic, you know?[23] . . . And you are like okay, great, but who's going to be a pediatrician or who's going to be the PCP? Not [USMDs]. So other people [non-USMDs] are finding their way and filling all those gaps." When asked why she thought USMDs were subspecializing so much, she replied simply, "Because this is how they are educated. Because this is what they teach them. . . . Some [of them] don't care; they will be PCPs. . . . But not a lot of them do. . . . Otherwise, you know, *why did I spend all this money and I have all these student loans?*" (emphasis added). Here the official made explicit the link between wanting to subspecialize and needing to make more money to pay off massive student loans. This sums up the US social contract. Because non-USMDs were socialized differently, even in the presence of considerable debt they did not come to expect subspecialty training (or at least they did not expect that it would come without many obstacles). They knew that going to medical school was going to be costly—financially and personally—but they had different expectations about the returns, perhaps stemming from a more intrinsic motivation in medicine, as I alluded to in chapter 1. This meant that unlike the USMDs at Stonewood, they were perhaps less motivated by earnings to subspecialize as a means of getting back their investment—and thus were less likely to be disillusioned by a profession that could not always deliver on its promises.

Definitions of Success

As the Legacy official hinted at earlier, USMDs were socialized to conceptualize success somewhat differently than non-USMDs did. As with residency, some Stonewood residents felt pressure to subspecialize in fellowship because that was where the game drove them—i.e., to the top, which generally involved subspecialization. This was a function, they argued, of the socialization process before and during medical school. As one PGY-2 resident put it during a focus group:

> There is this hidden curriculum in medical schools which promotes this. Everyone is always like, "Oh, they're a cardiologist," and so everyone internalizes that. And then what fifty years ago would have been the generalist being the smartest doctor has now subsequently become untrue because of the way that people are reimbursed . . . money become[s] equated with prestige and then competitiveness. It's difficult to be a cardiologist. So you do not only get prestige but you get this automatic CV. "Oh, I'm a cardiologist." "Oh, you must be brilliant!"

Subspecialty was considered the apogee of success for many USMDs, having been shaped by changing norms and incentive structures within the profession.

The drive to be the "best," however, sometimes led to the same tension that some USMDs experienced during residency applications: between reaching for the top and being happy. Some residents spoke about how prestige was equated with success for USMDs—a mentality that was inculcated early on, long before residency and even medical school. Cassandra, a PGY-1, captured this view nicely:

> Somebody explained to me: your whole life, everything has been based on *if you can, you should*. Leave every door open; keep everything open to yourself so that you never miss out on an opportunity because you didn't set yourself up for it. So each step along the way it's like, "I'll just do premed classes and excel in them *in case* I decide I do want to be a doctor after college." ... Then you get into med school, and you're like, "I'll just try to get the best grade in every class *just in case* there is a chance to be an AOA [Alpha Omega Alpha, an honors society] *just in case* that's going to help me get into a better residency. And then in residency, I'll just do well in every rotation and excel in the primary care end of things *just in case* I decide to go into a crazy fellowship like GI or cardiology *even though I don't really want to* but just in case. Or just in case I want to get into the best fellowship in something less popular like rheumatology, I should probably do really well and excel on every test." And then somebody explained, the right mentality is not *if you can, you should*. It's more *if you can, do you want to, and does that matter to you anymore?* (emphasis added)

The pressure to do something because one *could*, rather than because one *wanted to*, was the direct result of the process of getting into the profession and clearly constrained USMDs' decision-making surrounding their career plans. Interestingly, Miller came across a similar desire to keep as many doors open as possible in his study of Harvard interns from 1964. He called this kind of intern a "drifter": "He is looking for an internship that closes the door on no career and maximizes the number open to him."[24] For Miller, however, the drifter emerged out of indecision; at Stonewood, they came from a lifelong commitment to reaching for the top. In this way, choosing *not* to subspecialize (or to specialize in a less prestigious field) was as much a conscious decision for USMDs as choosing to subspecialize was for non-USMDs.

PLACEMENT

In 2014, approximately two-thirds (65.5 percent) of third-year categorical residents at Stonewood matched into the following fellowship areas: cardiology, endocrinology, GI, hematology and oncology, infectious diseases, nephrology, and pulmonary/critical care. In addition, 27.6 percent opted for careers in general internal medicine (as hospitalists, clinician-educators, or primary care practitioners), while another 6.9 percent became chief residents. Among residents who were on the primary care track, 40 percent pursued careers in general internal medicine, 30 percent became chief residents, and the remaining 30 percent continued their general internal medicine training in research and/or health policy (see table 5.2).

In 2012, only one-fourth of Legacy residents matched into fellowship. In 2013 and 2014, in contrast, exactly half of the graduating residents matched into comparatively less competitive fellowships in endocrinology, hematology and oncology, nephrology, pulmonary/critical care, rheumatology, and sleep medicine while the other half pursued careers in general internal medicine. One resident was selected per graduating class to become chief resident and went on to subspecialize thereafter.

These numbers were roughly commensurate with general trends in fellowship across the country. Nationwide in 2014, 87.2 percent of USMD applicants

TABLE 5.2 Placement After Residency (2014)

	Fellowship	General Internal Medicine	Chief Residency
Stonewood			
Categorical	65.5%[a]	27.6%	6.9%
Primary care	30%[a]	40%	30%
Legacy			
Categorical	50%[b]	41.7%	8.3%

[a]Stonewood residents generally matched into more-competitive specialties like cardiology, gastroenterology, and hematology and oncology.
[b]Legacy residents typically matched into less competitive specialties, like rheumatology, nephrology, and endocrinology. Exceptions include two residents who matched into pulmonary disease and critical care between 2011 and 2014.

matched into fellowship, whereas 74 percent of DO applicants, 66.4 percent of IMG applicants, and 63.9 percent of USIMG applicants matched.[25] Thus, even after residency at a US institution, inequalities persisted in match rates among graduate types, echoing disparities similar to those during the residency match.

Trajectories Into General Internal Medicine

Because of the severe shortage of primary care practitioners in the United States, generalist positions were easy to get for graduates from both programs.[26] For some Legacy residents, there was a sense that general internal medicine[27] was a safety net in case plans for fellowship fell through. Farha (IMG, PGY-2) was interested in endocrinology but knew that matching into fellowship from Legacy was going to be tough. She shrugged as she said, "So I mean I'm prepared that I won't get a fellowship position. I would probably work as hospitalist or primary care and then apply for fellowship maybe." Farha ended up accepting a position as a hospitalist at a small community hospital.

Other Legacy residents were so discouraged by the challenges of matching into fellowship that they decided to forgo applying altogether and instead chose primary care. Clark (USIMG, PGY-3) was a good example; after having little success securing cardiology research for fellowship applications, he decided that cardiology was "too much of a sacrifice" and opted instead for primary care. He found a practice with a "nice office" and "compliant patients." "It's a dream come true," he said, suggesting again that constraint did not always lead to dissatisfaction. Still others preferred general medicine, citing a better lifestyle and fulfilling work. Ricky (USIMG, PGY-3), for example, noted that being in his late thirties, he was "too old for this," referring to subspecialty training, suggesting that the generalist lifestyle may have been more attractive to Legacy graduates who tended to be older.

At Stonewood, in contrast, residents choosing careers in general internal medicine had to consciously hop off the "runaway freight train." They also had to take a significant pay cut compared to their peers, given that medical subspecialists make roughly $1.1 million more in lifetime earnings than primary care practitioners do.[28] Program support helped: one year a primary care resident and her program director created "Primary Care Is the New Black" buttons to draw attention to careers in general medicine. This encouragement, paired with an intrinsic passion for primary care, helped guide them toward careers as generalists. As one PGY-2 resident on the primary care track explained, "I think the more I've been exposed to specializing, the more I've said, 'Oh, wait, what about all that other stuff?' . . . If I only studied the heart, I think I would miss every other organ a lot!" Importantly, being in the primary care track did not restrict residents' options for subspecialty. As one PGY-1 noted, "[If] I suddenly was like, 'Hey, I want to do cardiology,' . . . there will be plenty of people to help guide me and help me achieve that goal . . . theoretically I could do anything within reason." This made primary care even more of a purposive choice for Stonewood residents.

Some Stonewood residents found positions in local practices or hospitals, others pursued fellowships in general internal medicine, and a sizable number joined the Stonewood teaching faculty every year. Most of the teaching hospitalists at Stonewood were former graduates of the program, and many had been offered the position right out of residency. Interestingly, no Legacy residents expressed interest in academic generalist positions. Perhaps this was because they did not have the strong academic role models that Stonewood residents did or because there were few positions available nearby, given that Stonewood almost exclusively hired its own graduates and Legacy staffed very few academic hospitalists.

Trajectories Into Fellowship/Subspecialty

Approximately half of Legacy's graduates successfully matched into fellowship despite the difficulties they faced while playing the game. Still, Fellowship Match Day at Legacy was more subdued than it was at Stonewood, just like Residency Match Day. No one at Legacy even mentioned the momentous occasion until the end of morning report, around 11 AM. "Good luck, guys," called out a PGY-2. Someone else replied that they find out only at noon. An hour later, instead of going to noon conference, the PGY-3s were upstairs in the resident's lounge, nervously checking their email, waiting to hear about fellowships. The first resident to enter the conference room announced he had matched into his first-choice program—hematology and oncology at Legacy. Everyone started clapping quietly, congratulating him. Moments later a different PGY-3 bounded into the room, declaring she had matched into pulmonary/critical care. Another announced she had matched into her first-choice nephrology program. One hundred percent of residents who applied matched into fellowship that year—the program's first perfect match.

By comparison, the excitement at Stonewood on Fellowship Match Day was palpable. The anticipation began three weeks prior, on Certify Day, when residents had to finalize their rank list of program preferences. I overheard one resident tell another that he was reconsidering one of the programs. When asked what made him change his mind, the resident replied, "Three consecutive calls from the program director will do that," referring to having been personally courted by a fellowship director so he would rank that program highly. Three weeks prior to Match Day, the experience of fellowship placement already looked different at Stonewood than at Legacy.

On Match Day itself, the mood was electric at Stonewood. A little before noon I entered the residents' lounge to find a bunch of residents milling around excitedly. I spotted one resident who had been hoping to match into a transplant center for cardiology. He ended up matching at Stonewood (which is not a transplant center). "I guess it beats not matching, right?" he said, with a twinge of disappointment. Like a blazing fire, the news spread that many residents had matched at Stonewood. One of them spluttered, "It's all coming to fruition—we're going to stay forever!" That year two-thirds of the cardiology positions at Stonewood went to Stonewood residents, as did two-thirds of the GI positions, half of the pulmonary/critical care positions, and two-thirds of the hematology and oncology positions, underlining the tremendous benefit of training for residency at a hospital with competitive fellowship programs. "I can't believe we're all staying," gushed another resident. Everyone had their phones out, texting frantically. Residents who were not around were being contacted to see where they matched. It was a joyous public occasion.

When fellowship applicants failed to match, they could try "scrambling" into unfilled positions, using a list of unfilled positions provided to them by the National Resident Matching Program. They were not always successful, however. Recall that Cody was the Legacy resident with aspirations of becoming an allergist/immunologist. But when Match Day rolled around, he did not match into allergy/immunology, despite his best efforts. He was also unable to scramble into an unfilled position in that specialty.

This outcome directly challenged the optimism exhibited by Legacy residents regarding their opportunity structure. It raised questions about whether there was anything more he could have done to overcome the barriers he faced as a USIMG from a community residency program. As one resident who was familiar with Cody's situation said, "I think it's very telling . . . in terms of someone who has all this research background and all this stuff but is essentially being hampered probably because of . . . the double whammy: [being an] international medical graduate and therefore the [Legacy] name following it." Cody was considered living proof that anything was possible at Legacy, but failing to match dampened much of that hopefulness.

Instead, Cody pursued a one-year fellowship in a related field as a stepping-stone toward an allergy and immunology fellowship, which he eventually obtained after completing his year-long fellowship. Stepping-stones like these were relatively common among Legacy residents who had ambitions of reaching more-competitive fellowships. A handful of Stonewood residents also took a so-called hospitalist year before applying for fellowship. This gave them extra time to do research and build connections.

One resident at Stonewood also failed to match. After the initial excitement had died down, a Stonewood official emerged from the leadership office with a look of consternation. "We're scrambling now," muttered the official. In addition to deeply affecting the resident in question, who was later described as "shell-shocked" and "humbled," this constituted a crisis for the residency program, which prided itself on a near-perfect matching record for fellowship. Previously, only residents with severe geographic restrictions had failed to match. This was not the case for this resident, who had applied widely but was known to have performance concerns. The program directors, however, fiercely advocated on behalf of the resident, who ended up successfully scrambling into a position.

That was the same day that Cody did not match at Legacy. Both residents tried to scramble for unfilled positions, but only the Stonewood resident was successful, despite having a flawed record. While it is impossible to know the exact reasons for this outcome, the evidence suggests that Cody's pedigree and limited access to resources played a significant role. He lacked the status and support associated with being a USMD resident at Stonewood.

CONCLUSION

The findings of this chapter suggest that the vertical separation of the elite (subspecialists) from the rank and file (generalists) is a process highly constrained by social structures, even though respondents heavily emphasized their agency. In fact, the same tensions between choice and constraint that led to the horizontal separation of medical graduates into different residency program tiers reappeared for fellowship and beyond, suggesting that educational pedigree has a lasting impact on physicians' career trajectories. Medical schooling determines residency opportunities, and residency largely determines fellowship, in part because graduates still have unequal access to the resources needed to play the game which a priori places stigmatized individuals at an additional disadvantage. Legacy residents were a lesser known quantity with greater doubt attached to their skills and thus had to prove themselves worthy of fellowship positions. And the very thing that put them at a disadvantage (training at a community hospital) was also what made it exceedingly difficult to overcome that disadvantage, as they lacked the research opportunities, mentors, connections, and prestige needed to prove themselves worthy. This "double whammy," as one resident put it, meant that Legacy residents were limited in the trajectories they could pursue, even after having trained for three years at a US hospital.

To further complicate matters, non-USMDs who had been denied opportunities all along because they were widely suspected to be subpar eventually ended up being weaker doctors than USMDs (at least as measured by exposure to certain pathologies and Board pass rates), thanks to inequalities between educational programs. This makes the game a self-fulfilling prophecy of sorts and reveals the extent to which merit is inextricably linked to widespread systematic inequality across what is otherwise supposed to be a level playing field.

But therein lies the rub. Inequalities in outcomes stem in large part from systemic differences in resources between residency programs, which constrain residents *implicitly* rather than officially. Residency training, in theory, is standardized across programs, and fellowship training is supposed to be open to any graduate; there is no rule that bars community residents' access to competitive fellowships. But (1) inequalities in training and professional development (lack of mentorship, research, and exposure), combined with (2) lower achievement levels in lower-quality training contexts, (3) considerable stigma associated with being a non-USMD community resident, and (4) harder rules of the game, make the jump from a place like Legacy to a competitive fellowship exceedingly difficult. Meanwhile, the officials who affirmed that Legacy residents "can go anywhere they want, they really can," created a false sense of self-determination among the housestaff, who sometimes blamed themselves when they didn't achieve their goals. Interestingly, rather than "cooling out" their residents (or helping them adjust their expectations), Legacy officials insisted that nothing was out of reach and encouraged them to become willful participants in a game where the odds were latently stacked against them.[29] Indeed, sometimes residents' strategies for advancement (such as doing outside electives at university hospitals rather than demanding better training at Legacy) only seemed to reinforce the extant structures contributing to their subordination, thereby helping reproduce inequality among residents.[30] In the next chapter, I explore why non-USMDs would participate in a profession that systematically subordinates them to USMDs.

CHAPTER 6

The Navy SEALs and the National Guard

On a sunny afternoon in October, I asked a group of third-year Stonewood University Hospital residents what was different about training at a place like Stonewood compared to a community hospital. One resident, Lucy, replied with a shrug, "We're like the Navy SEALs and community hospital is like [the] National Guard." She continued:

LUCY: [As US-trained medical graduates], you become very homogenous in the way that you learn, the way that you think, the way that you approach a problem, and that's a big difference between [us and] the [international medical graduates]. . . . I mean I think that's why people want to be here, because it's like *the* place to be, *the* top; you see *the* patients; you do *the* stuff. (emphasis in original)

TANIA: Does this resonate with others?

TED: Well, I like the homogenous [thing] you said. Although the argument is . . . we are learning how to practice medicine the *right* way. (emphasis in original)

LUCY: That's what the system is trying to do.

TED: Right but . . . Like in martial arts, there are two different schools, but do you still get the job done?

LUCY: There could very well be another way and we just don't know it. [*entire group laughs*]

The laughter after that last sentence is telling. The notion that there may be a different or better way of practicing medicine than the way graduates of US allopathic medical schools [USMDs] were taught in university hospitals was laughable. They understood there to be two kinds of internal medicine residents:

elite USMD "Navy SEALs," a "special breed of warrior" trained in tertiary hospitals to handle the most complicated of patients and situations, and a reserve army of non-USMD "National Guard" forces assigned to take on simpler roles in community hospitals.[1]

Lucy's words perfectly describe status separation in internal medicine. The Navy SEALs and National Guard metaphor not only captures horizontal hierarchies *within* internal medicine training—status separation—but also points toward the formal vertical hierarchies that emerge after graduation as many USMDs specialize and many non-USMDs remain generalists. Recall that Freidson had predicted the emergence of a formal vertical elite and a rank and file within the profession to help protect against external incursions (as I described in the introduction).[2] He never addressed, however, the existence of informal horizontal hierarchies *within* specialties or how they might precede those more formal vertical hierarchies. By now, it should be clear that in internal medicine, informal horizontal status distinctions exist along educational pedigree lines, with USMDs in university residency programs largely going on to constitute the formal elite and non-USMDs in community programs eventually comprising much of the formal rank and file.

Unsurprisingly, many at Stonewood fully expected their trainees to become future *leaders* in the profession, while community practitioners were expected to be the *followers*. One official said matter-of-factly, "At a second- or third-tier hospital, those residents are arguably needier because they didn't come with the credentials that other residents have. [They] will do less well. By that [I mean] they won't lead the field; they won't be as good a physician as somebody who trained here [at Stonewood]." He went on to say, "I just don't think that the less distinguished programs have the capability or the track record to train leaders . . . [they are not] going to turn out from their program people who will be [chairs] and deans." This perspective was shared by the Stonewood housestaff, who viewed themselves as so distinct from community trainees that several had never even heard of some of the other medical residency programs in the area, including Legacy Community Hospital. One afternoon a group of residents in their third postgraduate year (PGY-3s) was struggling to name the community programs in the area when one of them interrupted: "But I think it's almost like looking at a football team, you know, it's like 1A, 2A, whatever . . ." He went on to explain that "it's divisions; we are in our own division out here. So there may be other programs in the state, but for our scope of programs, I mean the next closest ones are [*he starts naming large cities in neighboring states*]." Thus, Stonewood residents were in a league of their own, untouched by the dozens of other residents training alongside them in nearby community hospitals.

For their part, non-USMD community hospital residents were widely considered gap fillers. One Stonewood faculty member put it rather bluntly:

> The Caribbean people [US citizens who trained in Caribbean medical schools], they are picking up the scraps, and the foreign medical grads are having a death match. There is a level of desperation—you've probably met some of these people—who were like *friggin' orthopedics professors in Tehran, ophthalmologists in Karachi.* It's crazy. And they come over here, and they go into the family med programs or internal medicine programs or psychiatry programs, give everything up . . . (emphasis added)

From his perspective, non-USMDs—even highly trained subspecialists—essentially plugged holes in the US health care system by competing fiercely over whatever undesirable positions were left over. Non-USMDs made it possible for the most desirable positions to go to USMDs because they filled the spots that no one else wanted, effectively constituting a rank-and-file workforce for USMDs to lead. This same official went on to stress the importance of that rank and file: "People need doctors. People don't need chief residents. . . . The pinnacle of success in American academia is the physician-scientist. The guy who's got lots of NIH funding, [for whom] seeing patients is . . . a total afterthought. . . . We need people who are going to be on the frontline doing nothing but seeing patients." Without people on the frontline, the physician-scientist would be superfluous.[3] Non-USMDs made it possible for USMDs to become leaders because they provided the workforce to be *led*.

Importantly, many non-USMDs also viewed themselves as gap fillers, both during residency and afterward. Farha, an international medical graduate (IMG) and a PGY-2, described community hospitals like Legacy as "the places where American medical graduates don't come. . . . These small programs—foreign medical graduates and Caribbean [graduates] come here." Clark, a US citizen who graduated from an international medical school (USIMG) and a PGY-3 at Legacy, understood segregation in residency programs in a similar way:

> I mean I hate to say it, but [community programs] they're probably like, "Well, we don't have enough US graduates [to fill our program], so we'll

take you." ... And then these high-paying fields, ... they fill them up with US grads. Not saying that there's no international medical graduates that have become radiologists; there are. But for the most part, that's the way it is.

Legacy residents thus understood that their role in the profession was to fill gaps toward the bottom of the medical status hierarchy—in lower-status specialties (like internal medicine) and in less prestigious hospitals (like Legacy) that USMDs did not want.

These residents might be thought of as the profession's equivalent to Bosk's "mop-up service"—a term used to describe how genetic counselors (who were physicians back in the early 1990s) would be called upon to do unpleasant work that others like obstetricians wanted to avoid, such as breaking terrible news to patients about genetic abnormalities.[4] Bosk's mop-up service, however, spanned several professional subspecialties within a single hospital, with one specialty (genetics) being subordinated to another (OB-GYN) and having to do the latter's dirty work. In the contemporary case of status separation in internal medicine, subordination spans a *single* specialty across the nation's hospitals. Also remarkable is the fact that Legacy residents did not experience the same kind of "status pain" that Bosk described as plaguing genetic counselors. Instead, most non-USMDs took on these lower-status, less desirable jobs willingly and even with enthusiasm—one could say they consented to this subordination or at least knew and accepted their place. This presents a puzzle: What beliefs sustain a system where a group of professionals willingly fills gaps for another group of professionals? In other words, to return to the earlier comment by a Stonewood faculty member, why are those orthopedics professors from Tehran and ophthalmologists from Karachi readily filling "National Guard" roles in community internal medicine programs rather than competing with USMDs for positions in orthopedics and ophthalmology?

In the previous chapters, I considered how structures and resources differentially shaped residents' trajectories into, during, and out of residency, segregating and separating USMDs from non-USMDs in status. In this chapter, I focus on how respondents made sense of this status separation by exploring the belief system that supported status inequalities between USMDs and non-USMDs within medicine, resulting in highly prestigious and highly stigmatized identities based on pedigree. I examine how shared status beliefs help frame USMDs as more competent and deserving of top positions while relegating ostensibly less competent and less deserving non-USMDs toward the bottom.[5] These beliefs were the product of both the game and the social contract of US medicine that I described in previous chapters and helped conceal the systematic structural inequalities that often passed for differences in merit.[6] These structures helped produce a "mental acceptance of a society's divisional structures," thereby making status distinctions between USMDs and non-USMDs seem natural and obvious.[7] As a result, non-USMDs *also* viewed USMDs as more meritorious, either because they thought USMDs worked harder or because they believed the country should prioritize its own. They therefore consented to occupying a subordinate status within the profession, and they counted themselves lucky to be part of it, given the tens of thousands of other applicants who would gladly take their place.

STATUS BELIEFS SUPPORTING USMD DOMINANCE

Overall, respondents felt that USMDs should have priority access to residency positions because they were better trained and more deserving than non-USMDs—meritocratic reasons that strongly resonated with the promises and expectations of the social contract. I discuss the complexities of these beliefs here, showing how some non-USMDs also subscribed to them and thereby contributed to USMDs' status dominance within the profession.

USMDs Are Better Qualified

The first belief supporting USMD dominance was that they were simply better doctors than non-USMDs. When I asked whether USMDs should be prioritized for residency positions, several USMDs thought that The Match should be an open competition and that residency programs should hire the best residents but that USMDs *were* the best. One USMD intern, for example, felt that resident selection should be based on merit but that USMDs were more meritorious anyway, so it "works": "Right now the marketplace aspect to the system seems to be doing a good job. It's a competition and the people who happen to be from here, who happen to go to US allopathic schools, happen to get the best spots for the most part. So for the most part, the system is working." From this intern's perspective, better outcomes were rightfully allocated to better candidates, therefore legitimating the system as highly meritocratic. Recall from chapter 2 that Stonewood leaders generally shared this intern's views. As one high-ranking official from Stonewood Medical School put it, "Well, I think that the approach that would be most consistent with delivery of high-quality care would be for US allopathic students to only get priority if it's clear that their preparation for residency is superior. Right now, in most cases, I think it is."

There are at least two problems with this perspective, however. First, the very people deciding what constitutes merit are USMDs themselves, like this official. Second, it overlooks the inherent inequalities in the game leading up to residency that systematically favor more-privileged USMDs (see chapters 1 and 2).[8]

Interestingly, very few Legacy residents decried the residency selection process as unmeritocratic (I'll elaborate on this later). Many of them felt that it made sense to prioritize USMDs according to current definitions of merit. Yasmin (IMG, PGY-2, Legacy) explained that certain residency opportunities were closed to her: "You can't come from [the Middle East] . . . and become an ENT [ear, nose, and throat] resident." She then rationalized this by pointing out that US residencies look for different markers of success than what she was used to: "I think it's somewhat unfair. It's fair if you think about the stuff they look for in your CV. I think people coming from my country and the other countries, we are hard workers." She went on to describe her strong clinical skills: "[Where I went to medical school,] we didn't have respiratory therap[ists], like [during] code blues [emergencies].[9] Whoever was there is going to intubate you, so *you better know how to intubate* because you are going to be by yourself intubating" (emphasis added). She noted, however, that these skills did not seem to matter when applying to residency programs: "So we have potential, but then you come here, and you start feeling like, oh my god, this is not even taken into consideration. They look for other stuff. That other stuff is very important, I do realize, because now I feel I need to improve myself in clinical research and those extracurricular activities I need to do."

While Yasmin was frustrated that her previous training was not fully "taken into consideration," she also understood that her CV lacked certain elements, such as research, which made USMDs more attractive. She did mention other strengths, like her intubation skills, but did not dwell on how those strengths were probably more clinically useful in a hospital than, say, having presented a poster at a conference. Instead, she and her colleagues at Legacy internalized the importance of research as a marker of merit in the game in the same way that USMDs did. She felt the game was legitimate in this way.

There were, however, a few non-USMDs who did not believe that residency selection was meritocratic. One was Liam, a Legacy USIMG intern who thought the system was rigged against non-USMDs. He explained that despite having rotated at Johns Hopkins during medical school and having worked there as a researcher prior to that, he knew that a Caribbean graduate like himself would never match there for residency: "There is absolutely no way in hell that Hopkins would ever even touch us *regardless of our numbers* [test scores], and they make that quite clear. Their program says we will not accept international medical graduates. Do not even bother applying or whatever" (emphasis added). When I asked why, he replied simply, "Well, elitist. Elitist, that's why. . . . I helped them publish their work! I reviewed their grants! I knew those doctors! But because of their elitist nature, they don't accept foreign medical graduates." Liam blamed Johns Hopkins for being exclusionary, but he was a notable exception. That so few non-USMDs shared these views, however, is reflective of the extent to which they internalized the belief in meritocracy, which helped legitimate status separation in the profession.

USMDs Are More Deserving

USMDs overwhelmingly expressed their belief that they were not only better qualified for but also more deserving of residency positions than non-USMDs were. After all, the term *merit* comes from the Latin *merere*, which means "to earn" *and* "to deserve."[10] Because of expectations built into the social contract between USMDs and the profession, USMDs felt that they were owed residency positions by virtue of having held up their end of the bargain. They really viewed it as a bargain, and even medical school officials viewed it that way. As one senior official at Stonewood University Medical School put it, "So the argument for [USMDs] getting priority [for residency] is one that relates to sort of the contract between medical schools and medical students. You know, we're charging a lot [in tuition]. . . . So there is this contract: we'll charge you a lot but you'll get something out of it." . . . Most [US] medical students go to medical school thinking the desired outcome here is for me to have the most gratifying career I can have." In exchange for their tuition, as well as years of hard work and deferred gratification, USMDs would come to expect "the most gratifying careers" possible upon graduation—which included top residency positions at places like Stonewood. Program officials (themselves USMDs) espoused a similar logic. When I asked a

Stonewood program official whether USMDs should get priority for residency, they often referred to their own efforts to get into medical school: "The rigor of the kind of application process and what I had to do to get into medical school helped to triage me into getting into an allopathic school, so I would say, for that reason, yes."

Beliefs about USMDs' deservingness were often strengthened by the widely shared—but inaccurate—myth that US graduates would soon outpace the number of available residency positions (see chapter 2 for more on this myth). Residents would point to the growth of allopathic and osteopathic medical schools in the past decade as a reason to be concerned that USMDs would get pushed out of residency positions.[11] Hunter (USMD, PGY-3, Stonewood), for example, explained, "We're seeing more and more that as we graduate more students, we don't have the residency spots for them. And I think there should be some element of a benefit of being someone who trained here, went to school here in the [United States]." Despite increased enrollments, however, the number of US doctors graduating (both Doctors of Medicine [MDs] and Doctors of Osteopathic Medicine [DOs]) is projected to remain well below the number of residency positions in the next decade.[12]

Nevertheless, the fear of running out of residency positions, combined with the belief in the social contract, engendered a shared sense of entitlement among USMDs, who were socialized to believe that because they survived the rigorous and cutthroat process of getting into a US allopathic medical school, they should be prioritized for residency positions. "You're earning your stripes so to speak," as one PGY-2 said. USMDs felt they had held up their end of the deal. In return, they expected the profession to hold up its end of the bargain by guaranteeing them residency positions—and thereby keeping the competition from outsiders at bay.[13] As one Stonewood intern put it, "We're all training with the idea and *we've been told* by our medical school that *we're going to get jobs afterwards* and now all those jobs are going to other people who aren't from the [United States]? . . . [If] all these programs now are only taking people from other countries because they have more experience, *where would that necessarily leave all of us?*" (emphasis added). Notice that merit took a backseat to entitlement in this explanation, with this intern feeling they were owed a residency position even more than someone with more experience.

Importantly, USMDs did not expect just *any* residency position. Most expected access to their *preferred* spots, particularly given the financial constraints they faced (as I described in chapter 5). When asked, for example, how they would have felt if they had matched into a community program instead of a place like Stonewood for residency after having accumulated all that debt, an intern shrugged and said, "I would be upset . . . because if you worked so hard." A PGY-3 elaborated:

> [It] depend[s] on your idea of what you want to do with your life. Maybe you don't want to see sick people, like really bad cases. [If] they don't want to subspecialize, they just want to do something small, yeah, then community is fine for them. But I think I find working at a tertiary care center also very personally fulfilling. Like there's this thought that somebody is going to die if you're not there, and that's a bit overdramatized . . . but how much of what we do every day can be outsourced? Really, hardly anything, and whereas if you are seeing the bread-and-butter cases in the small community center, there is much more there that can be . . . delegated, and your role is *less unique*. Where if you go through this many years of training and put all your life on hold, *you want to be something special*, and maybe that sounds silly, but that's part of our reality. (emphasis added)

In this way, being "something special" and getting top positions at university hospitals were considered an inherent reward—a status right for having played the game and deferred gratification for so long. Kamens, a sociologist of education, argued in 1977 that "schools symbolically redefine people and make them eligible for membership in societal categories to which specific sets of rights are assigned."[14] USMDs therefore felt that they had been assigned a set of rights associated with their trajectories into US allopathic medical schools. After all, remember that residency went from being considered a privilege to being a "right" for US doctors in the mid-twentieth century, when having an MD was no longer sufficient for practicing medicine.[15]

But also recall that USMDs had considerable help playing the game, yet that help was seldom acknowledged. Instead, the constant emphasis on USMDs' hard work playing the game (as the resident put it, "you go through this many years of training") helped obscure the privileges they received along the way and minimized the considerable efforts put in by non-USMDs, thereby further reinforcing their sense of deservingness compared to non-USMDs.

Another reason why respondents thought that USMDs were more deserving of residency positions than non-USMDs was that they had invested in the nation's health care system. As Dale (USMD, PGY-3, Stonewood) put it, "You have to accommodate the people that have put money into their education here before you outsource essentially, before you train outside physicians to do the job." Dale readily acknowledged that non-USMDs typically scored higher on standardized tests than USMDs did ("Oh, they're better"), but he felt that USMDs should still be prioritized because they had invested in the system. Here again merit (in the sense of being superior candidates) took a backseat to the deservingness argument.

The converse was also true; some believed that USMDs were more deserving because the system had invested so heavily in them. As Cassandra, a Stonewood intern, explained, "I do think that US students should be given preference. That's where the money is coming from [i.e., the United States]. Those are the people who probably are going to be doctors here." With student loans, subsidized public schooling, infrastructure supports, and the funding of residency positions nationwide by Medicare, the United States does invest considerable resources in training physicians, both US and foreign born.[16] Many respondents, however, were indignant to think about all those resources being spent on IMGs who might just end up going back to their home countries.[17] As Ken, a Stonewood PGY-3 who had immigrated to the United States as a child, put it:

> I think if you are an IMG and you apply to US schools [for residency], there should be some contractual obligation that after you finish your training, you have to spend a minimum of ten years practicing in the United States. Because if you come here and . . . you get a Medicare-funded residency and a fellowship position, you graduate and you get the fuck out of Dodge, that's not right because all of us taxpayers paid for your education that you just then took back to Greece or India.

Here Ken interestingly referred to medicine's social contract with *society* as a justification for prioritizing USMDs.[18] In exchange for the government's investment in their education, the residents offer their work and service to the public. In Ken's opinion, those doctors who could not or would not hold up their end of that bargain were not worthy of support. Some Legacy residents even adopted this view. For example, Trevor (USIMG, PGY-2) understood the preference for USMDs, given the United States' investment in residents: "Obviously you kind of have to take care of your own first, so it would reflect kind of badly on the

[United States] if you're graduating all these US grads but they're not finding spots. And these spots are funded by Medicare I believe, and Medicare is probably funded by our taxes, so it's kind of like there is a social aspect to it too."

Moreover, residents from both programs pointed out that other countries would do the same to retain their own doctors. As one Stonewood intern expressed, "I don't think I would feel upset if I were a US student applying to a foreign country and that country gave preference to their own citizens. I don't think I would feel that was unfair to me." Elliot, another Stonewood intern, put it in terms of a country having an obligation to its citizens who "did all the right things" and were promised success:

> There are a limited amount of positions . . . and for the same reason that I wouldn't expect to go to another country and take a spot that someone who grew up in that country and was part of that culture and has the expectations *that they do all the right things* that they'll be able to succeed in the way that they've been promised they could succeed. So in the same way that I wouldn't expect to go to that country and take a spot from someone who deserves it more than I do from that standpoint, I think it's reasonable for people from this country to not be denied opportunities. . . . You can't screw over your own people, you know? (emphasis added)

For Elliot, the country (or, rather, the profession because the US government is not directly involved in medical training or hiring) has an obligation to its own people who did all the right things—a further nod to the social contract. Most Stonewood residents agreed with this point of view, including those who were involved in global health initiatives and had experience training abroad. One such resident who traveled to Africa on elective said, "I have been that foreign medical grad reversely and it's equally hard. I suck at the system [in Africa]. I should necessarily be lower on the totem pole than the people who are used to that system." She went on to say that a lack of knowledge about the US medical system should also put IMGs lower on the totem pole than USMDs in the United States.

Several IMGs at Legacy sympathized with the US approach because similar processes occurred back home. One Lebanese PGY-1 resident admitted that foreign doctors had a lot of difficulty finding work in Lebanon: "[An] Indian guy who is coming to work in Lebanon as a doctor, [he] will not find a job, not even for a thousand dollars. We won't hire these people. . . . We are already kind of full.

Maybe [if] this guy was trained in the [United States] . . . we will *consider* hiring them, but still is he able to communicate with people? Is he able to be good?" (emphasis in original). Here the intern raised two important points. The first was that about being "full," suggesting that without a shortage of doctors, there would be no need for IMGs. The United States, however, is not full, which makes it reliant on IMGs. The second, however, was that about communication skills, which was a common justification for excluding IMGs from consideration at Stonewood (see chapter 2) and one that I will revisit. In other words, some IMGs shared concerns similar to those of many USMDs about foreigners practicing medicine in their own countries.

To support their views, several Stonewood residents gave examples of acquaintances who went to practice in other countries, like Australia, and who were placed in lower-tier training programs because they were foreign. Yet, unlike in Australia, where internship positions are awarded by priority group (with in-state Australian medical graduates assigned to Priority Group 1, the highest, and non–Australian citizen IMGs assigned to Priority Group 7, the lowest), the residency allocation process in the United States is far less transparent.[19] The US health care system relies on the globalization of medical human resources to staff its nursing departments and residency programs, but unlike in other countries, USMDs get prioritized *without* official policies to that effect, allowing the allocation of positions to operate under the guise of meritocracy. If USMDs were explicitly given priority in The Match, non-USMD applicants' aspirations could be tempered accordingly. Yet only a few USMDs (and virtually no non-USMDs) that I talked to denounced this lack of transparency in residency hiring practices. As one rare dissenting Stonewood resident, himself an immigrant, said, "If they [programs] know that they're just not going to rank them [non-USMDs] high enough to match there, there's really no reason to give them [non-USMDs] the hope or the incentive." He thought residency programs should be up-front about their practices to avoid giving false hope to applicants under a pretense of meritocracy. But such transparency would run counter to the dominant national ethos: the American Dream, which promises that with enough hard work and dedication, anything is possible, including a top residency spot. And as will become clearer, this logic was, in fact, essential for securing consent from non-USMDs for their own subordination.

Taken together, these beliefs about competence and deservingness provided support for elevating USMDs to a higher status within the profession—a position that even some non-USMDs felt was justified. In particular, the belief about USMDs' deservingness helped reinforce a system in which even the most skilled non-USMDs—the ophthalmologists from Karachi and the orthopedists from Tehran—did not provide real competition for USMDs, who felt they were more deserving of residency positions than even more experienced foreigners because of what they had sacrificed to enter the profession and what the nation had sacrificed to train them. The emphasis was squarely on putting USMDs first, so much so that only a small minority of respondents felt that the current recruitment practices, which seem to favor protectionism more than meritocracy, were not in the profession's best interest. One of these rare detractors was a Stonewood attending who said, "It's not part of the Constitution to . . . be employed as a resident," critiquing the notion that residency should be viewed a right by USMDs. The scarcity of these alternative views, however, speaks to just how widespread beliefs were about USMDs' entitlement to dominance within the profession.

BELIEFS SUPPORTING THE SUBORDINATION OF NON-USMDs

Non-USMDs Are Not as Good

While the beliefs just described served to elevate USMDs' status, a corresponding set of beliefs served to stigmatize non-USMDs as inferior—and thereby more deserving of lower-status positions. In addition to the Stonewood leaders who believed that non-USMDs were risky—because they lacked both medical knowledge and cultural competence (as detailed in chapter 2)—the Stonewood residents openly believed that non-USMDs were lazy and poor communicators. DOs and USIMGs, in particular, were widely perceived as not having worked as hard as USMDs to get into a US allopathic medical school and thus as not deserving the privileges associated with the social contract. As Elliot, (USMD, PGY-1, Stonewood) explained, "[As a USIMG], you're judged by default as being someone who doesn't deserve to be in med school and got in because you're paying a school that's trying to get as much money as it can. . . . The same as DO programs in that respect," referring to the widespread belief that DO and Caribbean schools operate under pay-to-play schemes. Many criticized DOs and USIMGs for not having been good enough to gain admission to US allopathic medical schools. In fact, several Stonewood residents were not admitted on their first try, but this was seldom discussed openly. Another intern spoke of a friend who went to medical school in Grenada: "He did not work as hard in college, which is why he didn't get into medical school, but he is probably every bit as smart as I am. Yeah, they [USIMGs] still have to take all the same tests, and a lot of times I'm sure they are a lot better [than USMDs] because they have a lot more to lose." Hard work was thus a critical aspect of merit—at least as important as intelligence for this intern. After all, IQ plus *effort* is thought to equal merit in a classic meritocracy.[20]

For their part, while most IMGs were praised for being very smart, they were almost uniformly criticized for lacking the cultural tools to adequately practice medicine in the United States—just as Stonewood program officials maintained in chapter 2. As Vivek (USMD, PGY-2, Stonewood), himself a first-generation immigrant, confided, "[When] I get something from a physician who I know has been trained abroad, I don't know what is going on with the patient. . . . They're brilliant; I ask them a medical question, [and they] know the answer right away. . . . But there's two parts to being a doctor," referring to knowledge and communication, which he had mentioned earlier in the conversation. Others made sweeping inferences about IMGs by referring to only a few individuals. For example, one intern said, "[IMGs] don't treat pain. A few people here that I have met are way less concerned about treating pain in procedures and stuff because they don't do that at home, so they just don't think to do it here."[21] As I will discuss later, this tendency to generalize may stem from the fact that Stonewood residents had only limited exposure to IMGs.

In addition to being characterized as lazy and culturally incompetent—and thus deserving lower-status residency positions in community hospitals—non-USMDs were stigmatized for training in those very community programs, which Stonewood residents widely viewed as less rigorous. These beliefs helped support the analogy of the dichotomy between the Navy SEALs and the National Guard introduced at the beginning of this chapter. Importantly, Stonewood residents rotated at three hospitals, two of which were community-based medical centers (only Stonewood was a tertiary university hospital), and some of them even felt that the ward rotations at the community hospitals were more challenging than the ones at Stonewood's flagship hospital were.

Still, negative perceptions of community-trained doctors abounded, to the point where some residents openly questioned their competence. After admitting that he would not want to be a patient at a community hospital—a sentiment widely shared by Stonewood residents—Logan, a PGY-2, said, "I'm not saying they're killing people over there or anything, [but], yeah, there's a lot of shitty doctors out there. I don't think people realize that there's a lot of shitty doctors out; we see it all the time. We get transfers from other [community] hospitals, and, you know, I'm a second-year resident and I can be like, this is ridiculous." Similarly, Gunther, a PGY-3, relayed a story about a friend in a community program: "They had a patient that came in with DKA [diabetic ketoacidosis] who died on the floor [wards].[22] . . . A patient shouldn't die from DKA. He was like thirty or something—a young person. But I just worry about what kind of training she's getting over there because I talk to her about stories, and she doesn't really, she doesn't get taught, [and] they work her like a dog, and I don't know if she's getting anything out of it." When I asked about the implications of having tiered residency programs, he replied, "I think it matters for the patients that you're going to care for." This resident felt that stratification within the profession could have alarming consequences for patient care. Similarly, Lynn, an intern, advised her father who had suffered a stroke to avoid his local community hospital: "Especially with time-sensitive things, like a stroke, where you can qualify for tPA,[23] I don't want any idiot who doesn't know what the window is for tPA greeting my dad at the door reading the wrong article that says it's a three-hour window as opposed to the new article that says it's safe to do it in four and a half hours. He didn't read that. I don't want that to be the difference between my dad using his hand again, you know what I mean?"

To be sure, some of these concerns are consistent with the findings in chapters 3 and 4 that there were considerable inequalities in training between Legacy and Stonewood residents. However, they also represent an important conceptual challenge to the presumed gap-filling function of non-USMDs in community hospitals; if their training is so poor, it could be hazardous to allow them to practice, creating a crisis for a profession that cannot staff all of those positions.

Perhaps for this reason, most respondents toed a fine line between believing that non-USMDs were less qualified than USMDs and believing that non-USMDs were dangerous: "They're probably trained enough, but I wouldn't say they're as well trained. I don't know," demurred one PGY-3 resident, echoing the same rhetoric used by Stonewood officials when pressed on the implications of pooling "risky" non-USMDs in community programs (see chapter 2). This professional doublethink ("not as good but good enough") came up during an interview with Dr. Taylor, one of the few non-USMDs on the faculty at Stonewood whom I introduced in the previous chapter. Despite having received a lot of pushback from the hospital leadership because of their pedigree, with one particular official even threatening to block their promotion simply because they were a non-USMD, Dr. Taylor was still considered one of the best doctors at Stonewood, and this sometimes led to awkward encounters: "The irony was . . . I remember being called down at least once to see one of this [official's] family members, being paged to come in." While this well-respected attending's pedigree was problematic from an institutional perspective, it did not seem to stop this official from paging Dr. Taylor directly to care for a family member who was sick. When I asked Dr. Taylor how they made sense of that, they shrugged and said with a laugh, "I think it's fascinating. You can't. And, obviously this individual, I think he had abject prejudice."

The truth was that Stonewood housestaff spent very little time working with non-USMDs, so their negative views were often based on limited knowledge or experience. One exception was at Tri-Hospital, where Stonewood residents spent at least two months rotating alongside non-USMD residents from nearby Solomon Community Hospital. At Tri-Hospital, patients were taken care of by four teams of residents: the red, white, and blue teams, which were composed of Stonewood residents, and the yellow team, which was composed of Solomon residents. The symbolism of these team labels could not have been more poignant—at once a nationalist nod to USMDs from Stonewood and a racist reference to the IMG housestaff at Solomon. A Stonewood intern who had yet to rotate at Tri-Hospital expressed surprise when she learned that the red, white, and blue teams were from Stonewood while the Solomon team was yellow. "What? No way, you have got to be kidding me!" Another intern replied innocently, "What? It's just a color. It's like this is a yellow room." The first intern repeated, "Red, white, blue, [and] yellow. Seriously?" The second replied, "One is the color of the flag, the other one is . . . [*trailing off*]." Yet another asked, "Would it be better if they were the *red* team?"

It was common for Stonewood residents to make fun of the yellow team. As Jerry (USMD, PGY-3, Stonewood) explained, "The majority of the residents here definitely kind of look down on [the yellow team]. . . . There's definitely a lot of snickering and condescension I think." Stonewood residents consistently complained that patient handoffs from the yellow team were sloppy—even though all four teams at Tri-Hospital were overseen by the same set of attendings, including a common chief resident from Stonewood. As Barbara, another PGY-3, relayed:

At [Tri-Hospital] we work with [Solomon] residents, and . . . we'll say, "Oh, who was on call today? Oh, it was the yellow team," and we know the yellow team is [the Solomon] team. If something goes wrong, it's like, "Oh, well, you know who was taking care of them." Or "Oh, obviously I didn't get a good sign-out because you know who it was." So that's definitely pervasive.

This perspective may have partly stemmed from the fact that Stonewood residents never actually worked on the same team with non-USMDs—they worked *alongside* the yellow team but in their own teams. In this way, segregation may have helped fuel stigmatization by making it easier to attribute negative outcomes to the lesser known other.[24]

In fact, those respondents who spent more time working with non-USMDs (outside of Tri-Hospital) tended to have a better perception of them. An Ivy League–trained preliminary USMD intern at Legacy admitted, for example, "For whatever reason, people don't think that those people who go to those schools are—I don't know if they don't think they are as smart or as prepared or whatever, [but] that's like the reputation. I have worked here [at Legacy] with pretty much all people that fit the category and I don't think that that's true, but *you don't really know unless you work with them*" (emphasis added). A PGY-2 Stonewood resident also conceded that his negative impressions of DOs had changed when he finally worked with them: "I had a lot of personal biases. I didn't think DOs were as good as MDs because I had never even heard of it until I was probably in medical school. . . . [During my rotations], most of the residents were DOs, and they were some of the best residents that I have worked with, some of the best mentors I have ever had. . . . I had thought they weren't as well trained, [when], in fact, they were better trained." If Stonewood residents had had more experience working with non-USMDs, their views of them might have been more positive, thereby helping attenuate status distinctions between USMDs and non-USMDs.

A few Stonewood residents acknowledged that these status distinctions were arbitrary or even "silly," as one resident put it. Several noted how distinctions boil down to minutiae—or minor details used to differentiate between equivalents.[25] One PGY-3 rolled his eyes and said, "I mean it's not like we're giving people antibiotics at this hospital and Solomon Hospital is telling them to take this root or herb to eat. You know we both have penicillin, we both have CT scans," suggesting that differences between university and community hospital trainees were likely overblown. Similarly, as Lorna (USMD, PGY-3, Stonewood) remarked about status differences between community and university programs, "I don't know, it's really weird. . . . I think everybody actually knows that it's kind of this nonthing that exists. . . . It's not actually a difference; it's just how things kind of polarize." Differences between USMDs and non-USMDs may have therefore been amplified to justify relegating non-USMDs to less desirable positions—not unlike how Stonewood officials justified excluding non-USMDs from the program's Match list in chapter 2—even though many believed that such differences were not hugely meaningful in practice.

Others went so far as to suggest that differences between USMDs and non-USMDs were completely made up. Elliot, a Stonewood intern, summarized this perspective: "I mean, there's no way around it: there are [non-USMD] students that are trained in an identical manner [to USMDs], that have the same potential, who are not allowed access to certain [residency] programs—that's sort of the definition of discrimination, you know?" Elliot's comment underlines an important reality: while the distinctions may have been (at least partly) artificial, they still had real implications for inequality.[26] Presumed differences between USMDs and non-USMDs, however arbitrary, were widely internalized as socially valid—and thus broadly influenced social behavior within the profession.[27] For example, Collette, a Stonewood intern who rotated at a hospital with non-USMD residents during medical school, described the mixed perception of those residents among her fellow medical students:

> It's so hard to explain. So I think everybody thought they were very good and were good teachers for the most part. One of the best teachers, she won the teaching award, was a Caribbean grad. . . . But the perception [among USMD medical students] is still, "I want to go to a place [for residency] where there is mostly US [MD] grads." . . . I don't know how to explain it other than just bias of "Oh, you went to a Caribbean school; there must be something that you couldn't get into US schools." . . . I guess, I don't know, that was my, all of my perceptions about them.

Despite having had very positive experiences with non-USMDs in medical school and seeing how competent they were, this intern still chose a residency program with mostly USMDs. Even though *her* perceptions of non-USMDs may have been positive, she knew that not everyone shared her view and that professional status is powerfully constructed around these negative assumptions. Put differently, she acted in accordance with those assumptions, making the beliefs real in their consequences. Her experience speaks to how ingrained the stigma has become, such that regardless of their performance or skills, non-USMDs will likely remain in subordinate positions because more powerful USMDs *believe* they belong there. As one rather perspicacious Stonewood intern pointed out, "[Medicine] has a culture of institutionalized perceptions about things that nobody's immune to."

Furthermore, these "institutionalized perceptions" were long-standing and regularly reinforced throughout USMDs' training, making them difficult to change. One preliminary intern at Legacy who went to an elite USMD school admitted how surprised they were at their non-USMD colleagues' competence, given how they were socialized to think negatively about them:[28] "It might sound like I'm an asshole and I really don't mean to, but I was surprised at how much a lot of them knew because I did think that I was going to know a lot more than everyone because of my background." USMD students and residents were repeatedly taught by peers and superiors—almost always informally—to believe that non-USMDs (and, by extension, the community programs staffing them) were second-rate. A Stonewood attending reflected, "I think *we tell ourselves* there is more variability at the other [at community hospitals], although ultimately we all have to pass the same Boards, right, to practice? . . . All I can say is I know we think that [about community hospitals], and I know that we kind of talk about that." Thus, whether or not USMDs were actually superior to non-USMDs was in some ways immaterial—what mattered was that USMDs (who held elite positions in the profession) *believed* they were.

Thus, arbitrary or not, USMDs systematically benefited from the social importance attached to the stigmatizing of non-USMDs because it helped make USMDs superior. As one Stonewood USMD intern thought aloud one day:

I just wonder overall if this whole issue is related to the [fact that] people who govern or who hold the power in medicine don't want to give that power up and they've always had it. So it's not necessarily [a matter of] do international grads deserve spots? It's not about that. That decision was made a long, long time ago, and now the people who benefit from it, like us, grew up in the [United States], went to school here, we know we have job security. *Why would we want to give that up, right?* . . . Once you have that advantage, I think it's really hard to get people to say someone's got to give. It's not going to be me: I'm in debt, I deserve a spot, I worked hard. So it's going to take some outside governing body to say this is how it should be. (emphasis added)

USMDs therefore gained considerable advantage from attributing lower status to non-USMDs—an advantage they were not likely to give up easily. Bolton and Muzio used a similar argument to explain gender inequality within the legal profession: "Gendered segmentation, which thrives on the ideology of women's difference, has become a defence mechanism of an embattled profession, ensuring that the elite segments can, in the context of a more hostile institutional environment, hold on to their traditional privileges and rewards."[29] Thus, even if the ideology of difference is sometimes based on thin evidence and arbitrary distinctions, the *benefits* it yields are invaluable to those who seek to protect their advantages, consciously or not.

CONSENTING TO SUBORDINATION

It makes sense that USMDs would espouse status beliefs that serve to elevate their own professional esteem. But I also found that many non-USMDs agreed with the beliefs I have discussed, particularly that the United States should prioritize its own graduates. These findings suggest that non-USMDs have come to embrace some of the very principles that lead to their own subordination. In fact, very few non-USMDs deplored the current system, in which the more elite segments of the profession cast them as second-rate. Only a handful of respondents at Legacy expressed outrage at the fact that they were systematically excluded from certain opportunities. One was Liam, the Caribbean graduate mentioned earlier who was angry at Johns Hopkins. Another was Faisal, an IMG who had already completed residency training in his home country before coming to the United States: "I was shocked. Because you heard always that [the United States] is a 'freedom country.' . . . Where's that freedom they are speaking about? I have said always, just give me a chance. Like just give me a chance to see me, test me, and then make a decision and [do] not say no just because I'm a foreigner. . . . They don't give you the chance to even go for an interview." Those who expressed such views, however, were definitely in the minority.

While the status beliefs described in the first part of the chapter are essential to the reproduction of USMD dominance, so is securing the implicit consent of those doctors being subordinated. After all, if non-USMDs refused to accept USMD dominance, the profession could face a serious revolt from non-USMDs demanding equal treatment for equal credentials (not unlike the deep split predicted by Freidson between the formal elite and the rank and file).[30] No such revolt has happened, however. Instead, as I have noted, many non-USMDs willingly took on lower-status positions in the profession. So why would trained professionals consent to such status subordination?

Belief in Hard Work (and Its Corollary, Self-Blame)

Non-USMDs consent to subordination in part because of their steadfast belief in the value of hard work and dedication. Despite being aware of the barriers associated with being non-USMDs, we have already seen how Legacy residents strongly believed that if they worked hard, they could overcome the stigma associated with their pedigree and be seen for their true worth. The emphasis on individual effort or agency, rather than on "circumstances of life," and the accompanying "belief in success among the unsuccessful" have long been major tenets of American managerial ideology—and the American Dream, more broadly.[31] I argue that this belief in agency helped legitimate the current social order in medicine, as it gave at least *the impression* that ascension to the elite was possible.[32]

Harvey (USIMG, PGY-2, Legacy) was a good example. Before accepting an offer from an offshore medical school, he asked alumni from that school about the prospects for residency. They told him:

> As long as you work hard, as long as you finish in the top half of your class, you're going to get a residency. Whether or not you get a *competitive* one, you know, that depends on how hard you work because obviously you're not going to get . . . like the chance of you getting dermatology or orthopedic surgery coming from [the Caribbean]? Doesn't look good. So you know, but *if you really want it, nothing is impossible.* (emphasis added)

Harvey's interaction with alumni is an example of how the belief in hard work and dedication can reproduce itself through peer networks. Legacy leaders also reinforced this belief when it came to fellowship applications. Recall how one internationally trained official said Legacy residents could match into any subspecialty, including highly competitive ones like cardiology: "So it's not like you can't; there is no can't; *it's just how much work you have to put into it. Do you really want it?*" (emphasis added).

Yet, when the belief in hard work is juxtaposed with the reality on the ground, it becomes apparent how misguided that belief was. No one matched into cardiology from Legacy, despite the official's optimism. And recall, for example, that when I asked a Stonewood official about the chances of *any* Caribbean graduate matching to Stonewood's internal medicine program, they replied, "Probably as close to zero as you can get. I don't even know if we've ever even interviewed someone" (see chapter 2). Stonewood did not openly advertise this position, however, so the lack of transparency in the residency selection process only helped stoke beliefs in a meritocratic process where hard work could unlock all doors.

The corollary to that belief, however, is that if non-USMDs did not attain their goals, it was because they did not work hard enough. This shared thinking led to a lot of self-blame, as we saw in chapter 1, particularly among USIMGs, many of whom took personal responsibility for their limited career options, despite facing severe structural constraints and harder work conditions than USMDs did. When describing his prospects for fellowship, Adrian (USIMG, PGY-2, Legacy) said:

> I want my fellowship program to be better than my residency. I want to improve on what I do. I got a late start in life and I procrastinated a lot. . . . *Can't blame anybody if you're in a shitty place.* . . . It's where you put yourself, and if what I've done in the past limits me, then I have to accept that. It sucks; it's hard not to look back and kind of kick yourself 'cause you knew if you did something better, you'd be in a better spot. (emphasis added)

Adrian and others would emphasize agency in this way, blaming themselves for their positions rather than explaining their struggles as a result of structural inequalities, like the fact that Adrian was the first to go to college in his family and had less support than most USMDs. The difference between Adrian and USMDs wasn't the *capacity* or even the desire to work—rather, it was that he lacked the blueprint for success that came with being born into privilege.

Harvey was in a similar position. About half an hour after he told me, "If you really want it, nothing is impossible," he admitted, "I was stupid. If I had to do it over again . . . but, no, I mean it was my own fault; I screwed up in college. I should have studied a little bit more. . . . I wish there was someone there like kind of like giving advice. I would tell my younger self like, 'Do this; do this instead.'" His comments are powerful; by emphasizing his role in going to the Caribbean, he obscured the structural obstacles (such as a lack of guidance), which he mentioned only in passing. In this case, lacking the early life and college support to get into a US medical school, Harvey and others (including many USMDs, as described earlier) viewed going to the Caribbean as a personal failure rather than (at least partly) the result of structural barriers.

These findings echo earlier work on medical education and the medical profession, which highlights how career trajectories are often believed to be the direct result of one's own decision-making.[33] Bourdieu and others have also written extensively about how educational institutions can produce a *habitus* that leads individuals to internalize the social order as legitimate (despite obvious structural inequality), which can help explain why non-USMDs were so quick to blame themselves for their struggles rather than a rigged system.[34] As Jewel has noted about American legal education, for example, "The myth of merit creates a habitus that causes law students to internally arrive at individual expectations and goals based on the legal profession's existing hierarchy. Through this process of objectification, students come to believe that status within the law profession is not arbitrary, but is instead based on principles of individual merit and intelligence."[35] Jewel goes even further to argue that such a habitus is more efficient than physical coercion at getting "the dominated to complicitly participate in their own domination," thereby making it a powerful tool for securing consent among the subordinated.[36]

Social psychologists also agree that for status beliefs to be effective, people in *both* the advantaged and the disadvantaged groups must agree (or at least concede) that people in the advantaged group are "better," despite the strong tendency toward in-group preference.[37] Thus, it is perhaps unsurprising that some Caribbean graduates felt they deserved to have a lower status compared to USMDs. For example, Allan (USIMG, PGY-2, Legacy) admitted, "Yes, the stigma is there [for Caribbean grads], and I think it's fair because the US graduate, for whatever they've done, they have proven themselves; they've overcome that obstacle already of getting to medical school. The Caribbean grads have not, so they have to get into residency, and then after that, I think it's all fair [equal] again." Interestingly, he felt that professional status normalized among USMDs and non-USMDs once they entered residency, even though the data presented in chapter 5 show otherwise. By finding the logic fair—or, at the very least, understandable—non-USMDs acquiesced to being considered inferior to USMDs, thereby helping perpetuate their status subordination within the profession.

The Reserve Labor Army

Internalized beliefs about merit are not the only reason why non-USMDs consented to take on lower-status positions in the profession. They also had to contend with more practical concerns. One such concern was the realization that
they were among the lucky few who made it. As Kamal (IMG, Legacy) put it,
"It's not an easy situation to get into residency in the [United States]." Similarly,
when I asked Rashad, an intern from the Middle East, how he felt about being
one of the IMGs who, in his words, were "filling the gap" in the United States,
he replied, "It doesn't bother me because there [are] already thousands of people
who want to be filling this gap, and they were not able to get here. So the point
is I am not looking at it as in, they took me because they were not able to [get]
anyone [else]. No, no, I'm good compared to my friends; everyone knows how
good I am. I'm happy." This intern was a willing participant because he knew how
hard it was to get a spot. He went on: "I mean for us [IMGs] being here by itself;
I'm not complaining, it's an accomplishment; I'm just fine, I'm happy. I'm not
like, ah shit! I ended up here. No, that's not the point. Being able to come here by
myself, it is an achievement." Remarkably, as others have found with (unskilled)
migrants, internationally trained physicians like Kamal and Rashad were willing
to take jobs that Americans viewed as undesirable partly because they knew that
they were quite fortunate compared to their compatriots back home.[38]

Indeed, several Legacy residents—including a few who were US citizens—
expressed gratitude for simply being able to practice medicine in the United
States. Some recounted stories about friends they knew who were not able to
match; for example, Trevor, a USIMG, said, "I have heard a lot of horror stories;
I have a friend that had double 99s [percentiles on his US Medical Licensing
Examination], applied to internal medicine. He didn't match actually." When
asked how he felt about having restricted opportunities for residency, Mathias,
a Canadian resident who studied in the Caribbean, replied, "I mean I think
that's fair. . . . It would have been really, really hard for me to become an MD
in Canada . . . so I'm thankful that this opportunity is here, and I think it's fair
because I guess there [are] more residency spots than there are med students.
So they can fill the gaps in that way." This intern had no objection to being
one of the physicians filling those gaps because he likely would have otherwise
been unable to continue his training in his home country. Georgina (another
Caribbean graduate), who initially aspired to become a surgeon, said, "I'm just

happy to be a doctor. And I changed my mind; I wanted to be a surgeon and I think if I really had tried, I could have done it, but now I'm happy being where I am, so I'm okay with it. I think the system is kind of the way it is, and I don't think it's going to change anytime soon. I think it's actually getting harder for foreign medical graduates, so for me I'm relieved I'm already in a spot." Georgina was glad to be part of the active labor force instead of part of the thousands in the large "reserve army" of unmatched applicants eager to take her place.[39] Like other historically marginalized workers, including women in male-dominated professions, non-USMDs understood that they ranked lower in the labor queue and filled positions only when the supply of more desirable workers (namely, USMDs) had been depleted.[40] In other words, non-USMDs were conscious that they benefited from the shortage of USMDs while also being acutely aware that up to half of all non-USMD residency applicants did not match.[41]

Residency Ready Physicians, a national Facebook group with more than five hundred members, reveals just how lucky these residents were. As Dr. Neviana Dimova, a Bulgarian-trained US citizen, wrote on behalf of the group, "According to the latest statistics, there may be as many as 6,000 U.S. citizens and permanent resident IMGs (International Medical Graduates) who have not been able to enter the required residency training. We want to work and are ready to serve where needed. We would consider it a privilege to work in a rural or inner-city area, just knowing that we have the opportunity to use our skills to help people."[42] Status pain—of the kind Bosk described among the "mop-up" genetic counselors— never materialized at Legacy because most non-USMDs had firsthand knowledge of how lucky they were to make it to front of the line compared to many of their colleagues who had not.

Pragmatic Acceptance

Some Legacy residents thought the system was unfair but felt resigned to accept things the way they were. As Allan, a Legacy PGY-2, explained, when he told attendings during clerkships that he went to a Caribbean school, "They automatically say you're at a disadvantage. And they know the system, that's how it is. It's not going to change anytime soon." This kind of "pragmatic acceptance" thus further allows for cohesion, rather than conflict, within the profession.[43] Mann studied social cohesion in liberal democracies and found that value consensus among societal strata is less important than *pragmatic* acceptance by subordinate classes of their limited roles in society. Similarly, Ridgeway and Correll found that people tend to accept negative beliefs about themselves, if only to manage the behavior and judgments of others, often resulting in a kind of self-fulfilling prophecy.[44] In this way, as long as non-USMDs accepted their treatment within the profession, even if they disagreed with USMD dominance, their subordination continued unfettered.

Ashley, an osteopathic medical student at Legacy with aspirations of becoming an orthopedic surgeon, espoused this pragmatic acceptance. She knew that despite having completed an excellent "audition rotation" in orthopedics prior to applying for residency, she would struggle to match because of her pedigree as a DO. When I asked her how she felt about that, she replied by telling me about her previous failed attempts at getting into an allopathic school: "Having that experience very early on of, like, *"Hey Sugar, this is life,"* [helped]. It's all about scores; there are way too many applicants for the number of spots and that's just how it is and deal with it; you're not going to be able to change it. . . . So I think now when I think about [how] it's going to happen again probably . . . it's not new to me because it's something I'm already over" (emphasis added). For this DO student, having lived through perceived injustices when applying to medical school helped condition her to accept unequal treatment later in her career.

Others felt it was just easier to be "at peace" with oneself and accept the current opportunity structure than to fight against it. Remember Trevor, the USIMG who went to medical school in Southeast Asia and used the term *foreigner* to refer to himself even though he was a US citizen. Trevor described the current situation for foreign-trained doctors like himself: "Foreigners are coming into the US system . . . so whether it's fair or not, like I said, it's inconsequential; you just have to play by the rules basically." Trevor's reference to himself as a foreigner speaks to just how internalized status distinctions along pedigree lines have become within the profession. He also felt compelled to accept his subordinate status as a foreigner if he wanted to be happy: "If you didn't know that coming into it, then it's almost like you were a little naïve and you didn't do your homework. So I think if you're aware of it and what to expect, I think it's a lot easier to be at peace with yourself instead of being grumpy about what could have been or wish it was more fair, wish I had the same opportunities."

Trevor raised an important point about being previously aware of how the system works. As I indicated in chapter 1, Legacy residents knew that they would face more limited opportunity when applying for residency; for example, one intern (a former surgeon in his home country) noted, "I knew that coming into this. I came into the whole thing with my eyes open." This perspective likely helped him feel more comfortable with having to start over as an intern after having completed residency in his home country. He was fully aware of the pitfalls, but his desire to practice medicine in the United States was stronger than whatever barriers he would face. In contrast, only a few others (like Faisal, the outraged resident I quoted earlier) had different expectations of the United States, thinking it was a land of opportunity and not expecting discrimination.

Lack of a Unified Perspective

A final possible reason why non-USMDs did not resist their own subordination is that they lacked a unified perspective. This was not for lack of opportunity, however. Segregation in residency programs actually offered the potential for a united front because non-USMDs were kept separate from USMDs. Legacy residents had access to "relational spaces," like the residents' lounge, which served as areas where they could discuss opinions and form a collective position away from superiors.[45] However, during the hundreds of hours I spent with them, they almost never discussed their status vis-à-vis USMDs, even though they would frequently discuss other injustices, such as the poor teaching at Legacy or Medicare cutbacks.

The diversity of the housestaff at Legacy may have been one factor preventing the formation of a united perspective. About half the residents had young families, which meant they spent less time socializing with those who did not have children. Age differences were also quite important, with some residents as young as twenty-five and others as old as forty-two, which meant they were in quite different stages of life. Cultural differences were perhaps the biggest barrier to unity. While almost every single resident expressed appreciation for working with such a varied housestaff, there were still visible distinctions between US and non-US residents. English, French, Spanish, and Arabic could be overheard simultaneously at any given time in the residents' lounge, and even though everyone got along, sometimes cultural references would be lost on those who were not from the United States. The US residents also sometimes teased the non-US residents, making fun of their accents or pronunciation. One day, for example, while playing a video game, a resident from Southeast Asia exclaimed, "He's malingaling!" referring to his avatar on the screen who just got injured. The other (US-born) residents began to laugh uncontrollably at the resident's attempt to

say *malingering*. "Malingaling?" one of them mocked jokingly. This comment elic-
ited good-natured laughter from everyone in the lounge, including the Southeast
Asian resident, suggesting that the housestaff actually got along well enough to
poke fun at one another. That said, the diversity of the housestaff likely made it
more difficult for them to form a unified perspective to challenge their subordinate status within the profession.

Also, not all non-USMDs had the same perspective on the issue of their place
in the profession, making it more difficult for them to join forces and create a
unified front. IMGs' experiences, for example, were quite different from those
of US citizens who studied in osteopathic or Caribbean medical schools. For
some IMGs, being a lower-status doctor in the United States was better than
being a high-status doctor in their home countries. As one IMG shared, "The
[United States] is giving you opportunities to live a better life." In contrast, some
USIMGs felt they should be prioritized over IMGs because of their citizenship
status, and some DOs and USIMGs heavily criticized IMGs' cultural and language skills. They were all underdogs—but for different reasons. This meant it was
more difficult to relate to one another and form alliances for collective action.

CONCLUSION

In sum, there is a widely shared and complex belief system supporting status
distinctions between USMDs and non-USMDs in internal medicine. USMDs
were generally believed to be more meritorious than other graduates; thus,
they were granted rightful access to elite positions within the profession under
a presumption of meritocracy. Perceptions of merit, however, were strongly
influenced by powerful expectations cultivated through a shared belief in a
professional social contract that nearly guaranteed certain privileges as *rights* to
USMDs. Meanwhile, non-USMDs were subordinated in status and stigmatized
through the reification of sometimes arbitrary distinctions that served to protect
the prestige of US medical graduates.

Non-USMDs, in turn, consented to this lower status either because they
counted themselves lucky to be part of the active labor force or because they
bought into the ideology that finds USMDs more meritorious to one degree or
another. In fact, USMDs at Stonewood were more likely to point out injustices in
the system than were the non-USMDs at Legacy. Put together, these beliefs make

it possible for non-USMDs to serve at the pleasure of USMDs, who rely on them to support USMDs' elite status and fill the positions they do not want to fill.

These findings support the theories of social psychologists who find shared status beliefs to be critical to the creation and maintenance of stratification because of the presupposed link between status and competence.[46] They also confirm the worst fears of Young, a British sociologist who published a satirical but cautionary monograph entitled *The Rise of the Meritocracy* in 1958. Referring to the book, Karabel notes:

> Perhaps worst of all, from Young's perspective, was the effect that meritocratic competition had on winners and losers alike. In the meritocracy, Young writes, "the upper classes are . . . no longer weakened by self-doubt and self-criticism," for "the eminent know that success is just reward for their own capacity, for their own efforts, and for their undeniable achievement. . . . As for the lower classes," they "know that they have had every chance" and have little choice but to recognize that their inferior status is due not as in the past to denial of opportunity, but to their own deficiencies.[47]

While Karabel was concerned with admission to elite colleges and Young was referring to a futuristic dystopian society, they might as well have been writing about the modern US medical profession. The myth of meritocracy in medicine, which emphasizes effort and achievement over structural inequality, helps grease the wheels of status separation between USMDs and non-USMDs, creating an entitled upper class of Navy SEALs and a humble underclass of National Guard members within the same specialty.

Conclusions and Implications

Elites are elites not because of who they are, but because of who they are in relation to other social actors and institutions. Elites are made.

—Shamus Khan, *Privilege*

T his book started out with a puzzle. How can the US medical profession rely so heavily on international and osteopathic graduates to fill undesirable health care positions without creating added competition for graduates of US allopathic medical schools (USMDs)? Put differently, how does the profession systematically ensure that non-USMDs end up training in places like Legacy Community Hospital and USMDs in places like Stonewood University Hospital without giving formal priority to US-trained graduates or even US citizens?

In theory, the residency selection process operates on a level playing field, with positions meted out through an "objective," "fair," and "transparent" process that ostensibly rewards the most meritorious among comparatively assessed applicants. Yet to assume that achievement and mobility in the profession are entirely the product of individual talent, hard work, and motivation—as emphasized by many residents and educators—is to overlook the informal structural processes of inequality that systematically advantaged USMDs.

It's not that individual merit didn't matter. Recall that Stonewood leaders could be convinced to consider the odd non-USMD applicant for residency if they scored two standard deviations above the national mean on the US Medical Licensing Examination (USMLE) and provided a ringing endorsement from a known faculty member who could vouch for their superiority over USMD trainees.

Far more systematically, however, I found that USMDs occupy elite positions compared to non-USMDs because USMDs, who are in relatively short supply, often received more help along the way in playing the game to get into medical school, residency, and the stages beyond.

A big difference in support came from the profession itself. USMDs viewed their participation in the profession in contractual terms: what I called the professional *social contract*, such that in return for playing the game successfully—which involved years of hard work, deferred gratification, and significant debt—USMDs would be nearly guaranteed safe passage by the profession through medical school into more or less the career of their choice. This support extended through medical school into residency for USMDs, such that Stonewood residents described themselves as "coddled," while non-USMDs were left to fend for themselves in terms of both their clinical training and their professional development. The result was bifurcated pathways of mobility within the same specialty: one more sponsored, for USMDs—albeit implicitly and unofficially—and the other more isolated, constrained, and contested, for non-USMDs. With fewer resources (and correspondingly lower status), non-USMDs unsurprisingly did not have as much choice about their career trajectories as USMDs, who viewed such *choice* as a cornerstone of the social contract. In fact, keeping "doors open" was a recurrent priority for USMDs, who sometimes felt that the social contract was more of a runaway freight train that trapped them in high-powered trajectories they did not necessarily want but felt obligated to pursue.

For their part, non-USMDs not only had less help playing the game than USMDs but also faced harder rules of the game because of the stigma associated with their pedigree. The former therefore often had to go above and beyond what the latter had to do in order to reach *lower*-status positions, even after residency. By training in lower-resource environments, non-USMDs, in turn, received poorer training and less supervision than USMDs did. The result was a kind of self-fulfilling prophecy, whereby many of the non-USMDs who had been denied opportunities all along because they were widely suspected to be subpar eventually became weaker doctors than USMDs—at least as measured by pass rates on the American Board of Internal Medicine (ABIM) Certification Examinations (Boards) and by fellowship match rates. Thus, a combination of stigma, fewer supports, and eventual differences in achievement—likely the result of structural inequalities in residency training—kept non-USMDs subordinated in status to USMDs.

Yet, despite these widespread sources of structural inequality, residents of all stripes still clung to strong beliefs in agency and meritocracy. These beliefs served to buttress USMDs' claims of superiority while simultaneously giving non-USMDs the illusion that with enough work and dedication, they could overcome the odds. In this way, non-USMDs embraced the game in ways that often served to reproduce, rather than resist, opportunity structures, thereby allowing the current system to perpetuate itself.

A THEORY OF STATUS SEPARATION IN MEDICINE

Decades ago Freidson and others theorized about the vertical restructuring of the medical profession into an elite and a rank and file to account for the way medicine has been able to maintain dominance over its own affairs, despite growing interference from extraprofessional actors.[1] This vertical restratification was predicated on *formal* knowledge-based or role-based divisions of labor within the profession, where the elite would create and enforce scientific and administrative standards among the rank and file, using legitimate authority vested in them by the profession.[2] There is little doubt that a version of such an elite and a rank and file exists today, with clinician-scientists and physician-managers taking on leadership roles in the knowledge and administrative elite. Although the degree of legitimate authority they wield may be questionable (particularly regarding the enforcement of scientific standards),[3] their presence likely contributes to the profession's ability to remain autonomous, despite important threats from *outsiders*: nonphysicians.

But formal vertical stratification does not capture the largely intangible inequality between residents at Stonewood and Legacy. Instead, I argue that informal horizontal stratification also exists in the profession between supposed equals—internal medicine residents—to help protect the profession's elite (USMD) core from *insiders*: i.e., other (non-USMD) physicians.[4] It is this horizontal stratification that allows the United States to import more than a third of its doctors every year from abroad—including some of the world's best and brightest—without posing additional competition for US-trained MDs. These horizontal status inequalities further have the potential to convert themselves into more formal vertical status hierarchies between specialists and general practitioners after graduation, as evidenced by the residents' trajectories after residency. But even among fully trained non-USMD attendings, like Dr. Taylor, whom we met in chapters 5 and 6, there was a sense that their second-class status in the profession never fully disappeared, suggesting that the stigma sustaining horizontal stratification may coexist alongside vertical stratification long after training is complete. Status is "sticky" in this way, with individuals often never fully able to get rid of the association with their former institutions.[5]

To account for these informal dynamics within the profession, I can now more formally develop the concept of status separation, which I defined in the introduction as *the process by which an ostensibly homogenous profession gets differentiated by pedigree into strata, according to their social worth (status)*. Much like separation in chemistry, whereby a mixture of two substances is reduced to its two component parts by external or natural forces (like gravity separating oil and water), there are invisible *social* forces in medicine helping USMDs float to the top and pushing non-USMDs toward the bottom within a single specialty. Meritocracy is widely believed to be the primary force separating out the proverbial cream of the crop, but I have shown that it is not the only, or even the most important, force at play (see figure C.1).

The first driver of status separation in internal medicine is *broader class inequality*. While USMDs were widely viewed as deserving, competent, and morally superior, they also came from more privileged backgrounds and thus had the resources and support they needed to successfully enter medicine in the United States.[6] Once in, they were able to parlay those resources into additional

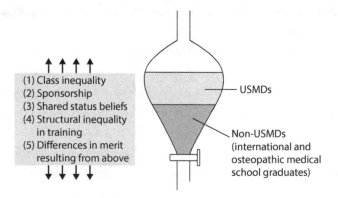

C.1 Status separation among medical residents by pedigree.

Source: "Diagram of a Separatory Funnel" by borb, used under CC BY-SA 3.0/adapted from original. See https://commons.wikimedia.org/wiki/File:SeparatoryFunnel.svg, licensed at https://creativecommons.org /licenses/by-sa/3.0/deed.en.

supports from the profession through the *social contract*, yet another driver of status separation in medicine. The sponsorship inherent in the social contract all but ensured USMDs entry into the medical elite, as I further explain later. Of course, USMD degrees differed in value depending on the medical school attended; a degree from Johns Hopkins University likely opened more doors for residency than, say, a degree from East Tennessee State University. But such differences paled in comparison to the categorical differences in support and opportunity between USMDs and non-USMDs. Non-USMDs mostly came from less-advantaged backgrounds and/or lacked the professional support needed to effectively play the game, thereby putting them at a systematic disadvantage compared to USMDs. Professional status hierarchies in medicine are therefore mired in larger social and even global inequalities.

Status separation is also driven by *strong status beliefs* within medicine. USMDs were widely assumed to be more competent and trustworthy because of their pedigree, helping them accumulate further advantage—a quintessential Matthew effect.[7] In contrast, non-USMDs were widely stigmatized, often regardless of their performance, with their pedigree constituting "a mark of disgrace" that counted against them as applicants to residency and fellowship and even beyond, effectively pushing them down in the profession.[8] The sources of stigma were multiple for these professionals, who comprised a heterogeneous group. Part of the stigma was xenophobic, rooted in assumptions and biases against people from other countries, as was the case with international medical graduates (IMGs), who were widely perceived to be intellectually brilliant but culturally incompetent. Part of the stigma had to do with upholding professional jurisdictions and inferring inferiority on that basis, as was the case with graduates of osteopathic medical schools (DOs), who were broadly viewed as failed MDs. Yet another part of the stigma was the result of biases and assumptions about US students who studied medicine abroad (USIMGs), who were generally pegged as being lazy or as having messed up along the way to a US medical education. While the various kinds of non-USMDs faced stigma from different sources, they had in common a shared experience of being treated as inferior within the profession. Stigma is a well-known mechanism for maintaining inequality between social groups, with more powerful groups subjugating less powerful groups on the basis of their stigma.[9] And those very same power dynamics are what can make stigma notoriously sticky, as we saw was the case for even top-notch non-USMDs at Legacy, like Cody.[10]

Next, stigmatized identities are reinforced by the *hierarchical field of residency programs*, which can represent a kind of "structural stigma," whereby "institutions perpetuate or exacerbate a stigmatized status."[11] Institutional status differences compounded existing prestige differences between USMDs and non-USMDs. Furthermore, institutional competitions over prestige and unequally distributed resources across training programs led to considerable differences in both the quality of training and the amount of support offered to residents. At the same time, through their recruitment practices and interactions with the housestaff, these institutions helped promote the widespread misidentification of structural advantages and disadvantages as differences in individual merit between USMDs and non-USMDs. This was even true at Legacy, where residents were constantly told that their success was a function of their own individual efforts even though that success was significantly constrained by institutional deficiencies.

And, finally, *differences in achievement and merit* helped distinguish USMDs from non-USMDs. But rather than being the straightforward product of individual variation, merit and achievement were tangled up with unequal life chances, very different opportunity structures, and dissimilar experiences with stigma and discrimination, leading to unequal outcomes. Put simply, the current structure of graduate medical education is designed to give USMDs a better education, making it unsurprising when they do better than non-USMDs on their Boards or outpace them in fellowship matches. Structural advantage and achievement therefore go hand in hand, muddling the distinction between merit and privilege.

Status Separation Ensures USMD Dominance

The skeptical reader might rightfully point out that a term already exists that describes polarization within the workforce: *segmentation*. Labor market segmentation theory emerged as a critique of neoclassical economists' portrayal of labor markets as unified when, in fact, there is at least an inner core (or primary market) characterized by highly stable workers and an outer periphery (or secondary market) composed of highly contingent workers.[12] The theory even accounts for segmentation *within* the primary sector, which perhaps more accurately describes what is going on in medicine right now. The theory becomes less useful, however, when explaining *why* segmentation—or what I call *separation*—is happening within the primary sector of medicine. As an economic theory, labor market segmentation is thought to protect capitalist hegemony by blocking opportunities for resistance within the labor force; in other words, it benefits *employers* rather than employees.[13] However, there is little evidence to suggest that capitalism is the primary driver of status inequalities within internal medicine. Instead, I have argued that status separation enables the profession to rely on an oversized pool of lower-status workers (which it can draw on as it pleases) and thus to shelter the upper echelons of the professional labor queue from larger fluctuations in the market related to supply and demand.[14] In this way, USMDs can continue to fill the most prestigious residency positions while relying on non-USMDs to fill gaps in lower-status areas such as primary care. Status separation therefore benefits an elite portion of the professionals themselves, who may (even unconsciously) be working to exacerbate and uphold horizontal separations in status to maximize rewards.

Importantly, status separation is widely taken for granted within medicine. The sorting of medical graduates on the basis of their medical school of origin has become a kind of standard operating procedure, to the point where Match statistics—even for postresidency fellowship positions—are reported along USMD/non-USMD lines.[15] Status separation is the process that leads to these taken-for-granted outcomes. Being taken for granted, however, should not be confused with being self-evident. Under the guise of unfettered meritocracy, USMDs broadly differentiate themselves as being better than non-USMDs when, in fact, the game is structurally designed to favor USMDs, sometimes *regardless* of their performance. Recall in chapter 1 that Greg, a USMD who failed his USMLE Step 1 exam, managed to secure a residency position at Stonewood anyway or in chapter 4 that problem residents at Stonewood were never allowed to "fall down." Meritocracy therefore serves as a well-worn cover for other social forces that contribute to status separation: namely, social reproduction, cumulative advantage, and sponsored mobility. As Young, the author of *The Rise of the Meritocracy*, has lamented, "It is good sense to appoint individual people to jobs on their merit. It is the opposite when those who are judged to have merit of a particular kind *harden into a new social class without room in it for others*" (emphasis added).[16] USMDs, who are more privileged from the outset, seem to have hardened into a social class of elites in medicine that prioritizes its own and allows very few others to join.[17] The uncomfortable reality is that if medicine operated as a true meritocracy, USMDs would have to make room for outsiders—an outcome that would likely threaten their dominance within the profession.[18]

USMD Dominance and the Social Contract

Ensuring USMD dominance is not merely a preference for the US medical profession—it is an imperative, I argue, given the current terms of the social contract with its trainees. USMDs have come to expect their choice of elite careers, both through a set of internalized expectations and through a series of promises made to them by their mentors, as described in previous chapters. Keeping USMD numbers low and relying on non-USMDs who are separated in status from USMDs help make this possible. As three USMD physicians advocating for the continued reliance on non-USMDs in US medicine recently opined:

> A cultural individualism resists being told where one can live and work. A sense of entitlement to "the good life" exists for students who have invested so much time and treasure into their education. A job market restricted to the less desirable areas could undermine the attractiveness of certain specialties and medicine in general. A concern that must be entertained is that greater numbers of US medical students could make admission less competitive as the supply of and demand for medical school admission slots come into greater balance.[19]

Tellingly, these writers explicitly make the case that IMGs help keep medicine appealing to Americans. In the absence of formalized policies prioritizing USMDs for residency, status separation allows a carefully controlled number of USMDs to have the life they have come to expect from the profession—a satisfying career, freedom of choice over geography and specialty, and an enviable living wage.[20] In this way, USMDs rely not only on non-USMDs to fill undesirable positions but also on non-USMDs' *subjugation in status* to fulfill their own dreams of greatness. Without status separation, USMDs would ostensibly compete with top-notch non-USMDs for elite positions, which would mean medicine could not consistently deliver on its promises to trainees. The profession, in turn, would run the risk of becoming less attractive to the next generation of young, brilliant minds. USMDs would have to fill positions in geographically and professionally undesirable areas and potentially embark on careers to which they did not aspire. Worse still, if the United States produced even a slight surplus of physicians, some USMDs might be left with no medical career at all. As the authors of an Institute of Medicine report warned, "In the event of a surplus, the time and money such prospective [USMD] medical students will have to spend on education and training may be a poor personal investment."[21] Status separation, when combined with efforts to keep USMDs sufficiently scarce, helps ensure that USMDs are unrestricted in their opportunities, making medicine still seem like a worthwhile investment.

To ensure that they meet USMDs' expectations, those in the medical profession still selectively rely on informal processes of sponsored mobility, where "upward mobility is like entry into a private club where each candidate must be 'sponsored' by one or more of the members."[22] In this case, the chosen few who gain entry into a US allopathic medical school (most of whom were already socially privileged) get sponsored into the medical elite by USMD mentors and leaders who preside over elite training programs. Back in 1948, Hall described how medical students entered the "inner fraternity" via informal sponsorship arrangements with elites:

> The sponsored protégé must be assisted and vouched for at each step in his career. This involves active intervention in his career by the established practitioner who has sponsored him. In some of the cases studied the encouragement originated long before the person went to medical school, then, later, in the form of aiding him over the crisis of securing a superior appointment as intern; it continued as the young doctor climbed up in the hierarchy of institutional positions, and was evidenced by the referral of patients by the sponsoring doctor.[23]

Hall could well have been writing about USMDs in the present day. I have presented concrete evidence that such sponsorship persists in the medical profession, despite its apparent demise in the 1950s with the advent of the national Match algorithm, which promises a "fair . . . [and] transparent" process, apparently leveling the playing field for all residency applicants.[24] It also continues despite efforts to standardize methods of admission into the profession dating back more than one hundred years to the Flexner Report, published in 1910.[25] As Marshall and colleagues found in 1978 in their study of how medical students get distributed into elite versus nonelite specialties, there is an informal "parallel order" that exists alongside the "formal [meritocratic] system" of medical education and that funnels certain students into the medical elite and others into the rank and file.[26] I find there to be a similar parallel order at play *within* specialties according to medical pedigree. These results echo similar processes between male and female physicians that Lorber identified in the 1980s when she argued that gender inequality is maintained through "sponsorship and patronage, and the tendency to offer opportunities for advancement to those most similar in background to the members of already established inner circles."[27] Put together, the sociological evidence is clear: elite status in medicine, so promised through the social contract, continues to be transmitted informally through sponsored mobility, even as the profession makes formal pledges to meritocracy, fairness, and inclusiveness.

The Informal Nature of Status Hierarchies Helps Ensure Their Reproduction

A key question is, How does this informal system of status separation sustain itself? After all, the social contract, to be tenable, requires not only buy-in from USMDs but also at least the passive consent of those it subordinates. Otherwise, the profession could have a revolt on its hands, with non-USMDs demanding equal treatment for equal credentials.

I argue that it is precisely by virtue of being *informal* that status distinctions between putative equals persist so robustly. As Karabel writes about admissions to elite universities, "The apparent openness of the system . . . gives credence to the American dream of upward mobility through education."[28] In the same way, the apparent openness of the system in medicine allows for the *belief*—however unsupported by the evidence—that ascension to the elite is, in fact, possible for anyone, regardless of pedigree. If there were policies prioritizing USMDs, it is unlikely that non-USMDs would subscribe so strongly to the notion that USMDs are better. Some non-USMDs might even reconsider applying to the United States for residency altogether, knowing that certain positions were explicitly off-limits to them, leaving the United States with an even worse doctor shortage. It could even have a ripple effect both locally and internationally, as US citizens interested in osteopathic or international medical training could be dissuaded from going to medical school altogether to avoid being at a formal disadvantage for certain positions compared to USMDs. Indeed, it is because restrictions were more informal and based on status rather than decreed by policy that the DOs, USIMGs, and IMGs in internal medicine at Legacy could (and did) aspire to match in orthopedics, anesthesia, and surgery—and when they did not succeed in those areas, they tended to blame themselves rather than the situation, thus aiding its reproduction.[29]

As I previously mentioned, implicit in this belief is the notion that USMDs worked harder for longer and are were more meritorious and deserving of their higher status. Khan writes about how the privileged increasingly espouse similar myths to account for their successes and to make the argument that anybody can reach their level of attainment with the right amount of work.[30] It is on this unproven belief that the social contract hinges: with enough work, one will get their just reward. By believing that USMDs were more deserving of top positions, non-USMDs consented to their subordination in the profession. Thus, by relying on informal status distinctions, rather than top-down formal policies, to prioritize USMDs, the profession secures the consent of the very non-USMDs whom it subordinates through status separation.[31]

IMPLICATIONS FOR MEDICINE

What Is Valued by the Profession May Not Translate Into the Best Doctors

My findings raise several implications for medicine. First, by sustaining the social contract and prioritizing medical pedigree in residency, the profession may not be recruiting the best candidates. While the definition of what constitutes a "good" doctor is up for debate, current selection processes may be excluding excellent physicians simply because of their pedigree or because of broader structural inequalities, such as class disparities. Given the current rules of the game, potential applicants often require years of advanced preparation to check off all the boxes to get into a US allopathic medical school; thus, it is little wonder that minorities continue to be grossly underrepresented within medicine, despite pressure on medical schools to diversify their ranks.[32] Physicians ought to question whether the processes of entry into the profession are equitable and whether they, in fact, yield the best results.

Another consequence of the social contract is that it may keep inadequate members in the profession longer than it should. The same social processes that give USMDs priority also ensure that once they enter the profession, there is little turning back. It is exceedingly rare to leave the profession during medical school or residency, which raises larger questions about how—or indeed whether—substandard physicians ever get filtered out. As noted in chapter 4, the fact that the profession closes ranks to protect its weakest links, so as not to "threaten the myth of elite omniscience," is a classic feature of sponsored mobility.[33] Even disciplinary action is notoriously rare among physicians. Studies find that the likelihood of being disciplined as an attending physician is linked to prior behavior during medical school, suggesting that early signs of trouble should be taken seriously.[34] More research is therefore needed on the long-term impacts of the social contract on the profession's self-governing abilities.

Relatedly, and perhaps more disconcertingly, the current system of medical education—which seems designed to maximize rewards for USMDs—may not yield the best results for society. Expanding on a quote in chapter 6 from a senior official from Stonewood University Medical School, "There's no public mandate to educate students to fulfill a specific need. . . . Most [US] medical students go to medical school thinking the desired outcome here is for me to have the most gratifying career I can have." But *should* medicine's larger priority be to fulfill physicians' expectations (i.e., fulfill the social contract), or should it be to satisfy the public need? Currently, "winning the game" in medicine often involves lucrative hyperspecialization, which has only worsened the country's shortage of primary care physicians. This is not a new concern, as scholars have been arguing for decades that medical education should be less inwardly focused and more concerned with the public interest.[35] The latest estimates, however, project shortfalls in primary care by 2032 ranging between 21,100 and 55,200 physicians—more than in any other specialty.[36] Of course, the profession largely relies on non-USMDs to help fill this gap, but is it fair or even desirable to saddle already marginalized members of the profession with this important work? And if so, what are the consequences of doing so?

The results presented in this book suggest that redressing the gap in primary care would ultimately require a fundamental shift in the bargain inherent to US medical education, which privileges subspecialty as the ultimate reward for USMDs' investment in the social contract. This could begin to happen if higher reimbursements were accorded to primary care or if the cost of medical school was reduced to lighten the debt burden on USMDs. In fact, several USMD schools have begun waiving tuition precisely in hopes of attracting more students to primary care specialties.[37] However, these arguably superficial modifications still will not change the early social origins of stratification in the medical profession, and they will not significantly equalize opportunities for non-USMDs, given that social beliefs surrounding merit would remain unchanged. Ultimately, the profession needs to do a better job of balancing its social contracts with society and with its trainees, as the two seem currently to be at odds with each other.

Physician Satisfaction

Paradoxically, for all the profession's efforts to hold up its end of the bargain and meet USMDs' expectations of high-status jobs upon graduation, the lower-status non-USMDs at Legacy expressed more satisfaction with their careers than the USMDs at Stonewood did. Studies have found that IMGs have higher personal growth scores than USMDs and lower rates of burnout, suggesting that, despite the obstacles they face, non-USMDs still thrive.[38] Perhaps Legacy residents' relative happiness was related to the fact that many of them were just happy to have jobs, as described in chapter 6. They may also have been more intrinsically motivated by medicine than some USMDs because they stuck with it despite considerable adversity.[39] As one Legacy intern said about his Caribbean training, "At the end, if you're left standing, you're there [because] you really want it." Alternatively, perhaps that same adversity helped temper non-USMDs' expectations, making them more content with fewer opportunities for career mobility.

In contrast, disillusionment smoldered among USMDs at Stonewood. Despite their relative advantages, several residents said they would advise people against entering the profession (see chapter 5). Many of them had received similar advice before pursuing medical training and were now echoing these sentiments themselves. Some regretted the debt, calling medical school a "$1 Million Mistake," while others bemoaned the loss of respect that physicians used to enjoy. As the game requires ever more from medical school applicants, it may be increasingly impossible for the profession to fully return that investment. These findings are on par with national trends: a 2012 survey found that 33.5 percent of doctors would choose a different career if they could go back in time (up from 27 percent in 2008) and that 57.9 percent would not recommend medicine as a career to their children.[40] Reasons for dissatisfaction include growing time pressures, excessive workload, erosion of the doctor-patient relationship, and decreasing reimbursements.[41] Some cope by choosing early retirement and/or cutting back patient hours, leaving the profession even more strapped for workers and worsening problems of access.[42] The profession will have to closely examine its priorities in the coming years as the shortage of doctors grows. Should the stakes remain so high to gain admission to US allopathic medical school in order to keep USMDs' numbers low and their value at a premium? Doing so has not kept the profession impervious to disillusionment. Or should it find new metrics of assessing merit and worth, potentially prioritizing those with less attractive pedigrees but higher levels of intrinsic motivation?

The Impact of Segregation and Disparities in Residency Training

Maintaining segregation along pedigree lines may not even be in the profession's best interest, despite ensuring USMD dominance. There are numerous benefits to having a diverse health care workforce, including enhanced cultural competence, improved access to care for the underserved, wider research agendas, and enhanced diversity in related workforces, such as among medical policy makers.[43] IMGs, in particular, bring much-needed diversity to training programs,[44] as well as their unique skills, such as advanced clinical experience,[45] which can be useful in teaching USMDs. At the same time, non-USMDs also experience unique professional challenges that could be mitigated by working alongside USMDs instead of in isolation from them.[46]

Segregation also has clear implications for differential treatment of trainees within the profession.[47] Like others, I found that USMDs, including the preliminary interns at Legacy, thought more highly of non-USMDs if they had experience working with them.[48] Desegregating residency programs or at least promoting more mixing between resident types could thus teach USMDs to be less biased against non-USMDs, who comprise a growing percentage of the workforce. One study found that biases against IMGs made USMD generalists less likely to refer patients to IMG specialists, which could lead to suboptimal referral decisions, especially if the IMG specialist is more qualified than the USMD specialist.[49] By working together, USMDs and non-USMDs would have the opportunity to revise their stereotypes and potentially minimize status differences between the two groups to the benefit of patients.[50] The Single Accreditation System, in effect in 2020, means that residency programs will no longer be separately accredited by either the Accreditation Council for Graduate Medical Education (ACGME) or the American Osteopathic Association. The effect that this new system has, if any, on MD-DO status relations in the profession remains to be seen.

In addition to desegregating residency programs, the medical profession needs to address worrisome disparities between training sites. For all the emphasis on standardization in residency training, training is not necessarily equal among all programs. My findings show systematic differences in the exposure and education offered to Legacy residents compared to those at Stonewood and invite further study into the benefits and drawbacks of these approaches for both clinicians and patients. In a separate study using national-level data, I find that USMD-dominated programs have higher ABIM Board pass rates, suggesting that educational experiences differ systematically between segregated settings in ways that have tangible impacts on graduates' careers.[51] Non-USMDs are also more likely to go on to staff underserved and more remote areas with low-socioeconomic-status populations, which could mean that differences in training could exacerbate social inequalities in health.[52] At the same time, studies dating back to the 1980s find no evidence that fully trained non-USMDs have worse patient outcomes compared to USMDs. This could suggest that any differences in the training they receive may not have long-lasting consequences for patients, even if these differences matter for residents' professional mobility.[53] Further research is therefore needed to parse whether and how inequalities among trainees (and their training environments) impact patient care. Research in the field of professions is exploring precisely this question by examining how professional inequalities can impact broader social inequalities, such as how marginalized fields of medicine, like complementary and alternative therapies, are relegated to the private sector, thereby making it difficult for certain segments of the population to access them.[54]

Another question to consider is, Why are such stark disparities among training programs even tolerated within the profession? After all, these are the exact differences in quality that physicians have been trying to eliminate since the Flexner Report appeared in 1910—in part to help maintain medicine's autonomy.[55] Their persistence may have to do with the very nature of standardization in medicine, which appears to be more symbolic than concrete. Indeed, it is not clear whether hospitals like Legacy would even violate current standards, given their symbolic compliance with the profession's guidelines.[56] For example, Legacy was affiliated on paper with a medical school, which helped keep the program in good standing with the ACGME. But simply having that affiliation did little to reduce training disparities between Legacy and Stonewood, especially because Legacy residents couldn't even access the medical school's electronic library resources. In this way, it may be that the *appearance* of standardized medical education is more important than actual standardization, at least for maintaining professional autonomy.

These findings also remind us that artifacts of standardization, like Board exams and program accreditation, should not be confused with indicators of *equality* in medical education.[57]

A final reason why variation among programs persists is likely pragmatic. The country needs doctors, hospitals like Legacy need workers, and non-USMDs are willing to take the jobs. There is little incentive to dismantle a system that fills such an important need on so many levels. We could question whether it is medically, and indeed ethically, responsible to exploit residents primarily for their labor, as appeared to be the case at Legacy.[58] But when I asked Trevor—the USIMG who studied medicine in Southeast Asia and referred to himself as a foreigner—what he thought, he said with a shrug, "You know, whether it's fair or not it's almost irrelevant because if you're coming here, you have to play by the, I don't want to say play by the rules, but it is what it is. You've got lemons? You got to make lemonade. You can't cry about not having fruit punch or whatever." In this way, unless the rules of the game, the social contract, or the readiness of non-USMDs like Trevor to take on positions in places like Legacy somehow changes, medicine will likely continue to rely on non-USMDs to fill jobs USMDs don't want.

LESSONS FOR OTHER PROFESSIONS

Medicine is not the only profession where status distinctions are drawn between putative equals according to educational pedigree. Currently, an underclass of attorneys is proliferating under a pretext of meritocracy when, in fact, elite reproduction in legal education is the product of very similar processes of cumulative advantage, class inequality, and misrecognized privilege.[59] Academia is another example. There is an oversupply of highly qualified PhDs (horizontal hierarchies) vying for an ever-smaller number of tenure-track positions, resulting in the expansion of contingent faculty (vertical hierarchies) without whom the tenure-track elite could not exist.[60] Graduates from top-tier institutions have less difficulty finding tenure-track jobs, while many graduates from second- or third-tier institutions end up having to take adjunct positions and live as "second-class citizens" if they remain in the profession at all.[61] Top-tier graduates also tend to have access to more resources during their training (such as fellowships), which often makes these candidates more competitive in the job market, while lower-tier graduates not only have fewer resources but also have to overcome the stigma associated with their degree when applying for jobs. In other words, like non-USMDs, they must do more with less to gain access to the least desirable positions in the academy. Academics even share similar beliefs in the ability of hard work and dedication to unlock the doors to success.[62] Thus, in academia, just like in medicine, assumptions about effort, privilege, and pedigree become entangled with notions of merit, thereby justifying and perpetuating systemic inequality across the profession. Future research should explore the parallels between medicine and professions like academia to further develop a more generalized theory of status separation among budding professionals.

While extensions to other professions are useful, it is also important to highlight the ways that medicine remains a profession apart. There continues to be a massive shortage of physicians, which helps ensure that even though non-USMDs are subordinated in status and fill less desirable positions, they still get to practice as fully licensed physicians with enviable job security. That's not true of many professions, where a surplus of talent has pushed many practitioners out of the profession altogether, creating an altogether different social contract between the profession and its members. Medicine also has yet to see some of the overt proletarianization that has occurred in other professions, as when lawyers are paid by the hour to do menial contract work and adjuncts are paid paltry sums by the course to replace a dwindling number of tenure-track faculty.[63] Instead, in medicine more than in other sectors, there is a growing reliance on paraprofessionals (like nurse practitioners and physician assistants) to take on the tasks physicians find more mundane rather than a movement toward hiring physicians to do contingent work per se.[64] Few professions also have the equivalent of residency training as an intermediate step between professional education and autonomous practice, with all the standardized testing that accompanies it, making comparisons between applicants for residency ostensibly more feasible than in other fields. Still, the findings herein may provide a useful starting point for understanding informal processes of internal stratification within professions more broadly.

Afterword

On February 12, 2020, the United States Medical Licensing Exam (USMLE) parent organizations (the Federation of State Medical Boards, FSMB, and the National Board of Medical Examiners, NBME) approved a major change in the USMLE Step 1 exam. The professional bodies have agreed to go from a three-digit score to making the exam pass/fail, effective January 1, 2022.[1] The decision was reached after a long consultative process initiated by the FSMB, NBME, and other professional bodies such as the American Medical Association, the Association of American Medical Colleges, and the Educational Commission for Foreign Medical Graduates to assess whether changes should be made to Step 1. To that end, they invited key stakeholders from graduate and undergraduate medical education institutions, state medical boards, medical students, and the public to a conference in March 2019 to discuss the relative benefits of numeric scoring options versus pass/fail scoring. In the end, they decided to make Step 1 pass/fail, but to keep the three-digit score for the Clinical Knowledge portion of Step 2 (CK).

IMPLICATIONS

What are we to make of this important change to the way trainees are being licensed?

Let me begin by first addressing the potential implications for non-USMDs. A three-digit Step 1 score undoubtedly contributed to the illusion that acceptance to residency was at least somewhat meritocratic—an illusion I spend much of this book critiquing. At the same time, for a small handful of non-USMDs, an astronomically high Step 1 score *could* help set them apart. Recall that one Stonewood leader said, "We don't automatically reject people. You know if someone [a non-USMD] is at the top of their class and has done 270s on Step 1 and 2, and . . . we know the people they've done an elective with and they say this kid is better than any American grad I've ever seen, we'll pay attention to that" (p. 97, this volume). Making Step 1 pass/fail could therefore restrict that (small but existent) pathway to competitive residencies for some non-USMDs and would likely place more emphasis on informal resources, such as social network ties to USMD attendings, which are more difficult for non-USMDs to come by, as I have argued herein.

Let us also not forget that the USMD residents in internal medicine at Stonewood already largely viewed Step 1 as a pass/fail proposition (see p. 46, this volume). According to the NRMP, scoring the passing grade on Step One is associated with an 80 percent probability of matching to internal medicine as a preferred specialty for USMDs.[2] (By comparison, for the same score among international and osteopathic medical graduates, the probability drops to 15 percent). With Step 1 becoming pass/fail, residency programs may be even more inclined to recruit lower-performing USMDs who might have otherwise been eliminated by their scores, over high-performing non-USMDs. Thus here again, the consequences of making Step 1 pass/fail may be felt much more strongly among non-USMD applicants, who will have to work to find new ways of getting noticed.

Of course, Step 2 Clinical Knowledge (CK)—which is not currently required by all residency programs prior to applying—might very well replace Step 1 as the main determinant of residency positions, leaving open a small window of opportunity for non-USMDs to outshine their USMD counterparts. But instead of two data points (and two opportunities for non-USMDs to shine), there would be only one exam for program directors to consider, meaning it could all ride on Step 2 CK for non-USMDs hoping to break into competitive residencies. Instead of being able to see growth and development between Steps, program directors would rely on a single standardized measure of competence. And if Step 2 CK does not become mandatory for all residency applicants, it is very likely that old and new signals of "ability" and "fit" will simply grow in importance—making things like medical school of origin, research experience, and honor society membership all the more important during recruitment, clearly favoring USMDs over non-USMDs. There may also be consequences for minority USMDs for the same reasons; in fact, there is an important sociological literature on how recruitment decisions based on "fit" often reproduce broader social inequalities along the lines of class, race, and gender.[3]

In terms of implications for USMDs, at least on the surface, there may be some tangible benefits to their mental health, as several studies have identified Step 1 as a specific determinant of USMD student burnout.[4] Because the exam is such an important determinant of matching to especially competitive fields—such as dermatology and orthopedic surgery—the stress surrounding Step 1 has led to significant mental illness among some test-takers. This anxiety, in fact, was a primary reason behind the decision to make Step 1 pass/fail.[5] Another reason had to do with the "parallel curriculum" that has emerged in medical schools surrounding the test. Students would rather invest considerable time and energy into acing this career-altering exam than focusing on other relevant subject matter, such as medical ethics or social determinants of health, which are often considered "low yield" topics because they are not on the test.[6] Making Step 1 pass/fail has therefore undoubtedly led many current and future medical students to breathe a collective sigh of relief as their dreams of matching no longer ride on a single, nail-biting eight-hour exam.

But that momentary relief was no doubt quickly followed by a more daunting uncertainty—if it is no longer Step 1 that determines how the most competitive residencies are meted out, then what will? Again, one obvious answer is Step 2 CK. As Step 2 CK becomes more relevant in the residency selection process, it is possible that it simply replaces Step 1 as the primary determinant of residency selection—and as the new stressor making medical students sick. And whatever currently constitutes high-yield topics will likely just shift from whatever is on Step 1 to whatever is on Step 2. For these reasons, making Step 1 pass/fail may not have the intended health and educational benefits that decision-makers hope.

MEANINGFUL CHANGE IN LIGHT OF ENDURING SOCIAL NORMS

Some members of the profession are hopeful that making Step 1 pass/fail will help encourage program directors to assess applications more holistically, rather than relying on a single three-digit score to cull applicants.[7] But making Step 1 pass/fail will only help increase the holistic review of applications if it is accompanied by sweeping changes in the professional norms and status beliefs surrounding non-USMDs. Programs still view it as a "badge of honor" to recruit exclusively USMDs. Changing Step 1 to pass/fail may only worsen this segregation, as programs will have less information about candidates' abilities and may be more inclined to worry about their reputations since they will not be able to plausibly justify the recruitment of non-USMDs as being due to astronomically high Step 1 scores.

If we really want to reduce stress and improve inequality between applicants, making Step 1 pass/fail is only an anodyne. To really help level the playing field, program directors could review applications blindly (without knowing the applicants' medical school of origin) and compare USMDs and non-USMDs "numbers to numbers," as one USIMG respondent put it (p. 97). That would, of course, require keeping Step 1 as a three-digit score—or perhaps, developing a new metric actually designed to measure applicants' suitability to residency instead of Step 1, which was designed to signal minimum proficiency for licensure.[8] Another approach could be to titrate recruitment to reflect the broader residency workforce, with American-trained allopathic physicians filling around 60 percent of residency positions nationwide. As for reducing stress among prospective residents, making Step 1 pass/fail does not address the broader hidden curriculum that paints some specialties as more desirable than others, nor does it attenuate the culture of having to constantly outperform one's peers in medicine; instead, it simply makes space for new markers of distinction for students to obsess over. In sum, to really tackle these critical problems will require far more wide-reaching, structural change in medicine than any one test can provide.

APPENDIX

On Being a "Second-Year Intern"

GETTING IN

To understand how and why the Legacy Community Hospital and Stonewood University Hospital residency programs became so segregated and how such segregation affected the lives of physicians-in-training, I needed to be there, on the hospital floor, examining the process as it unfolded. But, first, I had to negotiate access. I initially started fieldwork at Legacy through a class project. In retrospect, that fact probably helped me get over the initial hurdle of getting in because to gatekeepers I was a relatively harmless—if somewhat eager—graduate student whose time in the field was (initially) limited to the duration of the course. At the end of two months, however, I had begun to conceptualize the broader project, and because the housestaff and hospital leadership already knew me, they didn't mind letting me come back to do additional observations over the next two years. Toward the end of my time at Legacy, I had become such a fixture in the hospital that some fondly referred to me as a "second-year intern"—a play on words because interns, by definition, are first-year residents.

Gaining access to Stonewood, however, was far more challenging. In November 2012, I met with a high-ranking official at the Stonewood University Medical School who seemed interested in the project and vowed to help me gain access. Despite the official's best intentions, however, it proved difficult to convince the program directors at Stonewood University Hospital to allow me the kind of access I was requesting—namely, the ability to observe on rounds and interview residents as I had at Legacy. One program official told me that I would need to get approvals from no fewer than six different department heads, which was unlikely: "You're going to hear all about people's dirty laundry!" the official said while shaking their head. In January 2013, I met with the director of graduate medical education in charge of all the residency programs at Stonewood University Hospital. The director relayed concerns from the program directors about how overworked the residents were and how my presence might add to their already overloaded schedules. The director then urged me to consider Solomon Hospital, a community hospital affiliated with Stonewood University, as a less hectic alternative. Solomon, however, was not an appropriate case because it represented another hospital with mostly osteopathic medical graduates (DOs) and international medical graduates (IMGs); in other words, it was "DO- and IMG-friendly" like Legacy. I began to despair; Stonewood was the obvious comparison, and I was not making headway with access.

After five months of trying unsuccessfully to get into Stonewood University Hospital, I was contacted for a meeting with a high-ranking Stonewood official. To this day, I'm not fully certain what suddenly prompted the meeting; I'd been trying to meet with this official for months to no avail. During the meeting, the official explained that rounds were already saturated with too many people and reiterated concerns about duty hours. They didn't want an outsider disturbing the "sanctity of the rounds." For these reasons, the official could not allow me to interview or observe the residents while they were on the wards. However, they did offer me the opportunity to conduct focus groups with residents during their ambulatory block months (rotations during which residents spent time in didactic lectures and in clinic)—something the official would later admit to me was "just something I came up with on the spot." They also added that perhaps I could observe rounds a couple of times just to "color in some of the black and white." It was a foot in the door, and I accepted the offer eagerly.

A few months, and two rounds of tuberculosis testing later, I was credentialed at Stonewood as an intern (the way one might be an intern at Google) to lead the focus group discussions.[1] At the same time, I asked the high-ranking official if I could begin observing rounds before starting the focus groups, so I could get a sense of the context and players. The official agreed, as long as I tagged along with their team so as not to bother other attendings. By the end of the week—the agreed-upon duration of my observations—I met with the official to ask for another week or two of observing. The official paused for a moment and replied that they couldn't see why not: "The problem is, you on your own, you're fine. You're part of the team and you're not in the way. It's that these teams are so huge as it is." The official was right; my team that day had eight people in it. After that conversation, I had the implicit trust of this official, as well as the program's permission to observe and interview the housestaff as long as I remained unobtrusive.

As time went on and trust was established, my access at Stonewood expanded to the point where little was off-limits. The process unfolded slowly. First, program leaders would invite me to events by saying things like "You are welcome to attend, as with anything." Then, through conversations with the chief residents, I was invited to give a morning report lecture on the sociology of diagnosis. Regarding that lecture, the same high-ranking official who initially granted me access told me, "You know, when someone lets you drive their Ferrari, that's a real sign that they trust you," referring to the fact that morning report was the chiefs' responsibility, so they must have really trusted me to let me lecture. Eventually, through interviews with the teaching attendings, I learned about the Resident Selection Committee meetings at which the faculty discussed candidates. One attending offered to speak to the program director about granting me access to the meetings. When I eventually worked up the nerve to ask for permission, it was granted. Finally, toward the end of the fieldwork, I was invited by the chief residents (with permission from the leadership) to attend the Monday noon meetings, where the Clinical Competency Committee discussed residents' progress. These highly confidential meetings were sometimes restricted to the program directors, but I was still allowed to sit in and take notes. By the end of six months, I had managed to secure complete access to Stonewood, where only a year before, I was concerned that I might not even have a comparison case.

THE DATA

Table A.1 provides an overview of the methods I utilized in this study. The study received IRB approval.

Participant Observation

I spent twenty-three months over the course of three years observing daily life in these two residency programs. That usually meant arriving by 7:30 AM and accompanying teams of interns and residents as they treated patients, went on rounds, attended didactic sessions (e.g., noon conference, morning report, and

TABLE A.1 Overview of Methods

	Legacy Community Hospital	Stonewood University Hospital	Total
Date/frequency of fieldwork	• 2011–2012 (1 session per week); • 2012–2013 (3 sessions per week) 17 months total	• 2013–2014 (3 sessions per week) 6 months total	23 months in the field between 2011 and 2014
Method			
Participant observation	• 723 hours, 97 observation sessions • 20 different internal medicine teams	• 507 hours, 85 observation sessions • 11 different internal medicine teams	1,230 hours, 182 observation sessions 31 different internal medicine teams
In-depth interviewing	53 interviews	70 interviews	123 interviews
Focus groups	N/A	9 focus groups with a total of 37 individuals	9 focus groups

grand rounds), and admitted new patients. Wherever they went, I went; I even accompanied them during whatever leisure time they had during the day. I also asked brief but timely questions "on the fly" to clarify observations and gauge reactions to events.[2] While I was mostly there during normal daytime hours, I made a point of varying the time of my observations, such that I often spent twelve or more hours per day at Legacy during on-call days (even spending the night there once to observe the night shift) and arrived early in the morning at Stonewood to observe interns before rounds. I also varied the days of week I observed. These variations allowed me to get the broadest sense possible of what life was like in both settings, as certain events (like grand rounds) occurred only on certain days (see the section on "The Analysis" for more on the scheduling of fieldwork).

I spent more than 720 hours over the course of ninety-seven discrete observation sessions at Legacy between 2011 and 2013. In that time, I observed twenty different intern-resident pairs for five to sixteen hours per day between one and three times per week for up to four weeks at a time. I tried to work with as many residents as possible, such that by the end of the two years, I had observed thirty-five residents working with six medical students, three chief residents, and half a dozen teaching attendings. During the last eight months at Legacy, when my observations were more intense, I made a point of spending short and long call (until 6:00 and 9:00 PM, respectively) with my team, such that I averaged between thirty and forty hours per week at Legacy. I also had ample time for informal interactions with the housestaff, such as during morning coffee breaks in the cafeteria or in the car when residents generously offered to give me rides home.

At Stonewood, I spent more than five hundred hours over eighty-five observation sessions spanning six months. Although I spent fewer months overall at Stonewood, my observations were more intensive. It also helped that there were many things I had learned at Legacy that I did not need to relearn at Stonewood, such as basic medical jargon and the overall structure of internal medicine training. From October 2013 to March 2014, I spent three days per week, for two weeks at a time, observing a total of twelve different internal medicine teams on the teaching service. I would arrive before morning report to introduce myself to the patients and get their permission to observe while the medical team examined them later that morning (an IRB requirement). I would then attend morning report and join my team at 9 AM for rounds, which typically lasted between two to three hours. In the afternoons, I variously spent time doing more observations or interviewing residents. I was also invited to observe program meetings, such as the Resident Selection Committee meetings. Over the course of the six months, I observed a total of forty-two residents, working with nine attendings or program officials and five chief residents. I also observed their interactions with ten medical and pharmacy students and nurse managers.

Throughout my fieldwork, I continuously looked for ways to stay inconspicuous. This often meant trying to stay out of the way, especially when around patients. I was adamant about not interfering with the residents' work—a promise I had made not only to the program directors but also to myself. In addition to being physically unobtrusive, I had to be socially unremarkable. As Goffman put it, I needed to "socially shrink."[3] To that end, at Legacy, I wore blue scrubs to blend in with the housestaff because no one (except for patients or attendings) wore plain clothes.[4] At Stonewood, the teams were much larger, and plain clothes did not attract attention in the same way that they would have at Legacy. At the end of my fieldwork at Legacy, the program director told me, "I've never heard anything about you—negative or positive—in the past two years. . . . It's not like we even notice you." In some ways, this was the best praise an ethnographer could hope for.

Different residents reacted differently to the prospect of having someone tag along with them during their workday. Some people seemed to struggle to remember what species of social scientist I was, even though I reminded them frequently; I was variously called a social worker, a human behavioral specialist, and a socioanthropologist. Others envisioned more-interesting identities for me by musing that I must be a spy, a journalist, a reality TV producer, or a "mystery shopper" sent by the Accreditation Council for Graduate Medical Education. One afternoon in the Legacy residents' lounge, a group started to poke fun at me, joking that I was writing an exposé about medicine in the state. I replied good-naturedly that the state would not be identified in my findings. The housestaff then began to offer suggestions for titles of my book. "*Dysfunction Junction*," suggested one intern. "*Tiers of Pain*, with *tiers* spelled T-I-E-R-S," offered another with a laugh. When someone else asked what my comparison field site would be, another resident interrupted and replied that just as I would not reveal Legacy's identity, I could not reveal my comparison sites. Generally, the housestaff at both hospitals were very welcoming to me in this way. Only once during my three years of fieldwork did I notice a text message being sent between residents saying "OMG shoot the spy."

Occasionally, residents would give me menial tasks to do, like fetching charts. I readily obliged, happy to have something to do that was useful to the housestaff. It also helped mitigate some of the guilt I felt for watching *others* work without being able to help. More commonly, I was treated like a medical student, such that the staff would either ignore me or take great pains to explain what they were doing without giving me the benefit of using layman's terms.[5] This was perhaps because they had no other reference point for me; the only students who tagged along with them all day were medical students. It ended up being quite helpful, both because I could follow what was going on with patients and because it gave the staff a framework for dealing with me. Their explanations also gave them an opportunity to think out loud and put together diagnoses. For example, one morning a Legacy intern walked over to the telemetry screens by the nurses' station that tracked patients' heart rates. He pointed to a set of squiggly lines and said, "You see how the beat is irregular? How it doesn't occur at the same intervals? That's why we're concerned about this patient." Through these teachings, I came to learn a fair amount of medicine, which helped me make sense of my observations. One intern, in particular, would quiz me on my knowledge of medical jargon: epistaxis, hematochezia, cachexia. I would also look up terms while typing my fieldnotes, which helped expand my medical knowledge over time.

I took handwritten, nearly verbatim notes on what I saw and heard, endeavoring to keep straightforward observations separate from personal reflections, which I added only later to my typed notes.[6] While it was impossible to jot down everything, I especially focused on interactions involving resident education—namely, those between attendings and the housestaff—as well as interactions among the housestaff. I found that I was able to capture dialogue as accurately as possible by learning to write quickly and using my own form of shorthand, which drew heavily on the medical abbreviations I picked up during my fieldwork (e.g., hx for history).

Thankfully, hospitals are busy places where clipboards are ubiquitous, which meant I did not attract undue attention while taking notes. I purposely made my handwriting more difficult to read, although at the speed I was writing, it often was not especially legible anyway. Occasionally, when residents asked me what I was writing, I would truthfully answer that I was recording conversations and events as accurately as possible. For confidentiality reasons, I declined whenever someone asked to see my notes. I then transcribed handwritten jottings contemporaneously, usually within twenty-four hours of an observation, and expanded upon them with additional details from memory.

In-Depth Interviews

During the last ten months at Legacy and during six months at Stonewood, I interviewed residents and program officials intensively. A major benefit to doing the observations was that I was often physically present in the hospital, which meant that I could interview busy respondents, especially attendings, whenever they sporadically had pockets of free time. I also interviewed residents who generously shared their time with me after work or on their days off. I made handwritten jottings during the interviews, often to remember probes or to highlight an especially poignant quote, but I relied on a tape recorder to capture the bulk of the data. Interviews lasted from twenty-five minutes to over two hours, with the vast majority lasting roughly seventy-five minutes.

In total, I completed 123 interviews. At Legacy, I interviewed approximately 85 percent of the housestaff along with nearly every member of the program directorship, chief residents, and several key faculty members. Among the residents I interviewed, 17 percent were DOs, 27 percent were IMGs, 44 percent were international medical graduates who were US citizens (USIMGs), and 13 percent were graduates of US allopathic medical schools (USMDs), roughly commensurate with their representation on the housestaff (see table I.1 in the introduction). At Stonewood, I interviewed approximately 40 percent of the housestaff, in addition to about a dozen attendings and the entire program directorship, including chief residents. I aimed to capture the range of USMDs' and non-USMDs' trajectories and opinions, as well as the commonalities in their respective experiences while training at these two segregated institutions. Interviewing was completed only after thematic saturation was reached on both counts.[7]

The interview guide evolved substantially as the interviews progressed. While I used a list of questions as a starting point, I preferred to let the interviewees guide the interviews, which often meant departing from the schedule. Sometimes this resulted in covering a different range of topics with some respondents compared to others. The interview guide also evolved as I incorporated new ideas and questions from the emerging data. Often these new questions came from observations. For example, I recall attending my first Resident Selection Committee meeting at Stonewood and hearing repeatedly "Is this person worth the risk?" when discussing applicants (see chapter 2). This framing of resident recruitment in terms of relative risk prompted me to go back to my interview guide and include questions for the program leadership about what was meant by "risk" in the resident selection process.

In other cases, data emerging from the interviews themselves led me to revise my interview guide. For example, after interviewing Adrian, a Caribbean graduate at Legacy, early in my fieldwork, I realized the importance of exploring residents' social backgrounds as a starting point for understanding their professional trajectories. At the end of the interview, when I asked Adrian (as I did every respondent) whether there was anything else he wanted to add, he responded:

> Do you ask people how they grew up or what was in their life, like, "What did your parents do or your grandparents; what did this aunt do?" . . . I think that's a big question to ask. My mom's from a third world country. She moved to this country and had me. I was raised by my stepdad. His parents had a lot of money. They weren't educated. They made money in marketing and business. I wasn't really taught that you had to work really hard to get what you want.

After that interview, I changed my interview guide to cover the residents' social backgrounds. This took the form of a sociobiographical or life history approach, beginning with where they were born, what their parents did for a living, and how they first became interested in medicine.[8] I then would cover a range of topics: (1) the role of early socioeconomic status in achieving their current status, (2) the degree of choice versus constraint involved in reaching their current status, (3) understandings of tiers within residency training (and their opinions about the implications), (4) perceptions of self and others (e.g., USMD versus IMG), (5) understandings of segregation between residency programs (including beliefs about the value of USMDs versus that of non-USMDs and the fairness of the current system), (6) understandings of the quality of education (in community versus university hospitals, among USMDs versus non-USMDs), and (7) future goals/aspirations.

As I became increasingly interested in the social forces and stakeholders driving the sorting of medical graduates into different residency programs, I began to interview the key decision makers in the program's infrastructure, such as the chief residents, attendings, program directors, and chiefs of medicine. Questions focused on the decision-making process in resident recruitment, as well as broader goals for the residency program, perceptions of medical graduates from different backgrounds, and their thoughts about what ultimately makes a "good" doctor.

A common concern among interviewees was political correctness. This was especially true at Stonewood when I would ask respondents about their perceptions of non-USMDs or community residency programs. For example, when I asked one Stonewood attending about her perceptions of Caribbean graduates, she replied:

That's funny, I think the stigma might actually be worse than a DO. And again [it's] the same idea, the caliber of academic performance, rigor in getting accepted into medical school in the first place. I think there's definitely a sense that it's just not as strong, or as bright even as an applicant, which [*laughs*] *probably sounds terribly obnoxious and it's so funny that you're recording*, but I do think there's a general feeling you don't go to a medical school in the Caribbean if you can get right into medical school in the contiguous United States. (emphasis added)

This attending became self-conscious when relaying common perceptions about Caribbean graduates. To get around this, I would reassure respondents of their confidentiality and remind them that these were precisely the kinds of popular conceptions in which I was interested. Eventually, I learned to preface certain questions by saying "This is where political correctness goes out the window." In contrast, at Legacy, sensitive topics centered mostly on questions related to failed aspirations or disappointing trajectories. I learned to minimize ego threat by purposely avoiding the use of *choice* in my wording (e.g., I asked, "How did you end up at Legacy?" instead of "Why did you *choose* Legacy?"). Life history interviews were also helpful for putting respondents at ease, as I got to build rapport with them before asking sensitive questions later in the interview. At both hospitals, I also paraphrased responses to ensure I understood what they meant and used the same terminology as respondents to avoid imposing my own terms or my own meanings on their words.[9]

Despite these challenges, respondents at both hospitals were surprisingly open to being interviewed. Most were pleased by the idea of getting a chance to talk about their trajectories and opinions. Despite their busy schedules, even program leaders agreed to take one or two hours of their time to chat with me. I suspect this openness was partly the result of the nature of medical work. While most human beings are naturally inclined to talk about themselves, physicians spend the bulk of their time asking questions of *others*. An interview was an opportunity to be listened to and heard rather than always being the one doing the listening.

Focus Groups

Aside from being my only access to Stonewood at first, focus groups became a great supplement to the data, as they exposed me to an even wider pool of residents in a program that was more than three times the size of Legacy's and gave me insight into areas of consensus and disagreement among the housestaff. Residents were invited to participate in focus groups during their ambulatory block rotations, during which they spent their time alternating between didactic lectures and outpatient clinics. In total, I conducted nine focus groups stratified by postgraduate year (PGY-1, -2, and -3) and program type (categorical versus primary care) with thirty-seven residents. They each lasted approximately two hours and were transcribed verbatim.

THE ANALYSIS

As a social scientist, I believe that accounting for analysis is just as important as accounting for data collection, even though the former often gets brushed aside in methodological discussions. As the data were transcribed, I kept notes about the evolution of ideas, theories, and methods. These notes were divided into theoretical, and personal methodological, and personal notes.[10] An example of a theoretical note was one that resulted when the concept of risk was mentioned during the Resident Selection Committee meetings. Afterward, while transcribing my fieldnotes, I wrote, *"What constitutes more of a risk—someone who didn't do that well in medical school (but comes from a familiar place) vs. someone who did very well in medical school (but comes from a less familiar place)?"* Eventually, these in-process jottings evolved into coding memos, which helped inform the coding process.[11] I used methodological notes to keep track of logistical reflections. For example, one day I remarked out loud that they served only pancakes for breakfast at Legacy, and a resident replied that, no, they were served only on Fridays (the day I came in to do observations for the first few months at Legacy). This reflection prompted me to start coming in on different days to make sure I wasn't missing other important happenings during the week. Finally, personal notes were sparser but contained my personal reactions, thoughts, and feelings as an ethnographer. They helped me process the difficult scenes I sometimes encountered, like the first time a patient died. These theoretical, methodological, and personal notes were kept distinct from the data by using italic text and were woven in contemporaneously as the data were transcribed.

Once fieldwork was complete, I had the daunting task of sorting through thousands of pages of data. The fact that my fieldnotes were transcribed immediately after each observation helped with the analysis, as did my in-process notes, because they evoked vivid memories that transported me back to the events in question.[12] Using NVivo 10, I systematically analyzed the data line by line using open coding and asking "What is this an example of? What does this represent?"[13] This process resulted in over 150 codes, which were eventually divided by chapter, using a process known as focused coding. Then the coded segments for each chapter were further refined into subcodes.[14] Multiple rounds of coding ensured the reliability of my concepts because I would effectively test and then retest my understandings at different sittings. Finally, coded segments were selected for their representativeness or in some cases their uniqueness and then edited for length, relevance, readability, grammar, and confidentiality. Regarding this last point, in a handful of cases, I used different pseudonyms for the same respondent in different chapters to protect against deductive disclosure.[15] I did this particularly to prevent insiders from being able to identify respondents on the basis of public events reported in later chapters and connect them with more personal details about their trajectories into medicine from earlier chapters.

THE QUANDARIES

After spending over 1,200 hours in hospitals, I inevitably came across situations that tested my ethics as a researcher. One such instance happened during my first year of fieldwork at Legacy, the program characterized by inconsistent autonomy (see chapter 3). A resident tried to strong-arm a patient into changing her code status—which indicated whether or not she was to be resuscitated in the event of an emergency.[16] The patient—let's call her Gladys—was "Full Code" (i.e., she wanted to be resuscitated), but before going to see her, the resident told the intern that Gladys had stage three lung cancer and had been intubated twelve times in three months, so "it's time she stopped torturing herself," implying that she should change her code status to "Do Not Resuscitate." When we got to the bedside, however, despite the resident's implorations, Gladys remained steadfast in her decision, so the resident became more forceful:

> "You have stage 3 lung cancer—right? Stage 3?" confirmed the resident with the intern, who nodded. "And it has spread. Did you know that?" The patient responded worriedly that she didn't know it had spread, and now the resident seemed unsure about what he'd said. "Yeah, I mean I think it has spread. It said stage 3, right?" the resident asked the intern, who nodded again. [*Personal note: I was struck by how unfamiliar the resident seemed to be with the case and how nonchalantly they brought up the possibility of her cancer having spread without being absolutely sure. I suspect the resident said it to convince her of her own impending mortality and thus to get her to change her code status. This did not escape the patient, who became angry and asked us to leave her room.*]

The elderly patient reminded me of my grandmother, making it a difficult encounter to watch. As I wrote in a personal note, "*I suddenly and immediately felt a surge of sympathy for this poor patient, who was being strong-armed into a decision she had already made for herself. I felt like crying for this patient who, defenseless, had made her choice but that choice did not seem to be respected. I felt the sadness in her eyes, as she looked at me searchingly for support.*" I recall struggling with whether to report this encounter to the hospital leadership or to keep mum. As a relatively new ethnographer, I decided to keep quiet for fear of losing my access or rocking the boat. Despite this, a member of the Legacy leadership contacted me shortly afterward and asked for my fieldnotes on this particular resident. Once again, I had to make a decision that could jeopardize my access: deny the request (and risk being asked to leave by the leadership) or comply with the request (and risk losing the housestaff's trust). I opted for the former, replying that I was under an ethical obligation to keep all my fieldnotes confidential. The program official respected my decision.

A year or so later, after this resident had graduated, I learned that they had done something similar to a different patient, but this time the family had threatened to sue the hospital, which alerted the hospital administration to the residents' actions. My heart dropped when I heard this news; had I reported what I saw years prior, perhaps this second incident (and untold others) might never have happened. I still struggle with my decision, with whether or not I should have broken confidentiality and reported the behavior I witnessed. If I had, perhaps future patients could have been spared this indignity. On the other hand, I would have likely struggled to rebuild the kind of rapport I had established over the two years I spent at Legacy. Fieldwork, by definition, involves innumerable such decisions—like whether to follow a respondent into a private meeting, whether to ask a question or stay quiet, and whether to report unethical behavior—and all one can do is explain one's decision-making process and let the reader decide whether it was the right call.

That wasn't the only time I struggled with how much to be a *participant* versus an observer in the field.[17] One day an intern-resident pair at Legacy went to see a patient who was becoming hypoxic (lacking oxygen). They struggled to get the frail patient to sit up in the bed while I fixed my eyes on the oxygen saturation monitor, whose numbers started precipitously rolling backward. As the resident asked the patient to breathe deeply, the saturation dipped down to 81 percent.[18] Without thinking, I immediately called out, "Pulse ox 81!" The resident and intern jerked their heads toward the monitor and asked the patient to lie back down, but the figure kept going down: 78, 74, 71, 68, 67. It stopped at 67, the lowest saturation I had ever seen. An emergency code had been called earlier that day for a patient with a much higher pulse oximeter reading. The resident cranked the oxygen back on and pressed the oxygen mask to the patient's face.

Situations like these regularly made me question my role as an ethnographer. Was I to keep silent at all times and only strictly observe, or were there times when my participation was not only acceptable but also ethically indispensable? Then, of course, there were times when respondents directly asked me to weigh in on an issue. Once a patient made racist remarks to a resident, who later asked me as a sociologist, "How do you respond to that?" I shrugged and replied, "You don't. You just keep going." On more contentious issues, however, such as the Affordable Care Act, which was enacted during my fieldwork, I kept mum or deflected, not wanting to let my politics affect my relationship with respondents.

Another dilemma came in the form of what counts as data. Given the amount of informal time I spent with residents at both hospitals—in the residents' lounge, at social events, at graduation, during occasional car rides—there were times when I wondered whether my identity as a researcher was always salient. In other words, did what so-and-so told me in the car count as data? Did they tell me as a researcher or as a friend? Would they be upset if I used this information? Residents were quite open with me, especially during these informal interactions, and much of what they said was pertinent to the research. Unlike other field-workers, however, who might be more involved as *participants* in their field sites, I had no identity except as a researcher at Stonewood and Legacy. I could not be mistaken for a staff member or a fellow doctor because my role was primarily observatory and not participatory. For these reasons, I selectively made use of the information shared with me during these informal interactions, primarily when I was able to triangulate it with information obtained elsewhere. During one car ride, for example, a resident told me that Legacy was trying to recruit more USIMGs to give the program a more American feel. This information was corroborated by other respondents at a different time, so I elected to use it.

Several personal and professional traits made fieldwork easier for me. Being roughly of the same age and social background as many of the residents certainly helped me establish rapport.[19] The fact that I was relatively young meant that I was able to blend in inconspicuously and relate to the housestaff in ways that would have been much more difficult had I been a sixty-five-year-old university professor. My gender came in and out of salience throughout the fieldwork. Women at both hospitals were somewhat more distrustful of me than men, who often seemed amused by the idea of having a researcher study them. This could be because women have traditionally had to fight harder for acceptance within the medical profession.[20] As a Canadian, I was easily able to "pass" as American among the locals and play up my immigrant status among the foreigners. One European resident commented to me one day, "You're Canadian; you're not like all those Americans who just say things to be nice." I also made use of my language skills in French and Spanish to build rapport with residents from different countries. This helped win over a particularly recalcitrant resident from Latin America, who warmed up considerably upon hearing me speak Spanish.

Then there were the personal traits of mine that made fieldwork more challenging. I'm what you might call germ averse. I'm not clinically germaphobic, but I do have a stronger-than-normal fear of microbes, of which there is no shortage in hospitals. I also periodically experienced "medical student's disease," where I thought I had contracted the very diseases being discussed in didactic sessions.[21] Usually, my symptoms resolved once the lecture on vertigo or skin cancer or porphyria (or whatever) ended.

More seriously, a larger personal challenge I faced had to do with my professional identity. For over a decade, before I started in sociology, I had had a strong interest in medicine and even considered pursuing it as a career but decided against it. In this way, spending time in hospitals shadowing doctors during my fieldwork represented the road not taken. If Robert Frost wrote about reaching a fork in the road and being sorry he could not travel both paths, I was taking almost daily field trips to the other side, seeing what might have been. My continued interest in medicine was both helpful and harmful: helpful because it made thousands of hours of fieldwork not only bearable but also *exciting* and harmful because it caused me considerable anxiety about my choice to become a sociologist. I remember feeling uneasy about how much I enjoyed learning the various kinds of myocardial infarctions or being able to read an uncomplicated echocardiogram by the end of my fieldwork. Somehow I thought there was a direct correlation between how much I enjoyed medicine and how wrong my choice was to become a sociologist. It eventually became clear, however, that my interest in medicine did not negate my passion for sociology, which was undeniable. Luckily, as a hospital ethnographer, I could do both, in some measure.

Besides this, I experienced a whole range of emotions from boredom to shock (like during my first emergency code) to excitement to ambivalence. I never ceased being nervous before obtaining informed consent from a new team of residents at the beginning of each month—a feeling that sometimes made me strongly dislike the fieldwork. At both hospitals, there were individuals who were initially distrustful of me but who amazingly, over time, became some of my best informants. One such person at Stonewood barely tolerated me on their team at first, but by the end of my research, they agreed to spend over an hour being interviewed in what turned out to be a highly informative discussion. There were also memorable patients, like the flasher at Legacy who would expose himself to me and the medical student standing at the foot of his bed while the residents examined him and the patient who spread feces on the walls of his room. And I will never forget Gladys.

A final challenge I faced was how critical to be in my analyses, especially given how generous my respondents were with their time and candor. In the end, I elected to be critical of both hospitals, focusing on institutional structures and roles rather than specific persons.[22] In so doing, I aimed to be as balanced as possible in my portrayal of these two programs.

Notes

PREFACE

1. Verghese (2009, 490–91).
2. See, for example, Jauhar (2008).
3. *Allopathic* is a term used to describe "mainstream" medicine, often in juxtaposition to osteopathic medicine.
4. Compared to a Doctor of Medicine (MD), a Doctor of Osteopathic Medicine (DO) espouses distinct philosophical principles that recognize the body's self-healing abilities. Both types of doctors can practice medicine in the United States, but DOs maintain their own medical schools.

INTRODUCTION

1. I use pseudonyms throughout the book to protect individuals' and institutions' confidentiality.
2. National Resident Matching Program (2019b). The vast majority of USMDs are US citizens or permanent residents, with only 0.05% of all matriculating students in 2019–2020 listing their legal residence as being outside of the United States (AAMC, 2019b).
3. Jenkins and Reddy (2016).
4. National Resident Matching Program (2019b).
5. National Resident Matching Program (2019b).
6. National Resident Matching Program (2019b).
7. Undergraduate medical education refers to 4+ years of medical school (in the United States or elsewhere), whereas graduate medical education can refer to either residency or fellowship training after medical school.
8. American Medical Association (2019).
9. National Resident Matching Program (2019b).
10. National Resident Matching Program (2019b).
11. As of 2020, the American Osteopathic Association (AOA) and the Accreditation Council for Graduate Medical Education (ACGME) have fully merged osteopathic and allopathic residency programs into a single graduate medical education system, including

a single matching process. Several programs already merged prior to that date (American Osteopathic Association 2017).

12. National Resident Matching Program (2019b). In 2019 (the last year before the ACGME and AOA matching processes fully merged), 80 percent of all osteopathic training positions were accessible through the main National Resident Matching Program (NRMP) Match (American Osteopathic Association Staff 2019). The other 20 percent of positions were meted out through the AOA matching process, which occurred before the NRMP Match. Applicants who successfully receive a position through the AOA process are required to withdraw from the NRMP Match. The five-year rate cited for DOs—81.5 percent—includes only those who matched through the NRMP Match.

13. Ludmerer (2015).

14. IMG, USIMG, and DO are the acronyms commonly used in the medical literature. USMD is an exception; while many scholars refer to them as *US medical graduates* (or USMGs), this term should ostensibly include DOs who go to medical school in the United States, but it generally does not—a relic, perhaps, of the historical exclusion of DOs by the medical profession. Thus, to distinguish between American-trained MDs and DOs, I use the acronym USMDs throughout.

15. In 2019, for example, 213 (or 92 percent) of first-year positions in neurosurgery were filled by USMD seniors, while they represented only 78 percent of applicants. In contrast, 18 (or just under 8 percent) neurosurgery positions were filled by what the NRMP calls "independent applicants," including 6 USMDs who had already graduated from medical school, 4 DOs, and 8 IMGs. The remaining 1 position went unfilled (0.004%). For its part, internal medicine filled 41.5 percent of its spots with USMDs (who represented only 32 percent of applicants), while independent applicants (including DOs, USIMGs, IMGs, and USMDs who had already graduated) collectively filled 55.8 percent of positions, despite representing 68 percent of applicants. In addition, 2.8 percent of spots remained unfilled (National Resident Matching Program 2019b).

16. Jenkins, Franklyn, Klugman, and Reddy (2019).

17. In 2018, USMDs and international graduates (including USIMGs and IMGs) who matched into internal medicine (IM) as their preferred specialty have virtually the same mean scores (233 versus 232) on the United States Medical Licensing Exam (USMLE) Step 1 (National Resident Matching Program 2018d, 2018b). These scores are up from 226 and 225, respectively, in 2011 when I was conducting this study (National Resident Matching Program 2011). When the 2018 numbers are further disaggregated, on average, matched USIMGs scored lower than matched USMDs (225 versus 233), but matched IMGs—who outnumbered matched USIMGs two to one—scored significantly higher than matched USMDs (236 versus 233) (National Resident Matching Program 2018b). For their part, DOs who matched into IM as their preferred specialty had lower scores on average (226), but not all DO applicants take the USMLE; Step 1 scores are available for only 60.7 percent of DOs who agreed to share their scores with the NRMP (National Resident Matching Program 2018c).

18. In 2014, for example, non-USMDs who had already interviewed (and thus had been preselected) and were at the stage of ranking programs in The Match had to score approximately 60 points (three standard deviations) higher than USMDs on the same

USMLE Step 1 to have the same 80 percent probability of matching. This pattern extends to every specialty, such that with the same test scores, non-USMDs consistently have a much lower probability of matching than USMDs (National Resident Matching Program 2014a).

19. See, for example, http://www.blog.myresidencylist.com/img-friendly-residency-programs/ or https://forums.studentdoctor.net/threads/do-friendly-internal-medicine-university -programs.1008132/.

20. Based on analyses of data from the American Medical Association's Fellowship and Residency Electronic Interactive Database (FREIDA) (Jenkins et al. 2019).

21. "Integrated" programs are defined as those having between 30 and 65 percent USMDs, which represents one standard deviation of USMDs centered around the mean (Jenkins et al. 2019).

22. Nationwide, USMD-dominated programs have significantly higher Board pass rates by about 4 percentage points than USIMG and IMG-dominated ones (Jenkins, Franklyn, Klugman, and Reddy, 2019).

23. Matthews (2010); Skrentny and Novick (2018).

24. Anderson (2013).

25. Sabharwal (2008, 2011b, 2011a).

26. Cohen (2006).

27. Studies dating back to the 1980s have found no significant differences in the quality of care offered by USMDs versus international medical graduates (Saywell, Studnicki, Bean and Ludke 1979, 1980; Sang et al. 1986; Mick and Comfort 1997; Norcini et al. 2010). A recent Medicare study even found that patients treated by IMGs experienced lower mortality than patients treated by USMDs did (Tsugawa et al. 2017).

28. Olson (2013).

29. Palmer (2011).

30. American Medical Association (2013).

31. McGrath, Wong, and Holewa (2011). IMGs who train with J-1 (exchange) visas have to return to their home countries for two years after their training unless they complete a waiver. The waiver requires them to *work* (not train) for a minimum of three years in a designated underserved area (US Citizenship and Immigration Services, 2015), which restricts where IMGs can work after graduation.

32. Queensland Health (2015).

33. See Cullen (1931), McNamee (2018).

34. This is the description of The Match provided by the National Resident Matching Program (2019a). The NRMP is not involved in the residency selection process and does not take a stance on whether USMDs should be prioritized in recruitment decisions.

35. As Light writes, "Sociologists are best equipped to document and analyze medical education as a stratified institution that reproduces class relationships and promotes corporate medicine" (1988, 318).

36. Growe and Montgomery (2003, 23). See, for example, Armstrong and Hamilton (2013); Calarco (2018); Tyson (2011).

37. See also Bourdieu and Passeron (1990) and Jewel (2008) for more on how educational structures secure the consent of those they subordinate.

38. Ludmerer (2015); Stern and Markel (2004, 1). *House pupil, house officer,* and *housestaff* are all terms for interns and residents, so termed because they used to live "in-house" (the hospital) for the duration of their training.

39. Irigoyen and Zambrana (1979).

40. Stern and Markel (2004).

41. Stern and Markel (2004).

42. Ludmerer (2015, 137). See also Swanson (1973).

43. Hall (1948, 1949); Marshall, Fulton, and Wessen (1978); Miller (1970); Roth (2003).

44. Hall (1948, 336).

45. Hall (1948, 336).

46. Turner (1960).

47. Ludmerer (2015); Roth (2003).

48. Ludmerer (2015, 142), citing Council on Medical Education and Hospitals, 1955), *The Student and the Matching Program* (Chicago: American Medical Association), 9.

49. Ludmerer (2015, 144).

50. Roth (2003); Turner (1960, 855). See also Marshall, Fulton, and Wessen (1978).

51. The NRMP's mission is as follows: "To match healthcare professionals to graduate medical education and advanced training programs through a process that is fair, efficient, transparent, and reliable. To provide meaningful and accessible Match data and analysis to stakeholders" (National Resident Matching Program 2019a).

52. Abbott (1988); Bolton and Muzio (2007); Parkin (1974); Weber (1968).

53. Wu and Siu (2015).

54. Wu and Siu (2015).

55. Gevitz (2014, 487), citing J. H. Berge, J. M. Hutcheson, R. Ward, G. A. Woodhouse, and H. L. Pearson Jr., 1961, "Osteopathy: Special Report of the Judicial Council to the AMA House of Delegates," *JAMA* 177 (11): 775.

56. American Association of Colleges of Osteopathic Medicine (2014a).

57. Ludmerer (2015, 143).

58. Ludmerer (2015).

59. Irigoyen and Zambrana (1979); Mick (1978, 1987, 1993).

60. Irigoyen and Zambrana (1979).

61. Irigoyen and Zambrana (1979).

62. Ludmerer (2015, 143).

63. Irigoyen and Zambrana (1979).

64. Irigoyen and Zambrana (1979).

65. Feldstein and Butter (1978), Mick (1978, 1993), Roberts (1996).

66. Irigoyen and Zambrana (1979); Lohr, Vanselow, and Detmer (1996); Mick (1987); Roberts (1996).

67. Korcok (1979).

68. Between 1965 and 1985, the number of US medical schools increased from 88 to 127, with the total number of USMDs graduating annually growing from 7,574 to 16,191 (Mick 1987).

69. Wu and Siu (2015).

70. American Association of Colleges of Osteopathic Medicine (2014a).

71. Mick (1987).
72. Roberts (1996); see also Lohr, Vanselow, and Detmer (1996)
73. Irigoyen and Zambrana (1979).
74. Collins (1979, 156) makes a similar argument regarding the use of the bar exam by white elites in the legal profession to reaffirm their dominance over growing numbers of immigrants in the profession.
75. Perhaps the most effective obstacle was the direct screening of IMGs by the Educational Commission for Foreign Medical Graduates (ECFMG). From 1958 until 1976, it administered the American Qualification Examination as well as a basic English competency test to IMG applicants—in addition to carefully vetting all foreign credentials (e.g., transcripts and diplomas). The ECFMG then introduced the Visa Qualifying Examination (VQE), which IMGs were required to pass before even applying for a visa (Educational Commission for Foreign Medical Graduates 2015b; Mick 1987). The VQE was supposed to be equivalent to Parts I and II of the National Board of Medical Examiners Examination, which was taken by graduating USMDs, but it was actually much harder (Mick 1987). The resulting pass rate was approximately 25 percent in 1977, thereby curbing the influx of IMGs by 80 percent (Irigoyen and Zambrana 1979). In 1984, the VQE was replaced by the two-day Foreign Medical Graduate Examination in the Medical Sciences, which had an even more abysmal pass rate of 16 percent. (Mick 1987).
76. Mick (1987)
77. Eckhert (2010).
78. Irigoyen and Zambrana (1979).
79. The match rates have increased from 92.1 percent in 1982 to 95.1 percent in 2012 (the standard deviation is 0.6 percent). See National Resident Matching Program (2018e, 1985). I also consulted reports in between those dates to track the percentage of positions filled by USMDs.
80. Eckhert (2010); Hartocollis (2014).
81. American Association of Colleges of Osteopathic Medicine (2014b).
82. Educational Commission for Foreign Medical Graduates (2015a).
83. Educational Commission for Foreign Medical Graduates (2015a).
84. Educational Commission for Foreign Medical Graduates (2015a).
85. Pinsky (2017, 840).
86. Ludmerer (2015, 287–88).
87. Evetts et al. (2009).
88. Barber (1962); Blau and Scott (1962); Coser (1962); Goode (1957); Greenwood (1957); Merton, Reader, and Kendall (1957).
89. Freidson (1970, 135).
90. Abbott (1988); Evetts et al. (2009).
91. Abbott (1988, 2).
92. Abbott (1988).
93. See, for example, Becker et al. (1961); Bosk (2003); Coser (1962); Light (1980). See also Brosnan (2010).
94. Freidson (1970); Smith (1958).
95. Marshall, Fulton, and Wessen (1978).

96.   Mumford (1970).

97.   Freidson and Rhea (1972).

98.   Bucher and Strauss (1961, 332–33).

99.   Starr (1982).

100.   Hafferty and Light (1995); Halpern (1992); Light (2010); McKinlay and Marceau (2002).

101.   McKinlay and Marceau (2002).

102.   Hafferty and Light (1995, 135).

103.   Freidson (1970).

104.   McKinlay and Arches (1985).

105.   Freidson (1985, 1986b, 1986a).

106.   Freidson (1986b, 119).

107.   Freidson (1986a).

108.   Freidson (1985, 21).

109.   Timmermans (2008).

110.   Rothman (1991).

111.   Freidson (1985, 1986a).

112.   Hafferty (1988b).

113.   See Brooks (2011); Muzio and Ackroyd (2005).

114.   Annandale (1989); Hoff and Pohl (2017).

115.   Freidson (1985).

116.   Freidson wrote, for example: "By the power to allocate the total resources of the orga-
       nization, management is sharply distinguished from rank-and-file professional workers"
       (1986b, 154).

117.   Freidson (1984).

118.   Hafferty and Light (1995, 141).

119.   Hafferty and Light (1995). Lorber predicted a similar deep split among female physi-
       cians—another subordinated group in the profession—between "those who align with
       other physicians in the fight to maintain professional dominance, and those who align
       with other women health-care workers and consumers in the fight for a healthcare sys-
       tem with a flatter hierarchy and a holistic and self-help perspective" (1984, 28–29).

120.   See Hoff and Pohl (2017); Lorber (1984). Here I borrow the term *horizontal stratification*
       from the sociology of education, where it is used to refer to differences in the quality and
       prestige of education at the same level (Gerber and Cheung 2008, 300).

121.   Lorber (1984).

122.   Hoff (1998).

123.   A growing body of literature has explored horizontal stratification in the sociology of
       higher education (see, for example, Borgen and Mastekaasa 2018: Gerber and Cheung
       2008), but similar research has not yet been done in medical education.

124.   Hoff (2001).

125.   Weber (1968, 927).

126.   Davis and Allison (2013): Hoff, Sutcliffe, and Young (2017).

127.   Khan (2011).

128.   Rivera (2015).

129.   Brooks (2011); Cross and Goldenberg (2009); Jewel (2008).

130. See, for example, Anspach (1993); Bosk (2003, 1992); Coser (1962); Heimer and Staffen (1998); Light (1980); Miller (1970); Mumford (1970); Zussman (1992). Early hospital ethnographies focused on the distinct social world of the hospital and the complex relations between patients and staff, but the method became "largely moribund" in the 1990s (Zussman 1993, 167), partly due to a shift within the subdiscipline toward studying health instead of medicine. This book forms part of a growing resurgence of hospital ethnography as sociologists work to revive this research tradition (see, for example, Kellogg 2011; Menchik 2014; Oh and Timmermans 2013; Reich 2014; Szymczak and Bosk 2012).

131. In 2019, 41.5 percent of incoming internal medicine residents were USMDs. This number has declined every year since at least 2009, when USMDs filled 53.5 percent of positions (National Resident Matching Program 2009, 2019b).

132. American Board of Internal Medicine (2019). While I did not observe many gender differences in my findings, I do mention them where appropriate throughout the book.

133. Throughout the book, I use the terms *housestaff* and *residents* interchangeably. Generally speaking, *residents* is a collective term for postgraduate medical trainees in these two hospitals, including interns (first-year residents), junior residents (second-year residents), and senior residents (third-year residents). In certain instances, I use *residents* (i.e., second- and third-year trainees) in juxtaposition to *interns* (first-year trainees), but these instances should be obvious based on the context.

134. Residents could choose to specialize in primary care by selecting that track, which offered them additional months in the outpatient setting.

135. Internal medicine residents would seldom be the primary caretakers for these nonmedical patients, but learning how to coordinate care (or provide consultative services) for these patients can be an important aspect of an internist's training.

136. Legacy did have a telephone-based translation service, using a special telephone with two receivers. The residents did not like using that technology, however, and instead would often try to find informal translators (e.g., family members) to communicate with patients.

137. Loan forgiveness is guaranteed for federal loans under the Public Service Loan Forgiveness Program after loan recipients work for ten years, including residency, at a nonprofit (Federal Student Aid n.d.).

138. When a resident is "on call," they are responsible for admitting new patients until approximately 9 PM, after which a night resident comes on duty to handle overnight admissions.

139. Safety-net hospitals are defined by the Institute of Medicine as institutions that are designated to provide care for vulnerable, uninsured patients (Lewin and Altman 2000).

140. "When you hear hoofbeats, think of horses, not zebras," is a common medical axiom coined in the 1940s by Dr. Theodore Woodward.

141. American Medical Association (2018).

142. Middle-status conformity theory argues that only middle-status programs will try to improve their status by conforming with social expectations, such as recruiting USMDs, because the status positions are fixed for high-status and low-status programs (Dittes and Kelley 1956; Phillips and Zuckerman 2001). As will become clear in chapter 2, Stonewood and Legacy were both very concerned about increasing their status through recruitment,

which, according to middle-status convergence theory, suggests that they are both middle status, albeit at different points on the inverted U-shaped curve between status and conformity (Phillips and Zuckerman 2001, 385).

1. MEET THE RESIDENTS

1. Until 2015, the MCAT contained three sections, each worth a possible 15 points, making 45 the highest possible MCAT score. The mean score nationwide was 25.2 between 2012 and 2014 (Association of American Medical Colleges 2014d). Most students considered 30 to be a minimum "safe" score for getting into medical school.

2. The residents quoted here were asked what advice they would give to a twelve-year-old interested in pursuing a career in cardiology.

3. AAMC (2019c, 2019d). These figures do not account for earlier attrition during the premedical track (see, for example, Lin et al. 2014; Michalec et al. 2018).

4. Lin et al. (2014).

5. Bourdieu uses the metaphor of a "game" to describe how social actors in different positions compete for capital within a field (Bourdieu and Wacquant 1992). "Playing the game" in that context often means internalizing knowledge about how to act in order to secure more capital (Bourdieu 1998), such as how to dress or how to stand (Luke 2003) in order to "perform and progress within" a profession (Tomlinson et al. 2013, 259), otherwise known as *habitus*. But there's more to the game than just internalizing a sense of how to play; students must also learn the practical formal and informal rules that apply. Here I use "playing the game" to refer to both the development of cultural dispositions *and* the completion of the official and unofficial checklists of items that students must accomplish in order to gain admission to medical school, residency, fellowship, and beyond.

6. Clausen (1991).

7. Scholars have found similar processes among advanced degree holders in other elite professions such as law, banking, and consulting (Jewel 2008; Rivera 2015; Torche 2011).

8. Cruess and Cruess (2004).

9. This rate has remained stable from 1993–1994 to 2013–2014, the last data point available. See Association of American Medical Colleges (2014b).

10. Gravois (2007); Sowell et al. (2008).

11. In 2019, 93.9 percent of US medical school seniors matched into residency programs, up from 92.9 percent in 2004 (National Resident Matching Program 2014b, 2019b).

12. Davis and Moore (1944, 244).

13. Davis and Moore (1944, 243; emphasis added); see also Ludmerer (2015) and Swanson (1973) for more on residency as a right.

14. Persell and Cookson (1985).

15. Hall (1948, 336); see also Ludmerer (2015).

16. Turner (1960, 855). See also Marshall, Fulton, and Wessen (1978) and Roth (2003).

17. Kamens (1977); Persell and Cookson (1985).

18. See, for example, Rivera (2015, 93). Karabel (2005, 546), referring to elite college admissions, writes that "the quest to develop skills—athletic, musical, or artistic—that will later

serve as 'hooks' to attract the attention of elite college gatekeepers begins at ever-earlier ages, with expensive private lessons and summer camps viewed by many parents as indispensable."

19.   Tuition for the two-week program cost $2,795 in 2015 (Envision Experience 2014).

20.   See question 13 in Association of American Medical Colleges (2018b). Among those who reported receiving informal mentorship, 49.2 percent said that these informal mentors were "very important" as "a role model for me in terms of work/professional behavior that I would like to imitate" (see question 15).

21.   These findings echo broader national trends. In 2014, for example, USMDs who matched into internal medicine as their preferred specialty had an average of 2.6 research experiences and 6.7 volunteer experiences (compared to 1.8 and 3.8, respectively, for matched non-USMDs). Tellingly, non-USMDs who matched had an average of 4.3 work experiences prior to applying for residency, while USMDs had 2.7 (National Resident Matching Program 2014a).

22.   Kaplan Test Prep (2018).

23.   Simon (2012).

24.   Similarly, Rivera (2015, 77) describes careers in elite firms as "the path of least resistance" for elite students.

25.   Turner (1960, 858).

26.   In 2014, at the time of this interview, an MCAT score of 27 was in the 61st percentile; the test had a mean score of 25.4 and a standard deviation of 6.4 (Association of American Medical Colleges 2014d).

27.   Studies find that the medical school performance of initially rejected or wait-listed students is just as good as that of students who made the first cut (Devaul et al. 1987; Jardine et al. 2012; Paolo et al. 2006).

28.   Bourdieu (1986).

29.   This is a commonly used expression among medical students; see Knopes (2019), for example.

30.   Step 1 is a lot like the "golden doorstops" that Rivera (2015) described in her research on elite professional service firms, keeping the door open to future opportunity.

31.   Boulis and Jacobs (2008); Lorber (1984).

32.   According to the National Resident Matching Program (2014a), a score of 192 (the passing score) on Step 1 is associated with an 80 percent probability of matching to internal medicine as a preferred specialty for USMDs. For the same score among non-USMDs, the probability drops to 15 percent.

33.   National Resident Matching Program (2019b).

34.   From the PASS Program website: "Didn't pass the Exam? Come back for Free! . . . From your very first day, you will be working alongside the same instructors in a classroom size that is small enough for everyone's strengths to be isolated and reinforced. We can get to the bottom of why someone didn't pass" (PASS Program 2014).

35.   Only one USMD I interviewed ended up in internal medicine after a failed attempt at matching into a more competitive residency. He admitted he pursued that more difficult residency in part because of its elusiveness: "People said it was challenging and like you couldn't get into it, which I think was the appeal to me." When I asked how the process

of applying to internal medicine (his second-choice residency) went after a year off, he replied, "I found it much easier."

36. The very few USMDs who did apply to community programs (usually out of severe geographic constraint) were not always well received by these programs. Some were not offered interviews, and those who did were actively discouraged from ranking the program highly.

37. Binder, Davis, and Bloom (2016) similarly find that students at Harvard and Stanford come to value prestigious jobs in elite firms not only because they are available but also because they satisfy expectations for greatness imposed upon them by their university and because they keep doors open.

38. See Bourdieu (1996); Khan (2011); Lin et al. (2014); Rivera (2015).

39. Not all USIMGs I interviewed went to Caribbean schools. Four of twenty-three were US citizens who studied internationally in other places, like Southeast Asia. Their stories closely resembled those of the Caribbean graduates except that their medical school experience more closely resembled that of IMGs.

40. Most did not seriously consider osteopathic options, as they strongly believed that getting an MD was better than getting a DO.

41. One respondent, for example, witnessed his friends spend $100 per US application and decided to apply to the Caribbean instead, where his cousin had recently been accepted.

42. See, for example, Hartocollis (2008).

43. Turner (1960, 863).

44. See, for example, Lorin (2013).

45. See National Resident Matching Program (2014a). Because of the open-ended nature of my interviews and the fact that I let respondents shape the course of our conversations, only about a third of the USIMGs whom I spoke to disclosed their Step 1 scores to me. The scores for all applicants to internal medicine residency were in the 85th percentile or above, except for one that was toward the bottom of the interquartile range in internal medicine (National Resident Matching Program 2011). Had they graduated from US medical schools, Caribbean graduates with scores in the 80th percentile could have likely matched into much more competitive specialties and/or programs.

46. National Resident Matching Program (2019b).

47. Most respondents agreed that internal medicine, pathology, and family medicine were more within reach for non-USMDs. Georgina's perceptions about OB-GYN, however, are not borne out by Match data, with match rates below 50 percent for non-USMDs (compared to 91 percent for USMDs) (National Resident Matching Program, 2014a).

48. This difference in average number of programs also represented an important difference in cost. In 2014, the Electronic Residency Application Service charged $95 total for application to the first 10 programs, $10 for each of the next 11 to 20 programs, $16 for each of the next 21 to 30 programs, and $26 per program thereafter (Association for American Medical Colleges 2014a). The average USMD applying to 15 programs therefore paid only $145 ($95 + $10 × 5) in application fees, while a USIMG applying to between 40 and 250 programs could pay anywhere from $615 ($95 + $10 × 10 + $16 × 10 + $26 × 10) to $6,075 ($95 + $10 × 10 + $16 × 10 + $26 × 220).

49. Prematches were available only to non-USMDs (i.e., IMGs, USIMGs, and DOs). Until 2012, residency programs could choose to extend prematch offers to non-USMD candidates of their choice, take part in The Match, or use some combination thereof. As of the 2013 Match, however, the National Resident Matching Program's All In Policy required that programs either exclusively use The Match or some other nationally recognized matching system or exclusively choose their candidates outside The Match through prematch offers (National Resident Matching Program 2018a).

50. Goffman (1952).

51. Colby College (2014).

52. In 2018, 22 percent of internal medicine residency programs, including one-third of all programs based at university hospitals, required all applicants to take the USMLE (American Medical Association 2018).

53. Hasty et al. (2012).

54. Hilsenrath (2006).

55. Turner (1960, 857).

56. After I completed my fieldwork, the allopathic Accreditation Council for Graduate Medical Education and the American Osteopathic Association merged into a single accreditation system for residency programs, so there are no longer "DO-only" programs. As of 2020, all programs are open to all applicants (American Osteopathic Association 2019).

57. National Resident Matching Program (2019b).

58. National Resident Matching Program (2018b, 2018d).

59. National Resident Matching Program (2019b).

60. In 2014, around the time of this interview, the Electronic Residency Application Service charged $95 for application to the first 10 programs, $10 for each of the next 11 to 20 programs, $16 for each of the next 21 to 30 programs, and $26 per program thereafter (Association for American Medical Colleges 2014a). This respondent therefore would have paid $2,955 to apply to 130 programs ($95 + $10 × 10 + $16 × 10 + $26 × 100).

61. Association of American Medical Colleges (2015c); Gruppuso and Adashi (2017).

62. See Bourdieu (1996); Khan (2011); Persell and Cookson (1985); Rivera (2015); Turner (1960).

63. See Hall (1948, 1949); Marshall, Fulton, and Wessen (1978); Miller (1970).

64. Turner (1960).

65. Indeed, as Jewel (2008, 1194) has noted about inequalities in legal education, "The myth of merit excludes the possibility that a poor performance might result from a dearth of social and economic capital."

2. THE MATCH LIST

1. H-1 visas are congressionally capped work permits that allow non-US residents to work in specialty occupations, including medicine. They are more desirable than J-1 visas, which are less expensive but require non-US residents to return to their home countries after completing their work or studies. Waivers exist but require that IMGs work in underserved areas for a period of time after residency in order to stay in the United States. For more information, see http://www.uscis.gov/.

2. I use *officials* throughout this chapter as a collective term for the program directors, associate program directors, and assistant program directors who constituted the programs' leadership. While the residents often simply referred to these individuals as program directors—regardless of rank—I use the terms *officials* and *leaders* instead to avoid confusion and maintain confidentiality.

3. National Resident Matching Program (n.d.). The National Resident Matching Program (NRMP), which provides national-level data on the main residency and specialties (fellowship) matches, is not involved in the selection process; it simply reports aggregate-level data on the decisions made by individual programs. The NRMP does not take a stance on whether USMDs should be prioritized in recruitment decisions.

4. National Resident Matching Program (2015a). One exception is the applicants to advanced specialties that require a preliminary internship year, such as dermatology and radiology. They simultaneously apply for their "prelim" position and their advanced specialty, which means they often receive two legally binding offers: one for the internship and the other for the advanced residency.

5. Few social scientists have been able to observe recruitment decisions as they unfold because of access restrictions and confidentiality concerns (Rivera 2015, 211). In this chapter, I draw on in-depth interviews with key decision makers at Stonewood and Legacy, as well as participant observations of resident selection committee meetings at Stonewood.

6. As Bourdieu notes, "To think in terms of field is to *think relationally*" (as quoted in Wacquant 1989, 39; emphasis in original), with prestige existing only in relation to other institutions within the field. He defined *field* as an arena for struggle over resources or "capital." See Brosnan (2010) and Naidoo (2004) for examples of how medical schools and universities, respectively, use admissions policies to strategically maintain or gain symbolic capital in the field of higher education.

7. See Bowen et al. (1999). In 2014, the online physician network Doximity released the Residency Navigator, a tool designed to rank residency programs by reputation. The survey sample was not nationally representative, however, so Doximity's results did not represent official rankings (see https://health.usnews.com/health-news/blogs/second-opinion/2014/09/10/doximitys-residency-navigator-injects-transparency-into-gme; Harder 2014).

8. In a world full of rank-ordered lists for everything from restaurants to dog walkers, the absence of rankings in residency might suggest a certain veneer of equality within graduate medical education, when, in fact, I argue it helps obscure the classificatory power of residency training.

9. American Board of Internal Medicine (2014).

10. As one Stonewood University Medical School official explained, "The leaders in the institution would always look at the places [our students matched to] to know how many of our students are going to Harvard-affiliated hospitals? How many are going to Hopkins? How many are going to Stanford? That's what the medical school committee would want to know."

11. See Corley and Gioia (2000), Deephouse and Carter (2005), and Fombrun and van Riel (1997) for more on how observers interpret social "signals" emitted by organizations to eventually form a reputation.

12. For more on the bias against programs that are heavily staffed by non-USMDs, see Manthous (2012).

13. Given the small number of decisionmakers involved in recruitment at Legacy, I have intentionally chosen to use gender-neutral pronouns here to protect their identities.

14. Bourdieu (1986, 1998).

15. The very fact that Legacy tried to conform to the industry-wide norm of hiring USMDs as a way of improving its status made it more comparable to Stonewood than some of these other nearby hospitals, which were perhaps more resigned to their status position. Middle-status conformity theory argues that high- and low-status social actors are more likely to defy social norms because they are more secure in their positions at the top and bottom of the status hierarchy. Middling actors, however, are more insecure and are thus more likely to conform to widely accepted norms and behaviors—such as hiring USMDs, in this case—in the hopes of increasing their status. See Dittes and Kelley (1956); Phillips and Zuckerman (2001).

16. Previous studies of hiring practices in firms have found that a dearth of "qualified" workers can lead employers to search for nontraditional employees. See Reskin (1993).

17. National Resident Matching Program (2018a).

18. Given the very small number of individuals charged with selecting interviewees at Stonewood, I have intentionally chosen to use gender-neutral pronouns here to protect their identities.

19. Association of American Medical Colleges (2018a).

20. Preference- or taste-based discrimination occurs when employers rely on prejudices as shortcuts to exclude certain groups of applicants, even when more information is available about those applicants' qualifications, resulting in discrimination (Becker 1957).

21. Elites are known to "say" meritocracy and often do something else. See Khan and Jerolmack (2013), for example.

22. Not all DO applicants take the USMLE, but they are all required to take the Comprehensive Osteopathic Medical Licensing Examination, an equivalent three-step licensing exam that measures medical knowledge.

23. Rivera (2015, 89) found a similar pattern among executives at elite service firms who viewed the decision to go to nonelite, lower-ranked schools as a mark of both intellectual and *moral* failure.

24. See, for example, National Resident Matching Program (2018d, 2018b, 2018c). See also note 17 in the introduction.

25. Neckerman and Kirschenman (1991, 435).

26. Norcini, van Zanten, and Boulet (2008); Weber and Mathews (2012).

27. Lorber (1984).

28. Podolny (2005, 13).

29. Podolny (2005).

30. Podolny describes how status "leaks" between institutions and individuals, making it difficult to fully escape one's association with low-status entities, despite stellar performance. See Podolny (2005, 14) for an example of this process involving high-end jewelers.

31. Blau (2017); Podolny (2005).

32. Mick and Comfort (1997); Norcini et al. (2010); Sang et al. (1986); Tsugawa et al. (2017).

33. Iglehart (2013).

34. Mullan, Salsberg, and Weider (2015).

35. Jenkins and Reddy (2017).

36. This is true even net of other factors correlated with race, such as crime rates (Emerson, Chai, and Yancey 2001).

37. Stonewood, like Legacy (see note 15), is exhibiting middle-status conformity, where a social actor (in this case, an organization) is anxious to increase its social status and does so by conforming to conventional behavior—hiring prestigious USMDs (see Dittes and Kelley 1956; Phillips and Zuckerman 2001). Higher-status actors, like Harvard, are more secure in their status and therefore may be more comfortable deviating from the norm without fear of losing status.

38. See Bourdieu (1984); Rivera (2015, 48).

39. In 2014, the mean USMLE Step 1 score nationwide for US seniors who matched to internal medicine as a preferred specialty was 231 (National Resident Matching Program 2014a). The mean USMLE Step 1 score that same year for US and Canadian test takers was 229, with a standard deviation of twenty points (National Board of Medical Examiners 2015). A score of 270 is therefore two standard deviations above the mean.

40. This echoes studies in surgery and family medicine that found internationally trained applicants (including USIMGs) were less likely to receive residency interviews than equally qualified US-trained applicants were, and they were expected to have higher qualifications for the same positions (Desbiens and Vidaillet 2010; Moore and Rhodenbaugh 2002; Nasir 1994).

41. The out-of-pocket costs, however, were steep: there was a $175 application fee (US students paid $150), and tuition cost $4,000, excluding living expenses. Students from US allopathic institutions, in contrast, could rotate tuition-free. IMGs were also forbidden from doing an elective at Stonewood if they had already obtained their medical degree, which barred many those who had already graduated from gaining crucial US clinical experience at Stonewood.

42. Rivera (2015, 224) found something similar in her study of hiring in elite professional service firms: "The same errors made by candidates from groups not negatively stereotyped in these domains were oftentimes explained in terms of situational factors (e.g. a bad day) and excused."

43. This is what Podolny calls making a "disclaimer"—i.e., when a high-status social actor does something considered "deviant" (like hiring non-USMDs) and it draws a distinction between itself and others who regularly deviate in this way to control the narrative.

44. See Bolton and Muzio (2007); Rivera (2015).

3. A DAY ON THE WARDS

Portions of this chapter were published in Jenkins (2018).

1. To be "on call" means that the resident is responsible for admitting new patients until approximately 9 PM, after which a night resident comes on duty to handle overnight admissions.

2. See Brosnan (2010); Jenkins (2018).

3. American Medical Association (2015).

4. See, for example, Manthous (2012, 290), who, upon joining the faculty of an IMG-friendly program, was warned by colleagues that he "would be throwing away [his] career on 'missionary work.' "

5. Two accounts of medical training in community versus university settings from the late 1960s reveal that hospital characteristics, such as the case mix and whether residents are supervised by busy physician-scientists at a large academic medical center, can impact residents' autonomy. See Miller (1970); Mumford (1970). These studies considered only interns (first-year residents), however, and are now outdated, as graduate medical education has changed considerably since the late 1960s.

6. Medical students and pharmacy students were also part of the team.

7. Teams were generally composed of one intern and one resident at Legacy, with an occasional medical student. Teams were not assigned a specific attending at Legacy, instead working for several attendings at once.

8. Legacy's conference room also had black-and-white photographs on the walls, but these were of older generations of doctors from the period when the hospital still belonged to Stonewood University.

9. The Maddrey discriminant function is a measure of disease severity and mortality risk in hepatitis (or liver inflammation) associated with excessive alcohol consumption. A score of 32 or higher is thought to reflect a high likelihood of short-term mortality (Friedman 2019).

10. Giving steroids to patients with infections is generally inadvisable because they lower the body's immune response.

11. One attending quipped, for example, "Some people say our patients walk off the wards and onto the Boards. So I like to look at stuff we've seen [on the wards] and reinforce it by looking at [a MKSAP] question."

12. Legacy did employ two full-time hospitalists who worked on alternating weeks, admitting patients without a primary care physician. Although they were in-house and thus slightly more accessible, these hospitalists had teaching loads similar to those of the community-based attendings.

13. This diverges from other ethnographic accounts of attending supervision, which primarily took place in university hospital settings. See, for example, Becker et al. (1961); Bosk (2003); Light (1980); Stelling and Bucher (1972). The findings at Legacy suggest that there is more variation in medical training than we might otherwise have gleaned from previous studies of single institutions.

14. Guidelines recommend transfusions only when Hgb = 7–8g/dL (a range lower than this patient's hemoglobin level). See Carson et al. (2016).

15. See, for example, Coburn, Rappolt, and Bourgeault (1997); Knaapen (2014).

16. See, for example, Frosch et al. (2012).

17. Bush (2010).

18. Jenkins (2015).

19. Endocarditis with the bacterium *strep bovis* is highly suggestive of colon cancer—to the point where physicians typically suspect colon cancer until proven otherwise (Galdy and Nastasi 2012).

20. US National Library of Medicine (2017).

21. Allen (2013).

22. The ACGME requires internal medicine residents to spend at least 130 half-days over the course of their training in an outpatient continuity clinic devoted to "longitudinal care" (Accreditation Council for Graduate Medical Education 2013).

23. Association of American Medical Colleges (2004). This is likely a vestige of the fact that Medicare pays for residency positions and thus does not pay for outpatient work—it provides only inpatient reimbursements. See Ludmerer (2015, 145).

24. Legacy residents were frequently asked to care for surgical, orthopedic, and psychiatric patients on evenings and weekends when attendings on those services were less available—further evidence of the hospital's dependence on their labor. While Legacy residents frequently "babysat" (as they called it) other services' patients, Stonewood had entire departments (with their own specialized residents) to care for those patients.

25. Residents at Legacy could complete elective rotations at nearby Stonewood; see the next chapter for more details about the role of electives in the Legacy curriculum.

26. Rounds were scheduled from 9 AM to 12 PM, which meant that teams had roughly thirteen minutes to discuss and examine each patient before noon conference.

4. GROOMING

1. In legal contexts, contracts require the exchange of one consideration (or thing promised) for another. See https://www.law.cornell.edu/wex/consideration.

2. See Becker et al. (1961); Bosk (2003); Coser (1962); Fox (1957); Haas and Shaffir (1987); Hafferty (1988a, 1991); Light (1980); Mumford (1970); Merton, Reader, and Kendall (1957); Underman (2015); and Underman and Hirshfield (2016) for examples of research on socialization. As Brosnan writes, "Despite repeated calls for the sociology of medical education to move beyond the focus on student socialization, very few studies have examined medical education at a more macro or structural level. Almost all studies have been conducted within a single medical school, and have tended to take for granted the medical school itself as an institution, thereby ignoring medical schools' relationships to the healthcare system, the bioscientific research enterprise and the state" (2009, 54). See also Hafferty (2006) for more on the need to consider training environments to better understand differences in professionalism.

3. Bourdieu (1996); Brosnan (2009, 2010).

4. As Brosnan notes, "Medical education involves the development of lasting dispositions which imbue trainees with a practical sense of how to succeed in the field and could potentially be seen as the production of a habitus." (2009, 58) See Brosnan (2009, 58–61) for more on the medical habitus. See also Stern (1998) for more on how the learning environment has a direct bearing on the professionalism of residents.

5. Bourdieu (1996); Brosnan (2009, 2010).

6. Hafferty (1998, 404). Before the hidden curriculum concept really took over the medical education literature in the 1990s, sociologists like Light had been calling for more attention to the unspoken messages being communicated to students. In 1988, Light wrote: "The structure of a training program—the sequence of experiences, the organization of work, the trainers' background and orientation, the hierarchy of values—constitutes a

latent curriculum that affects the residents' clinical habits and perspectives as strongly as the manifest curriculum" (1988, 313).

7. Hafferty (1998, 405).

8. Swick (2000, 614).

9. Chen et al. (2011); Chen et al. (2010).

10. This includes approaches to treating pain, for example. See Meghani and Rajput (2011).

11. Porter et al. (2008); Whelan (2006); Zulla, Baerlocher, and Verma (2008).

12. To be sure, Stonewood's program had three times the number of residents spread across three hospitals, which meant that there was considerably more to cover during orientation. Even so, Stonewood's approach to orientation as a process, rather than a discrete event like at Legacy, illustrates how Stonewood really shepherded its housestaff through residency.

13. Networks are a known determinant of labor market inequality, especially among gender and ethnic minorities, who tend to have fewer network ties than individuals in more privileged groups (Gerxhani and Koster 2015; McDonald 2011; Petersen, Saporta, and Seidel 2000).

14. Since at least 1993, in internal medicine, the ACGME has required evidence of participation in some kind of "scholarly activity" before graduation, defined as "original research, comprehensive case reports, or review of assigned clinical and research topics" (Alguire et al. 1996, 321). However, the extent to which programs actually implement research requirements varies widely, such that in 2011 the ACGME issued 402 citations for noncompliance with required scholarly activities across all specialties—amounting to 6.5 percent of all citations issued that year (Grady et al. 2012).

15. Clinical research for physicians can include case reports on interesting/unique patients (often considered low-hanging fruit), retrospective chart reviews, and randomized controlled trials (generally the most prestigious kind of publication).

16. According to the ACGME's Program Requirements for Graduate Medical Education in Internal Medicine, "II.B.5. The faculty must establish and maintain an environment of inquiry and scholarship with an active research component. . . . II.B.5.b). Some members of the faculty should *also demonstrate scholarship* by one or more of the following: II.B.5.b).(1) peer-reviewed funding; II.B.5.b).(2) publication of original research or review articles in peer reviewed journals, or chapters in textbooks; II.B.5.b).(3) publication or presentation of case reports or clinical series at local, regional, or national professional and scientific society meetings; or, II.B.5.b).(4) participation in national committees or educational organizations" (2013, 9; emphasis added).

17. Many Legacy-based teaching attendings had pro forma affiliations with Carter Medical College but had little contact with the medical school.

18. Categorical residents at Stonewood had one less elective month per year than the residents at Legacy (two in PGY-1, three in PGY-2, and four in PGY-3). Legacy residents had three in PGY-1, four in PGY-2, and five in PGY-3.

19. Bosk (2003, 1980).

20. Accreditation Council for Graduate Medical Education (2013).

21. The head of infectious diseases came to a different noon conference to announce the new hospital policy but did not attend the M&M where the residents discussed how the error occurred.

22. See Bosk (2003).

23. While I was able to observe the Clinical Competency Committee meetings at Stonewood for three months, I was not privy to them at Legacy, meaning that I could have been unaware of the committee's disciplinary efforts. The data for this section of the chapter come from interviews with and observations of the Legacy residents and program directorship.

24. The use of a gender-neutral pronoun here is intentional to protect this individual's confidentiality.

25. Stonewood's three-year average Board pass rate in 2012–2014 was about half a standard deviation above the national mean (American Board of Internal Medicine 2014).

26. Andriole et al. (2008); Association of American Medical Colleges (2014b).

27. Turner writes: "In sponsored mobility, the unpromising recruit reflects unfavorably on the judgments of his sponsors and threatens the myth of elite omniscience; consequently, he may be tolerated and others may 'cover up' for his deficiencies in order to protect the unified front of the elite to the outer world" (1960, 860).

28. Hafferty (2006, 2151). Medical professionalism "consists of those behaviors by which we— as physicians—demonstrate that we are worthy of the trust bestowed upon us by our patients and the public, because we are working for the patients' and the public's good" (Swick 2000, 614).

29. Stonewood was not one of these programs.

30. Studies find, for example, that decreasing duty hours can reduce burnout among residents (Gopal et al. 2005).

31. When I asked an internist colleague about the significance of this lab value (before explaining the context), her reaction was telling: "This is a very sick patient and needs to be seen as soon as possible."

32. The use of a gender-neutral pronoun here is intentional to protect this individual's identity.

33. Lockwood, Jordan, and Kunda (2002).

5. GRADUATION

1. These include allergy and immunology, cardiovascular disease, endocrinology, gastroenterology, hematology, infectious disease, nephrology, oncology, pulmonary disease/critical care medicine, and rheumatology. Residents can also match into fellowships in associated subfields within these subspecialties, such as sleep medicine in pulmonary disease/critical care medicine or hepatology in gastroenterology; see https://www.acponline.org/about-acp/about-internal-medicine/subspecialties.

2. Fried, Muchmore, and Sundstrom (2012).

3. Association of American Medical Colleges (2015a).

4. Patients requiring angioplasty to remove blockages around their heart (known as ST-elevation myocardial infarctions or STEMIs) were transferred to hospitals with "cath" labs for heart catheterization. Legacy residents thus had very restricted exposure to complex cardiac cases and cardiologists as mentors, which made pursuing a fellowship in cardiology more difficult.

5. National Resident Matching Program (2015b).

6. While technically true that cardiology fellows would learn to do catheterizations during fellowship, many fellowship programs want to see that applicants have the relevant practical experience to know that they actually want to pursue that subspecialty. Certainly, applicants from places like Legacy without cath labs would be competing against applicants from places with cath labs, thereby likely putting them at a disadvantage.

7. See Binder, Davis, and Bloom (2016) for more on how definitions of success are shaped by elite educational institutions.

8. Clausen (1991).

9. As Marshall, Fulton, and Wessen noted as early as the 1950s, getting the "right" internship was important "not because they necessarily involve less 'drudge work,' but because they place the young physician in a place with desirable sponsorship lines to future career opportunities. Participants in these programs are likely to establish strong collegial specialty bonds, and to become committed to scientific norms as well as to research" (1978, 127).

10. Podolny (2005) argues that status leaks in this way between institutions and individuals, making it difficult to recover from such a loss of prestige even long after the individual separates from the institution.

11. The use of gender-neutral pronouns here is intentional to protect this individual's confidentiality.

12. For example, only twenty positions in oncology (not hematology and oncology, which is a much more popular fellowship) were available nationwide in 2015 (National Resident Matching Program 2015d).

13. National Resident Matching Program (2015d).

14. The National Resident Matching Program, which provides national-level data on the main residency and specialties (fellowship) matches, is not involved in the selection process; it simply reports aggregate-level data on the decisions made by individual programs.

15. Podolny (2005).

16. American Board of Internal Medicine (2014). These results are generally consistent with national trends; USMD-dominated programs have higher Board passage rates on average compared to integrated, DO-dominated, and IMG-dominated programs (Jenkins, Franklyn, Klugman, and Reddy, 2019).

17. National Resident Matching Program (2014c). Ranking refers to candidates who have interviewed and have reached the point of ranking programs in The Match process.

18. Association of American Medical Colleges (2014b).

19. Jauhar (2014); Rotenstein et al. (2018). West, Shanafelt, and Kolars's (2011) study of internal medicine residents found that burnout was associated with higher debt and was more likely to occur among USMDs compared to IMGs.

20. Kristof (2013).

21. Eckhert (2010).

22. Residents with federal loans were entitled to loan forgiveness after spending ten years working at a nonprofit institution, which included residency (Federal Student Aid n.d.).

23. Because cystic fibrosis is a rare disease in adults, this respondent is making the point that USMDs specialize in niche areas while non-USMDs fill important gaps in more general medicine.

24.   Miller (1970, 87).

25.   National Resident Matching Program (2014c).

26.   Association of American Medical Colleges (2015a).

27.   General internal medicine comprises careers in both outpatient primary care and inpatient hospital medicine.

28.   Leigh et al. (2012).

29.   Goffman (1952).

30.   Tomlinson et al. (2013) found similar results among female and minority lawyers whose strategies for advancement often resulted in the reproduction, rather than the transformation, of opportunity structures.

6. THE NAVY SEALs AND THE NATIONAL GUARD

1.   National Navy UDT-SEAL Museum (2019).

2.   Freidson (1985).

3.   Light (1988) noted as early as the mid-1980s that there was a disconnect between institutional incentives and rewards in medical education, with those at the top getting large grants and doing obscure research when hospitals needed more generalists to care for regular patients (see pp. 309, 311).

4.   Bosk (1992, 63) writes: "The genetic counselors are in the basement of the prestige hierarchy, and it is to the basement that other physicians go to find help to 'mop up,' messy situations," such as counseling bereaved parents and coordinating complex care for patients.

5.   Ridgeway et al. (1998).

6.   As Jewel writes about legal education, "Schools reinforce the theme that success is a product of individual merit or an innate gift, rather than any sort of inherited capital, economic or symbolic" (2008, 1166).

7.   Jewel (2008, 1168). See also Bourdieu and Passeron (1990).

8.   As Jewel similarly notes about legal education in the United States, "The myth of merit . . . causes advantaged law students to believe that their success is based on their individual merit, gaining the 'supreme privilege of not seeing themselves as privileged' " (2008, 1195, citing Bourdieu and Passeron 1990, 210). She goes on to write: "Thus, American legal education, with its emphasis on symbolic prestige and merit, enables the privileged classes to 'appear to be surrendering to a perfectly neutral authority the power of transmitting power from one generation to another, and thus to be renouncing the arbitrary privilege of the hereditary transmission of privileges' " (Jewel 2008, 1195, citing Bourdieu and Passeron 1990, 167).

9.   In most US hospitals, when a "code blue," or cardiopulmonary emergency, occurs, a code team composed of nurses, physicians, and respiratory therapists is dispatched to the bedside, where the respiratory therapists—i.e., nonphysician specialists in pulmonary disease—handle or assist with intubation.

10.   *Merriam-Webster* (n.d.).

11.   Iglehart (2013).

12.   Mullan, Salsberg, and Weider (2015).

13. As Turner writes, "Under sponsored mobility, the objective is to indoctrinate elite culture in only those presumably who will enter the elite, lest there grow a dangerous number of angry young men who have elite skills without elite station" (1960, 863). This speaks to how angry USMDs would be if they did not get a residency position after graduation.

14. Kamens (1977, 217–18).

15. Ludmerer (2015).

16. Association of American Medical Colleges (2015b); Iglehart (2011).

17. While there is a lack of national data documenting how many IMGs return to their home countries after residency, very few IMGs at Legacy chose to leave the United States. With the exception of a handful of Canadian-born residents who pursued fellowships in Canada, the vast majority stayed in the United States to continue their training and/or establish a practice.

18. See Cruess and Cruess (2004).

19. Queensland Health (2015).

20. See Young's (1958) satirical account of meritocracy.

21. Anecdotal studies have found differences in the pain management approaches of IMGs (Meghani and Rajput 2011).

22. DKA, a serious complication of diabetes, is typically managed in the intensive care unit rather than on the general medical floors.

23. Tissue plasminogen activator (tPA) is a time-sensitive medication used to break down blood clots.

24. This is the main premise of intergroup contact theory (see Pettigrew 1998). Reeves and Burke (2009), for example, found more negative perceptions of DOs among MDs in the Deep South who had had little previous contact with DOs, suggesting that adequate representation of graduate types in training programs could help reduce status differences among graduates.

25. See Larson (1980).

26. As Thomas and Thomas famously argued, "If men [or women] define situations as real, they are real in their consequences" (1928, 572).

27. Ridgeway and Correll (2006).

28. The use of a gender-neutral pronoun here is intentional to protect this individual's identity.

29. Bolton and Muzio (2007, 48).

30. Freidson (1984).

31. Bendix (1956, pp. 261, 262); Cullen (1931).

32. See Alon and Tienda (2007); Bourdieu (1984); Bourdieu (1996); Bourdieu and Passeron (1990); Jewel (2008); Khan (2011, 15); Rivera (2015).

33. "Whether one is 'sponsored up,' 'cooled-out [discouraged from high-status positions],' or thrown into a contest for success, all this is done in a way that makes the experience one that seems *self-generated*" (Marshall, Fulton, and Wessen 1978, 127; emphasis added).

34. See, for example, Bourdieu (1996); Bourdieu and Passeron (1990); Jewel (2008); Khan (2011).

35. Jewel (2008, 1194).

36. Jewel (2008, 1162).

37.   Ridgeway and Correll (2006); Ridgeway et al. (1998).

38.   See, for example, Waldinger and Lichter (2003) for similar patterns among unskilled labor.

39.   Bolton and Muzio (2007) similarly argue that gendered segmentation in the British legal profession ensures that the current legal elite can maintain their status, while creating a female "reserve army of legal labor with lesser terms and conditions" (47).

40.   Labor queues represent employers' prioritization of candidates based on their desirability and the number of positions available (Thurow 1972). For example, see Reskin et al. (1990) for more on how women constitute a surplus labor force and enter professions only when more desirable workers—namely, men—are no longer available or interested. See also Lorber (1984).

41.   National Resident Matching Program (2015c).

42.   Edwards (2016).

43.   Mann (1970).

44.   Ridgeway and Correll (2006). See also Steele and Aronson (1995, 797) for more on stereotype threat, or the "risk of confirming, as self-characteristic, a negative stereotype about one's group."

45.   Kellogg (2009).

46.   Ridgeway (2014); Ridgeway and Correll (2006); Ridgeway and Erickson (2000); Sennett and Cobb (1972).

47.   Karabel (2005, 556, citing Young 1958, 106-8).

CONCLUSIONS AND IMPLICATIONS

1.   Freidson (1983, 1984, 1985, 1986a); Hafferty and Light (1995).

2.   Freidson (1983).

3.   Timmermans and Oh (2010).

4.   For more on how professional elites rely on internal social closure, see Bolton and Muzio (2007)

5.   Podolny describes how, unlike reputation, which is based on a previous track record of performance, status can *leak* between institutions and individuals, becoming sticky and making it difficult for individuals to ever recover from the status loss associated with their pedigree (2005, 14).

6.   Merton (1968). Lorber (1984) found similar evidence of a Matthew effect for male physicians versus female physicians.

7.   Link and Phelan (2001, 364). Goffman (1963, 4) conceptualized stigma as "a special kind of relationship between attribute" (in this case, pedigree) "and stereotype" (in this case, the view that non-USMDs are subpar doctors).

8.   Bos et al. (2013).

9.   See Groysberg et al. (2016).

10.   Bos et al. (2013, 4).

11.   Reich, Gordon, and Edwards (1973).

12.   "Segmentation divides workers and forestalls potential movements uniting all workers against employers" (Reich, Gordon, and Edwards 1973, 364).

13. See Jenkins and Reddy (2016). Bolton and Muzio (2007) examined similar instances of gendered social closure within the legal profession. They refer to the process whereby female lawyers are confined to lower-prestige jobs as "segmentation," when traditionally that term refers to a labor market arrangement that benefits *employers*. See Reich et al. 1973. I argue instead that status separation describes horizontal processes of social closure among professionals designed to benefit elite portions of the *profession*.

14. See, for example, National Resident Matching Program (2019b, 2019c).

15. Young (2001).

16. Hall (1948, 335) similarly described the medical profession's inner elite core as difficult to penetrate, even back in 1948: "Outside the core are doctors who are attempting by their individual efforts to break into the central core. However, as the core has its own specific mechanisms for recruiting and legitimating its members, the would-be intruders gain admittance only with the greatest difficulty." The main difference is that Hall was referring to an inner core of specialists and a periphery of general practitioners—a vertical hierarchy. I am interested in the horizontal hierarchy within internal medicine, characterized by an inner core primarily composed of USMDs and a periphery of non-USMDs.

17. A similar thought experiment was discussed in a *New York Times* op-ed about Harvard's relative paucity of Asian Americans, who tend to have very high scores on exams and standardized tests: "The real problem is that, in a meritocratic system, whites would be a minority—and Harvard just isn't comfortable with that" (Mounk 2014).

18. Allman, Perelas, and Eiger (2016, 894).

19. Jenkins and Reddy (2016).

20. Lohr, Vanselow, and Detmer (1996, 748).

21. Turner (1960, 856).

22. Hall (1948, 336).

23. Hall (1948); National Resident Matching Program (2019a).

24. See Flexner (1910); Marshall, Fulton, and Wessen (1978).

25. Marshall, Fulton, and Wessen (1978, 135).

26. Lorber (1984, 7).

27. Karabel (2005, 549).

28. Lorber (1984) similarly found that women are also blamed for being less productive—or less interested in career advancement—to explain their absence from the upper echelons of the profession.

29. Khan (2011).

30. See also Bourdieu and Passeron (1990) and Jewel (2008) for more on how educational structures secure the consent of those they subordinate.

31. The numbers of Hispanic and black doctors have actually *decreased* in the last thirty years (Sánchez et al. 2015; Silverman 2015), but a new study points to a slow increase in the diversity of medical school classes since 2012 (Boatright et al. 2018).

32. Turner (1960, 860).

33. Papadakis et al. (2005).

34. See Lewis and Sheps (1983); Swanson (1973).

35. Association of American Medical Colleges (2019a).

36. Adams (2018); Goodnough (2019); Hassan (2019).

37.   Gozu, Kern, and Wright (2009); West, Shanafelt, and Kolars (2011).

38.   Hall (1948, 329) found something similar when comparing a lower-socioeconomic-status physician to a higher-socioeconomic-status physician: "The initial drive was presumably greater in the first than in the second, but the latter was continuously assisted by groups who had an inside knowledge of the profession."

39.   Physicians Foundation (2012).

40.   Landon, Reschovsky, and Blumenthal (2003); Patel et al. (2018).

41.   Patel et al. (2018).

42.   Cohen, Gabriel, and Terrell (2002); Silver et al. (2019).

43.   Andriole, Klingensmith, and Schechtman (2005); Cohen, Gabriel, and Terrell (2002).

44.   Chen et al. (2010).

45.   Chen et al. (2011).

46.   See Reskin (1993, 241).

47.   Reeves and Burke (2009) found similar results: MDs in the Deep South had more negative perceptions of DOs when they had had little previous contact with DOs, suggesting that adequate representation of graduate types in training programs could help reduce bias.

48.   Kinchen et al. (2004).

49.   For more on how contact between different social groups reduces prejudice, see Pettigrew (1998).

50.   See Jenkins et al. (2019).

51.   American Medical Association (2010); Fordyce et al. (2012); Hagopian et al. (2004).

52.   See, for example, Mick and Comfort (1997); Norcini et al. (2010); Sang et al. (1986); Saywell et al. (1980); Tsugawa et al. (2017). Tsugawa et al.'s recent study (2017) using Medicare data determined that elderly patients treated by IMG hospitalists had slightly *lower* mortality rates than those treated by USMD hospitalists did. Data specific to *trainees* is elusive, however. Patients are never treated solely by trainees, and the myriad other clinicians involved make it difficult to isolate the impact of the trainees' education on patient outcomes.

53.   Saks (2015).

54.   Jenkins (2018).

55.   Edelman (2016).

56.   Ludmerer (2015, 177) makes a similar argument about heterogeneity among residency programs in the 1960s; structurally, programs were similar, but learning environments differed importantly (by including things like role modeling and discussions), thereby leading to significant differences in Board passage rates between community and university hospitals.

57.   Interestingly, the earliest residency positions primarily emphasized the extraction of labor; for example, the job criteria for a house officer position at Massachusetts General Hospital in 1897 were "Subordination, Capacity for Labor, Conduct" (Ludmerer 2015, 7).

58.   Brooks (2011); Jewel (2008).

59.   Childress (2019); Cross and Goldenberg (2009); Kendzior (2013). Without adjuncts, tenured and tenure-track faculty would likely be unable to focus so much on their research (a more prestigious task within the academy) because universities would need them to teach.

60. Saideman (2013).

61. Petersen (2019) has written about her own pursuit of a tenure-track job as a media studies professor: "Thousands of PhD students clung to the idea of a tenure-track professorship. And the tighter the academic market became, the harder we worked. We didn't try to break the system, since that's not how we'd been raised. We tried to *win* it. I never thought the system was equitable. I knew it was winnable for only a small few. I just believed I could continue to optimize myself to become one of them."

62. See Brooks (2011); Cross and Goldenberg (2009).

63. Hoff, Sutcliffe, and Young (2017).

AFTERWORD

1. United States Medical Licensing Exam (2020) "Change to Pass/Fail Score Reporting for Step 1." https://www.usmle.org/inCus/#decision.

2. National Resident Matching Program (2014a).

3. See for example Lorber (1984); Quadlin (2018); Rivera (2012, 2015).

4. Jenkins et al. (2018).

5. See United States Medical Licensing Exam (2020) "The Issue." https://www.usmle.org/inCus/#appreciating.

6. Knopes (2019).

7. See for example https://thesheriffofsodium.com/2020/02/13/usmlepassfail-a-brave-new-day/.

8. United States Medical Licensing Exam (2020) "The Issue." https://www.usmle.org/inCus/#appreciating.

APPENDIX: ON BEING A "SECOND-YEAR INTERN"

1. The credential, of course, was highly confusing in a hospital setting, where an intern is usually a first-year resident. My badge was a different color from the housestaff badges but likely still helped me gain access to certain spaces (such as areas behind nursing stations) that would have otherwise required more explaining.

2. These were what Mumford (1970) called "situational interviews."

3. Goffman (2014, 237).

4. Jenkins (2014).

5. This is not uncommon for hospital ethnographers. See, for example, Bosk (2003).

6. Mumford (1970).

7. Guest, Bunce, and Johnson (2006).

8. Tomlinson et al. (2013).

9. Gorden (1998).

10. Schatzman and Strauss (1973).

11. Corbin and Strauss (1990).

12. Emerson, Fretz, and Shaw (2011).

13. Lofland et al. (2006).

14. Emerson, Fretz, and Shaw (2011); Lofland et al. (2006).

15. Tolich (2004).
16. See Jenkins (2015) for more about this particular incident.
17. Smith (2014).
18. Pulse oximetry measures the amount of oxygen in the bloodstream. Normal values range from 95 to 100 percent.
19. Light (1980); Lofland et al. (2006).
20. Lorber (1984).
21. Lerner (2013).
22. Bosk (1992).

Works Cited

Abbott, Andrew. 1988. *The System of Professions: An Essay on the Division of Expert Labor*. Chicago: University of Chicago Press.

Accreditation Council for Graduate Medical Education. 2013. "ACGME Program Requirements for Graduate Medical Education in Internal Medicine." http://www.acgme.org/acgmeweb /Portals/0/PFAssets/2013-PR-FAQ-PIF/140_internal_medicine_07012013.pdf.

Adams, Susan. 2018. "NYU Makes Medical School Tuition Free." *Forbes*. https://www.forbes .com/sites/susanadams/2018/08/16/nyu-makes-medical-school-tuition-free/#7d639a28a9d8.

Alguire, P. C., W. A. Anderson, R. R. Albrecht, and G. A. Poland. 1996. "Resident Research in Internal Medicine Training Programs." *Annals of Internal Medicine* 124 (3): 321–28.

Allen, Marshall. 2013. "Why Doctors Stay Mum About Mistakes Their Colleagues Make." *ProPublica*. https://www.propublica.org/article/why-doctors-stay-mum-about-mistakes-their -colleagues-make.

Allman, Richard, Apostolos Perelas, and Glenn Eiger. 2016. "POINT: Should the United States Provide Postgraduate Training to International Medical Graduates? Yes." *CHEST* 149 (4): 893–95.

Alon, Sigal, and Marta Tienda. 2007. "Diversity, Opportunity, and the Shifting Meritocracy in Higher Education." *American Sociological Review* 72 (4): 487–511.

American Association of Colleges of Osteopathic Medicine. 2014a. "The Evolution of Osteopathic Medical Education." https://www.aacom.org/docs/default-source/default-document-library /infographic-osteo13.pdf?sfvrsn=c3094897_18.

American Association of Colleges of Osteopathic Medicine. 2014b. "Trends in Osteopathic Medical School Applicants, Enrollment and Graduates." http://www.aacom.org/docs/default -source/data-and-trends/2014-trends-COM-AEG-PDF.pdf?sfvrsn=26.

American Board of Internal Medicine. 2014. "Exam Pass Rates." http://www.abim.org/about /examInfo/data-pass-rates.aspx.

American Board of Internal Medicine. 2019. "Percentage of Third-Year Internal Medicine Residents Who Are Female." https://www.abim.org/about/statistics-data/resident-fellow -workforce-data/third-year-residents-female.aspx.

American Medical Association. 2010. "International Medical Graduates in American Medicine: Contemporary Challenges and Opportunities." http://www.slideshare.net/drimhotep /internationalmedicalgraduatesinamericanmedicinecontemporarychallengesandopportunities.

American Medical Association. 2013. "Match Results Highlight Growing Shortage of Residency Slots."http://web.archive.org/web/20130420133316/http://www.ama-assn.org/ams/pub/meded/2013-april/2013-april.shtml.

American Medical Association. 2015. "FREIDA Online®." http://www.ama-assn.org/ama/pub/education-careers/graduate-medical-education/freida-online.page.

American Medical Association. 2018. "FREIDA Online®." http://www.ama-assn.org/ama/pub/education-careers/graduate-medical-education/freida-online.page.

American Medical Association. 2019. "Practicing Medicine in the U.S. as an International Medical Graduate." https://www.ama-assn.org/education/international-medical-education/practicing-medicine-us-international-medical-graduate.

American Osteopathic Association. 2017. "The Single GME Accreditation System." http://www.osteopathic.org/inside-aoa/single-gme-accreditation-system/Pages/default.aspx.

American Osteopathic Association. 2019. "Single GME Student FAQs." https://osteopathic.org/students/student-resources/single-gme/single-gme-student-faqs/.

American Osteopathic Association Staff. 2019. "Final DO Match Day Produces More than 500 Primary Care Residents." The DO. https://thedo.osteopathic.org/2019/02/final-do-match-day-produces-more-than-500-primary-care-residents/.

Anderson, Stuart. 2013. "The Importance of International Students to America: National Foundation for American Policy Brief." http://www.nfap.com/pdf/New%20NFAP%20Policy%20Brief%20The%20Importance%20of%20International%20Students%20to%20America,%20July%202013.pdf.

Andriole, D. A., D. B. Jeffe, H. L. Hageman, M. E. Klingensmith, R. P. McAlister, and A. J. Whelan. 2008. "Attrition During Graduate Medical Education: Medical School Perspective." *Archives of Surgery* 143 (12): 1172–77.

Andriole, D. A., M. E. Klingensmith, and K. B. Schechtman. 2005. "Diversity in General Surgery: A Period of Progress." *Current Surgery* 62 (4): 423–28.

Annandale, Ellen. 1989. "Proletarianization or Restratification of the Medical Profession—The Case of Obstetrics." *International Journal of Health Services* 19 (4): 611–34.

Anspach, Renée R. 1993. *Deciding Who Lives: Fateful Choices in the Intensive-Care Nursery*. Berkeley: University of California Press.

Armstrong, Elizabeth A., and Laura T. Hamilton. 2013. *Paying for the Party: How College Maintains Inequality*. Cambridge, MA: Harvard University Press.

Association of American Medical Colleges. 2004. "Assessing the Scope of Medical Practice." https://www.aamc.org/download/84554/data/scopeofpracticev4.pdf.

Association of American Medical Colleges. 2014a. "The Cost of Applying for a Medical Residency." https://www.aamc.org/download/94416/data/applyingformedicalresidency.pdf.

Association of American Medical Colleges. 2014b. "Graduation Rates and Attrition Factors for U.S. Medical School Students." https://www.aamc.org/download/379220/data/may2014aib-graduationratesandattritionfactorsforusmedschools.pdf.

Association of American Medical Colleges. 2014c. "Medical Student Education: Debt, Costs, and Loan Repayment Fact Card." https://www.aamc.org/download/152968/data/debtfactcard.pdf.

Association of American Medical Colleges. 2014d. "Percentile Ranks for MCAT Total and Section Scores for Exams Administered from January 2012 Through September 2014." https://

aamc-orange.global.ssl.fastly.net/production/media/filer_public/5f/16/5f169a91-12b7-42e0
-8749-a17f3bebe7a4/finalpercentileranksfortheoldmcatexam.pdf.

Association of American Medical Colleges. 2015a. "The Complexities of Physician Supply and Demand: Projections from 2013 to 2025." https://www.aamc.org/download/426248/data/thecomplexitiesofphysiciansupplyanddemandprojectionsfrom2013to2.pdf.

Association of American Medical Colleges. 2015b. "Medicare Direct Graduate Medical Education (DGME) Payments." https://www.aamc.org/advocacy/gme/71152/gme_gme0001.html.

Association of American Medical Colleges. 2015c. "Table C-4: Residency Applicants from U.S. M.D.-Granting Medical Schools by Specialty, 2010–2011 Through 2015–2016." February 17. https://www.aamc.org/download/321564/data/factstablec4.pdf.

Association of American Medical Colleges. 2018a. "Electronic Residency Application Service—How Filters Work." https://www.aamc.org/download/446202/data/howfilterswork.pdf.

Association of American Medical Colleges. 2018b. "Matriculating Student Questionnaire: 2018 All Schools Summary Report." https://www.aamc.org/download/494044/data/msq2018report.pdf.

Association of American Medical Colleges. 2019a. "2019 Update: The Complexities of Physician Supply and Demand: Projections from 2017 to 2032." https://www.aamc.org/system/files/c/2/31-2019_update_-_the_complexities_of_physician_supply_and_demand_-_projections_from_2017-2032.pdf.

Association of American Medical Colleges. 2019b. "Matriculants to U.S. Medical Schools by State of Legal Residency, 2010-2011 through 2019–2020." http://www.aamc.org/download/159534/data/table4-facts2010slrmat-web.pdf.

Association of American Medical Colleges. 2019c. "Table A-7.1: Applicants, First-Time Applicants, Acceptees, and Matriculants to U.S. Medical Schools by Sex, 1999–2000 Through 2008–2009." https://www.aamc.org/download/321470/data/factstablea7_1.pdf.

Association of American Medical Colleges. 2019d. "Table A-7.2: Applicants, First-Time Applicants, Acceptees, and Matriculants to U.S. Medical Schools by Sex, 2009–2010 Through 2018–2019." https://www.aamc.org/download/492954/data/factstablea7_2.pdf.

Barber, Bernard. 1962. *Science and the Social Order*. New York: Collier Books.

Becker, Gary. 1957. *The Economics of Discrimination*. Chicago: University of Chicago Press.

Becker, Howard S., Blanche Geer, Everett C. Hughes, and Anselm L. Strauss. 1961. *Boys in White: Student Culture in Medical School*. Chicago: University of Chicago Press.

Bendix, Reinhard. 1956. *Work and Authority in Industry: Ideologies of Management in the Course of Industrialization*. Berkeley: University of California Press.

Binder, Amy J., Daniel B. Davis, and Nick Bloom. 2016. "Career Funneling: How Elite Students Learn to Define and Desire 'Prestigious' Jobs." *Sociology of Education* 89 (1): 20–39.

Blau, Peter M. 2017. *Exchange and Power in Social Life*. 2nd ed. New York: Routledge.

Blau, Peter M., and Richard W. Scott. 1962. "The Organization and Its Publics." In *Formal Organizations: A Comparative Approach*, 59–86. San Francisco: Chandler.

Boatright, Dowin H., Elizabeth A. Samuels, Laura Cramer, et al. 2018. "Association Between the Liaison Committee on Medical Education's Diversity Standards and Changes in Percentage of Medical Student Sex, Race, and Ethnicity." *JAMA* 320 (21): 2267–69.

Bolton, Sharon C., and Daniel Muzio. 2007. "Can't Live with 'Em; Can't Live Without 'Em: Gendered Segmentation in the Legal Profession." *Sociology* (British Sociological Association) 41 (1): 47–64.

Borgen, Nicolai T., and Arne Mastekaasa. 2018. "Horizontal Stratification of Higher Education: The Relative Importance of Field of Study, Institution, and Department for Candidates' Wages." *Social Forces* 97 (2): 531–58.

Bos, A. E. R., J. B. Pryor, G. D. Reeder, and S. E. Stutterheim. 2013. "Stigma: Advances in Theory and Research." *Basic and Applied Social Psychology* 35 (1): 1–9.

Bosk, Charles L. 1980. "Occupational Rituals in Patient Management." *New England Journal of Medicine* 303 (2): 71–76.

Bosk, Charles L. 1992. *All God's Mistakes.* Chicago: University of Chicago Press.

Bosk, Charles L. 2003. *Forgive and Remember.* 2nd ed. Chicago: University of Chicago Press.

Boulis, Ann K., and Jerry A. Jacobs. 2008. *The Changing Face of Medicine: Women Doctors and the Evolution of Health Care in America.* Ithaca, NY: Cornell University Press.

Bourdieu, Pierre. 1984. *Distinction: A Social Critique of the Judgement of Taste.* Cambridge, MA: Harvard University Press.

Bourdieu, Pierre. 1986. "The Forms of Capital." In *Handbook of Theory and Research for the Sociology of Education,* ed. J. Richardson, 241–58. New York: Greenwood.

Bourdieu, Pierre. 1996. *The State Nobility: Elite Schools in the Field of Power,* trans. Lauretta C. Clough. Stanford, CA: Stanford University Press.

Bourdieu, Pierre. 1998. "The Economy of Symbolic Goods." In *Practical Reason: On the Theory of Action,* 92–123. Stanford, CA: Stanford University Press.

Bourdieu, Pierre, and Jean-Claude Passeron. 1990. *Reproduction in Education, Society and Culture,* trans. Richard Nice. 2nd ed. London: Sage.

Bourdieu, Pierre, and Loïc Wacquant. 1992. *An Invitation to Reflexive Sociology.* Cambridge: Polity.

Bowen, J. L., L. E. Leff, L. G. Smith, and S. D. Wolfsthal. 1999. "Beyond the Mystique of Prestige: Measuring the Quality of Residency Programs." *American Journal of Medicine* 106 (5): 493–98.

Brooks, Robert A. 2011. *Cheaper by the Hour: Temporary Lawyers and the Deprofessionalization of the Law.* Philadelphia: Temple University Press.

Brosnan, Caragh. 2009. "Pierre Bourdieu and the Theory of Medical Education." In *The Handbook of the Sociology of Medical Education,* ed. Caragh Brosnan and Bryan S. Turner, 51–68. London: Routledge.

Brosnan, Caragh. 2010. "Making Sense of Differences Between Medical Schools Through Bourdieu's Concept of 'Field.'" *Medical Education* 44 (7): 645–52.

Bucher, Rue, and Anselm Strauss. 1961. "Professions in Process." *American Journal of Sociology* 66 (4): 325–34.

Bush, Roger. 2010. "Supervision in Medical Education: Logical Fallacies and Clear Choices." *Journal of Graduate Medical Education* 2 (1): 141–43.

Calarco, Jessica. 2018. *Negotiating Opportunities: How the Middle Class Secures Advantages in School.* New York: Oxford University Press.

Carson, J. L., G. Guyatt, N. M. Heddle et al. 2016. "Clinical Practice Guidelines from the AABB: Red Blood Cell Transfusion Thresholds and Storage." *JAMA* 316 (19): 2025–35.

Chen, Peggy Guey-Chi, Leslie Ann Curry, Susannah May Bernheim, David Berg, Aysegul Gozu, and Marcella Nunez-Smith. 2011. "Professional Challenges of Non-US-Born International Medical Graduates and Recommendations for Support During Residency Training." *Academic Medicine* 86 (11): 1383–88.

Chen, Peggy Guey-Chi, Marcella Nunez-Smith, Susannah Bernheim, David Berg, Aysegul Gozu, and Leslie Curry. 2010. "Professional Experiences of International Medical Graduates Practicing Primary Care in the United States." *Journal of General Internal Medicine* 25 (9): 947–53.

Childress, Herb. 2019. *The Adjunct Underclass: How America's Colleges Betrayed Their Faculty, Their Students, and Their Mission.* Chicago: University of Chicago Press.

Clausen, John S. 1991. "Adolescent Competence and the Shaping of the Life Course." *American Journal of Sociology* 96 (4): 805–42.

Coburn, D., S. Rappolt, and I. Bourgeault. 1997. "Decline vs Retention of Medical Power Through Restratification: An Examination of the Ontario Case." *Sociology of Health and Illness* 19 (1): 1–22.

Cohen, Jordan J. 2006. "The Role and Contributions of IMGs: A US Perspective." *Academic Medicine* 81 (12): S17–S21.

Cohen, Jordan J., Barbara A. Gabriel, and Charles Terrell. 2002. "The Case for Diversity in the Health Care Workforce." *Health Affairs* 21 (5): 90–102.

Colby College. 2014. "Colby Graduate Admission Statistics." http://www.colby.edu/careercenter /students/healthprofessions/stats/.

Collins, Randall. 1979. *The Credential Society: An Historical Sociology of Education and Stratification.* New York: Academic Press.

Corbin, Juliet, and Anselm Strauss. 1990. "Grounded Theory Research: Procedures, Canons, and Evaluative Criteria." *Qualitative Sociology* 13 (1): 13–21.

Corley, Kevin, and Dennis Gioia. 2000. "The Rankings Game: Managing Business School Reputation." *Corporate Reputation Review* 3 (4): 319.

Coser, Rose Laub. 1962. *Life in the Ward.* East Lansing: Michigan State University Press.

Cross, John G., and Edie N. Goldenberg. 2009. *Off-Track Profs: Nontenured Teachers in Higher Education.* Cambridge, MA: MIT Press.

Cruess, Sylvia R., and Richard L. Cruess. 2004. "Professionalism and Medicine's Social Contract with Society." *Virtual Mentor* 6 (4). http://virtualmentor.ama-assn.org/2004/04/msoc1-0404 .html.

Cullen, Jim. 1931. *The American Dream: A Short History of an Idea That Shaped a Nation.* Oxford: Oxford University Press.

Davis, Georgiann, and R. Allison. 2013. "White Coats, Black Specialists? Racial Divides in the Medical Profession." *Sociological Spectrum* 33 (6): 510–33.

Davis, Kingsley, and Wilbert E. Moore. 1944. "Some Principles of Stratification." *American Sociological Review* 10 (2): 242–49.

Deephouse, David L., and Suzanne M. Carter. 2005. "An Examination of Differences Between Organizational Legitimacy and Organizational Reputation." *Journal of Management Studies* 42 (2): 329–60.

Desbiens, N. A., and H. J. Vidaillet. 2010. "Discrimination Against International Medical Graduates in the United States Residency Program Selection Process." *BMC Medical Education* 10:5.

Devaul, R. A., F. Jervey, J. A. Chappell, P. Caver, B. Short, and S. Okeefe. 1987. "Medical School Performance of Initially Rejected Students." *JAMA* 257 (1): 47–51.

Dittes, James E., and Harold H. Kelley. 1956. "Effects of Different Conditions of Acceptance Upon Conformity to Group Norms." *Journal of Abnormal and Social Psychology* 53 (1): 100–107.

Eckhert, N. L. 2010. "Perspective: Private Schools of the Caribbean: Outsourcing Medical Education." *Academic Medicine* 85 (4): 622–30.

Edelman, Lauren B. 2016. *Working Law: Courts, Corporations, and Symbolic Civil Rights*. Chicago: University of Chicago Press.

Educational Commission for Foreign Medical Graduates. 2015a. "Certification." http://www .ecfmg.org/certification/index.html.

Educational Commission for Foreign Medical Graduates. 2015b. "History." http://www.ecfmg .org/about/history.html.

Edwards, Dali. 2016. "The Plight of an International Medical Graduate Physician Who Is an American Citizen." *Women in Medicine*. http://www.womeninmedicinemagazine.com/profile -of-women-in-medicine/the-plight-of-an-international-medical-graduate-physician-who -is-an-american-citizen.

Emerson, Michael O., Karen J. Chai, and George Yancey. 2001. "Does Race Matter in Residential Segregation? Exploring the Preferences of White Americans." *American Sociological Review* 66 (6) :922–35.

Emerson, Robert M., Rachel I. Fretz, and Linda L. Shaw. 2011. *Writing Ethnographic Fieldnotes*. Chicago: University of Chicago Press.

Envision Experience. 2014. "National Youth Leadership Forum: Medicine." http://www .envisionexperience.com/explore-our-programs/nylf-medicine.

Evetts, Juali, Charles Gadea, Mariano Sanchez, and Juan Saez. 2009. "Sociological Theories of Professions: Conflict, Competition and Cooperation." In *The ISA Handbook in Contemporary Sociology: Conflict, Competition, Cooperation*, ed. Devorah Kalekin-Fishman and Ann B. Denis, 140–54. Los Angeles: Sage.

Federal Student Aid, U.S. Department of Education. n.d. "Public Service Loan Forgiveness (PSLF)." Accessed April 12, 2015. https://studentaid.ed.gov/repay-loans/forgiveness-cancellation /public-service#what-is-pslf.

Feldstein, Paul J., and Irene Butter. 1978. "The Foreign Medical Graduate and Public Policy: A Discussion of the Issues and Options." *International Journal of Health Services* 8 (3): 541–58.

Flexner, Abraham. 1910. *Medical Education in the United States and Canada*. New York: Carnegie Foundation for the Advancement of Teaching.

Fombrun, Charles, and Cees van Riel. 1997. "The Reputational Landscape." *Corporate Reputation Review* 1 (1): 5–13.

Fordyce, Meredith A., Mark P. Doescher, Frederick M. Chen, and L. Gary Hart. 2012. "Osteopathic Physicians and International Medical Graduates in the Rural Primary Care Physician Workforce." *Family Medicine* 44 (6): 396–403.

Fox, Renée. 1957. "Training for Uncertainty." In *The Student-Physician*, ed. Robert K. Merton, George G. Reader, and Patricia Kendall, 207–41. Cambridge, MA: Harvard University Press.

Freidson, Eliot. 1970. *Professional Dominance*. New York: Atherton Press.

Freidson, Eliot. 1983. "The Reorganization of the Professions by Regulation." *Law and Human Behavior* 7 (2–3): 279–90.

Freidson, Eliot. 1984. "The Changing Nature of Professional Control." *Annual Review of Sociology* 10: 1–20.

Freidson, Eliot. 1985. "The Reorganization of the Medical Profession." *Medical Care Review* 42 (1): 11–35.

Freidson, Eliot. 1986a. "The Future of the Professions." *Journal of Dental Education* 51 (3): 140–44.

Freidson, Eliot. 1986b. *Professional Powers: A Study of the Institutionalization of Formal Knowledge*. Chicago: University of Chicago Press.

Freidson, Eliot, and Buford Rhea. 1972. "Processes of Control in a Company of Equals." In *Medical Men and Their Work: A Sociological Reader*, ed. Eliot Freidson and Judith Lorber. Chicago: Aldine Atherton.

Fried, Ethan, Elaine Muchmore, and Carina Sundstrom. 2012. "Preparing for the New Fellowship Recruitment Timeline." Alliance for Academic Internal Medicine. www.im.org/d/do/4707.

Friedman, Scott L. 2019. "Management and Prognosis of Alcoholic Hepatitis." UpToDate. https://www.uptodate.com/contents/management-and-prognosis-of-alcoholic-hepatitis?search=alcoholic%20hepatitis&source=search_result&selectedTitle=1~85&usage_type=default&display_rank=1.

Frosch, Dominick L., Suepattra G. May, Katharine A. S. Rendle, Caroline Tietbohl, and Glyn Elwyn. 2012. "Authoritarian Physicians and Patients' Fear of Being Labeled 'Difficult' Among Key Obstacles to Shared Decision Making." *Health Affairs* 31 (5): 1030–38.

Galdy, Salvatore, and Giuseppe Nastasi. 2012. "Streptococcus Bovis Endocarditis and Colon Cancer: Myth or Reality? A Case Report and Literature Review." *BMJ Case Reports* bcr2012006961. https://doi.org/10.1136/bcr-2012-006961.

Gerber, Theodore P., and Sin Yi Cheung. 2008. "Horizontal Stratification in Postsecondary Education: Forms, Explanations, and Implications." *Annual Review of Sociology* 34 (1): 299–318.

Gerxhani, K., and F. Koster. 2015. "Making the Right Move: Investigating Employers' Recruitment Strategies." *Personnel Review* 44 (5): 781–800.

Gevitz, Norman. 2014. "From 'Doctor of Osteopathy' to 'Doctor of Osteopathic Medicine'": A Title Change in the Push for Equality." *Journal of the American Osteopathic Association* 114 (6): 486–97.

Goffman, Alice. 2014. *On the Run: Fugitive Life in an American City*. New York: Picador.

Goffman, Erving. 1952. "On Cooling the Mark Out: Some Aspects of Adaptation to Failure." *Psychiatry* 14 (4): 451–63.

Goffman, Erving. 1963. *Stigma: Notes on the Management of Spoiled Identity*. New York: Simon and Schuster.

Goode, William J. 1957. "Community Within a Community: The Professions." *American Sociological Review* 22 (2): 194–200.

Goodnough, Abby. 2019. "Kaiser Permanente's New Medical School Will Waive Tuition for Its First 5 Classes." *New York Times*. https://www.nytimes.com/2019/02/19/health/kaiser-medical-school-free-.html.

Gopal, R., J. J. Glasheen, T. J. Miyoshi, and A. V. Prochazka. 2005. "Burnout and Internal Medicine Resident Work-Hour Restrictions." *Archives of Internal Medicine* 165 (22): 2595–600.

Gorden, Raymond L. 1998. *Basic Interviewing Skills*. Long Grove, IL: Waveland Press.

Gozu, Aysegul, David E. Kern, and Scott M. Wright. 2009. "Similarities and Differences Between International Medical Graduates and US Medical Graduates at Six Maryland Community-Based Internal Medicine Residency Training Programs." *Academic Medicine* 84 (3): 385–90.

Grady, Erin C., Adam Roise, Daniel Barr et al. 2012. "Defining Scholarly Activity in Graduate Medical Education." *Journal of Graduate Medical Education* 4 (4): 558–61.

Gravois, John. 2007. "Graduate Schools Reduce Ph.D. Attrition Rates." *Chronicle of Higher Education* 54 (17): A12.

Greenwood, Ernest. 1957. "Attributes of a Profession." *Social Work* 2 (3): 45–55.

Growe, Roslin, and Paula S. Montgomery. 2003. "Educational Equity in America: Is Education the Great Equalizer?" *Professional Educator* 25 (2): 23–29.

Groysberg, Boris, Eric Lin, George Serafeim, and Robin Abrahams. 2016. "The Scandal Effect." *Harvard Business Review* 94 (9): 90–122.

Gruppuso, Philip A., and Eli Y. Adashi. 2017. "Residency Placement Fever: Is It Time for a Reevaluation?" *Academic Medicine* 92 (7): 923–26.

Guest, Greg, Arwen Bunce, and Laura Johnson. 2006. "How Many Interviews Are Enough? An Experiment with Data Saturation and Variability." *Field Methods* 18 (1): 59–82.

Haas, Jack, and William Shaffir. 1987. *Becoming Doctors: The Adoption of a Cloak of Competence*, ed. Jaber F. Gubrium. Contemporary Ethnographic Studies 2. Greenwich, CT: JAI Press.

Hafferty, Frederic W. 1988a. "Cadaver Stories and the Emotional Socialization of Medical Students." *Journal of Health and Social Behavior* 29 (4): 344–56.

Hafferty, Frederic W. 1988b. "Theories at the Crossroads—A Discussion of Evolving Views on Medicine as a Profession." *Milbank Quarterly* 66: 202–25.

Hafferty, Frederic W. 1991. *Into the Valley: Death and the Socialization of Medical Students*. New Haven, CT: Yale University Press.

Hafferty, Frederic W. 1998. "Beyond Curriculum Reform: Confronting Medicine's Hidden Curriculum." *Academic Medicine* 73 (4): 403–7.

Hafferty, Frederic W. 2006. "Professionalism—The Next Wave." *New England Journal of Medicine* 355 (20): 2151–52.

Hafferty, Frederic W., and Donald W. Light. 1995. "Professional Dynamics and the Changing Nature of Medical Work." *Journal of Health and Social Behavior* 35 (Special issue): 132–53.

Hagopian, Amy, Matthew Thompson, Emily Kaltenbach, and L. Gary Hart. 2004. "The Role of International Medical Graduates in America's Small Rural Critical Access Hospitals." *Journal of Rural Health* 20 (1): 52–58.

Hall, Oswald. 1948. "The Stages of a Medical Career." *American Journal of Sociology* 53 (5): 327–36.

Hall, Oswald. 1949. "Types of Medical Careers." *American Journal of Sociology* 55 (3): 243–53.

Halpern, Sydney A. 1992. "Dynamics of Professional Control—Internal Coalitions and Crossprofessional Boundaries." *American Journal of Sociology* 97 (4): 994–1021.

Harder, Ben. 2014. "Doctors Name America's Top Residency Programs." https://health.usnews.com/health-news/top-doctors/articles/2014/02/20/doctors-name-americas-top-residency-programs.

Hartocollis, Anemona. 2008. "New York Hospitals Create Outcry in Foreign Deal." *New York Times*. https://www.nytimes.com/2008/08/05/nyregion/05grenada.html.

Hartocollis, Anemona. 2014. "Second-Chance Med School." *New York Times*. https://www.nytimes.com/2014/08/03/education/edlife/second-chance-med-school.html

Hassan, Adeel. 2019. "Cornell's Medical School Offers Full Rides in Battle Over Student Debt." *New York Times*. https://www.nytimes.com/2019/09/16/us/weill-cornell-free.html.

Hasty, Robert T., Samuel Snyder, Gabriel P. Suciu, and Jaclynn M. Moskow. 2012. "Graduating Osteopathic Medical Students' Perceptions and Recommendations on the Decision to Take the United States Medical Licensing Examination." *Journal of the American Osteopathic Association* 112 (2): 83–89.

Heimer, Carol A., and Lisa R. Staffen. 1998. *For the Sake of the Children: The Social Organization of Responsibility in the Hospital and the Home*. Chicago: University of Chicago Press.

Hilsenrath, Peter E. 2006. "Osteopathic Medicine in Transition: Postmortem of the Osteopathic Medical Center of Texas." *Journal of the American Osteopathic Association* 106 (9): 558–61.

Hoff, Timothy J. 1998. "Same Profession, Different People: Stratification, Structure, and Physicians' Employment Choices." *Sociological Forum* 13 (1): 133–56.

Hoff, Timothy J. 2001. "Exploring Dual Commitment Among Physician Executives in Managed Care." *Journal of Healthcare Management* 46 (2): 91–109.

Hoff, Timothy J., and Henry Pohl. 2017. "Not Your Parent's Profession: The Restratification of Medicine in the United States." In *The Healthcare Professional Workforce: Understanding Human Capital in a Changing Industry*, ed. Timothy J. Hoff, K. M. Sutcliffe, and G. J. Young, 23–46. Oxford: Oxford University Press.

Hoff, Timothy J., Kathleen M. Sutcliffe, and Gary J. Young, eds. 2017. *The Healthcare Professional Workforce: Understanding Human Capital in a Changing Industry*. Oxford: Oxford University Press.

Iglehart, John K. 2011. "The Uncertain Future of Medicare and Graduate Medical Education." *New England Journal of Medicine* 365 (14): 1340–45.

Iglehart, John K. 2013. "The Residency Mismatch." *New England Journal of Medicine* 369 (4): 297–99.

Irigoyen, Mathilde, and Ruth E. Zambrana. 1979. "Foreign Medical Graduates (FMGs): Determining Their role in the United States Health Care System." *Social Science & Medicine* 13A (6):775–83.

Jardine, D. A., T. Dong, A. R. Artino et al. 2012. "Alternate List Matriculants: Outcome Data from Those Medical Students Admitted from the Alternate List." *Military Medicine* 177 (9): 7–10.

Jauhar, Sandeep. 2008. *Intern: A Doctor's Initiation*. New York: Farrar, Straus, Giroux.

Jauhar, Sandeep. 2014. *Doctored: The Disillusionment of an American Physician*. New York: Farrar, Straus, Giroux.

Jenkins, Tania M. 2014. "Clothing Norms as Markers of Status in a Hospital Setting: A Bourdieusian Analysis." *Health* 18 (5): 526–41.

Jenkins, Tania M. 2015. "'It's Time She Stopped Torturing Herself': Structural Constraints to Decision-Making About Life-Sustaining Treatment by Medical Trainees." *Social Science & Medicine* 132: 132–40.

Jenkins, Tania M. 2018. "Dual Autonomies, Divergent Approaches: How Stratification in Medical Education Shapes Approaches to Patient Care." *Journal of Health and Social Behavior* 59 (2): 268–82.

Jenkins, Tania M., Franklyn, Grace, Klugman, Josh, and Reddy, Shalini T. 2019. "Separate but Equal? The Sorting of USMDs and Non-USMDs in Internal Medicine Residency Programs." *Journal of General Internal Medicine*. doi:10.1007/s11606-019-05573-8.

Jenkins, Tania M., and Shalini Reddy. 2016. "Revisiting the Rationing of Medical Degrees in the United States." *Contexts* 15 (4): 36–41.

Jenkins, Tania M., and Shalini T. Reddy. 2017. "Unmatched U.S. Seniors and Residency Placement Fever." *Academic Medicine* 92 (11): 1510.

Jewel, Lucille. 2008. "Bourdieu and American Legal Education: How Law Schools Reproduce Social Stratification and Class Hierarchy." *Buffalo Law Review* 56 (4): 1155–224.

Kamens, David H. 1977. "Legitimating Myths and Educational Organization: Relationship Between Organizational Ideology and Formal Structure." *American Sociological Review* 42 (2): 208–19.

Kaplan Test Prep. 2018. "MCAT Course Options." http://www.kaptest.com/mcat.

Karabel, Jerome. 2005. *The Chosen: The Hidden History of Admission and Exclusion at Harvard, Yale, and Princeton*. New York: Houghton Mifflin.

Kellogg, Katherine. 2009. "Operating Room: Relational Spaces and Microinstitutional Change in Surgery." *American Journal of Sociology* 115 (3): 657–711.

Kellogg, Katherine. 2011. *Challenging Operations: Medical Reform and Resistance in Surgery*. Chicago: University of Chicago Press.

Kendzior, Sarah. 2013. "Academia's Indentured Servants." Al Jazeera. http://www.aljazeera.com /indepth/opinion/2013/04/20134119156459616.html.

Khan, Shamus Rahman. 2011. *Privilege: The Making of an Adolescent Elite at St. Paul's School*. Princeton, NJ: Princeton University Press.

Khan, Shamus Rahman, and Colin Jerolmack. 2013. "Saying Meritocracy and Doing Privilege." *Sociological Quarterly* 54: 9–19.

Kinchen, K. S., L. A. Cooper, N. Y. Wang, D. Levine, and N. R. Powe. 2004. "The Impact of International Medical graduate Status on Primary Care Physicians' Choice of Specialist." *Medical Care* 42 (8): 747–55.

Knaapen, Loes. 2014. "Evidence-Based Medicine or Cookbook Medicine? Addressing Concerns Over the Standardization of Care." *Sociology Compass* 8 (6): 823–36.

Knopes, Julia. 2019. "Yields and Rabbit Holes: Medical Students' Typologies of Sufficient Knowledge." *Medical Anthropology*. https://doi.org/10.1080/01459740.2019.1640220.

Korcok, Milan. 1979. "Caribbean Medical Schools, Part 2: Entry to Mainland Teaching Hospitals Is Tough." *Canadian Medical Association Journal* 121: 1299–1301.

Kristof, Kathy. 2013. "$1 Million Mistake: Becoming a Doctor." CBS News. http://www.cbsnews .com/news/1-million-mistake-becoming-a-doctor/.

Landon, B. E., J. Reschovsky, and D. Blumenthal. 2003. "Changes in Career Satisfaction Among Primary Care and Specialist Physicians, 1997–2001." *JAMA* 289 (4): 442–49.

Larson, Magali Sarfatti. 1980. "Proletarianization and Educated Labor." *Theory and Society* 9 (1): 131–75.

Leigh, J. P., D. Tancredi, A. Jerant, P. S. Romano, and R. L. Kravitz. 2012. "Lifetime Earnings for Physicians Across Specialties." *Medical Care* 50 (12): 1093–1101.

Lerner, Barron H. 2013. "When Med Students Get Medical Students' Disease." *Well* (blog), *New York Times*. http://well.blogs.nytimes.com/2013/09/05/when-med-students-get-medical -students-disease/?_r=0.

Lewin, M. E, and S. Altman, eds. 2000. *America's Health Care Safety Net: Intact but Endangered*. Washington, DC: National Academies Press.

Lewis, Irving J., and Cecil G. Sheps. 1983. *The Sick Citadel: The American Academic Medical Center and the Public Interest*. Cambridge, MA: Oelgeschlager, Gunn and Hain.

Light, Donald W. 1980. *Becoming Psychiatrists*. New York: Norton.

Light, Donald W. 1988. "Toward a New Sociology of Medical Education." *Journal of Health and Social Behavior* 29 (4): 307–22.

Light, Donald W. 2010. "Health-Care Professions, Markets, and Countervailing Powers." In *Handbook of Medical Sociology*, ed. Chloe Bird, Peter Conrad, Allen M. Fremont, and Stefan Timmermans, 270–89. Nashville, TN: Vanderbilt University Press.

Lin, Katherine Y., Renée R. Anspach, Brett Crawford, Sonali Parnami, Andrea Fuhrel-Forbis, and Raymond G. De Vries. 2014. "What Must I Do to Succeed? Narratives from the US Premedical Experience." *Social Science & Medicine* 119: 98–105.

Link, B. G., and J. C. Phelan. 2001. "Conceptualizing Stigma." *Annual Review of Sociology* 27: 363–85.

Lockwood, Penelope, Christian H. Jordan, and Ziva Kunda. 2002. "Motivation by Positive or Negative Role Models: Regulatory Focus Determines Who Will Best Inspire Us." *Journal of Personality and Social Psychology* 83 (4): 854–64.

Lofland, John, David Snow, Leon Anderson, and Lyn H. Lofland. 2006. *Analyzing Social Settings: A Guide to Qualitative Observation and Analysis.* 4th ed. Belmont, CA: Thomson/Wadsworth.

Lohr, Kathleen N., Neal A. Vanselow, and Don E. Detmer. 1996. "From the Institute of Medicine: The Nation's Physician Workforce Options for Balancing Supply and Requirements." *JAMA* 275 (10): 748.

Lorber, Judith. 1984. *Women Physicians: Careers, Status, and Power.* New York: Tavistock.

Lorin, Janet. 2013. "Caribbean Medical Schools Would Face U.S. Loan Hurdle Under Bill." Bloomberg. http://www.bloomberg.com/news/print/2013-12-11/caribbean-medical-schools -would-face-u-s-loan-hurdle-under-bill.html.

Ludmerer, Kenneth M. 2015. *Let Me Heal: The Opportunity to Preserve Excellence in American Medicine.* Oxford: Oxford University Press.

Luke, Haida. 2003. *Medical Education and Sociology of Medical Habitus: "It's Not About the Stethoscope!"* Dordrecht: Kluwer Academic Publishers.

Mann, Michael. 1970. "The Social Cohesion of Liberal Democracy." *American Sociological Review* 35 (3): 423–39.

Manthous, Constantine A. 2012. "Confronting the Elephant in the Room: Can We Transcend Medical Graduate Stereotypes?" *Journal of Graduate Medical Education* 4 (3): 290–92.

Marshall, Robert J., Jr., John P. Fulton, and Albert F. Wessen. 1978. "Physician Career Outcomes and the Process of Medical Education." *Journal of Health and Social Behavior* 19 (2): 124–38.

Matthews, Christine M. 2010. *Foreign Science and Engineering Presence in U.S. Institutions and the Labor Force.* Washington, DC: Congressional Research Service.

McDonald, S. 2011. "What's in the "Old Boys' " Network? Accessing Social Capital in Gendered and Racialized Networks." *Social Networks* 33 (4): 317–30.

McGrath, Pam, Anne Wong, and Hamish Holewa. 2011. "Canadian and Australian Licensing Policies for International Medical Graduates: A Web-Based Comparison." *Education for Health* 24 (1): 452.

McKinlay, J. B., and J. Arches. 1985. "Towards the Proletarianization of Physicians." *International Journal of Health Services* 15 (2): 61–95.

McKinlay, J. B., and L. Marceau. 2002. "The End of the Golden Age of Doctoring." *International Journal of Health Services* 32 (2): 379–416.

McNamee, Stephen J. 2018. *The Meritocracy Myth.* 4th ed. Lanham, MD: Rowman and Littlefield.

Meghani, S. H., and V. Rajput. 2011. "Perspective: The Need for Practice Socialization of International Medical Graduates—An Exemplar from Pain Medicine." *Academic Medicine* 86 (5): 571–74.

Menchik, Daniel. 2014. "Decisions About Knowledge in Medical Practice: The Effect of Temporal Features of a Task." *American Journal of Sociology* 120: 701–49.

Merriam-Webster. n.d. S.v. "merit (*n.*)." Accessed January 11, 2019. https://www.merriam-webster .com/dictionary/merit.

Merton, Robert K. 1968. "The Matthew Effect in Science:" The Reward and Communication Systems of Science Are Considered." *Science* 159 (3810): 56–63.

Merton, Robert K., George G. Reader, and Patricia Kendall, eds. 1957. *The Student Physician.* Cambridge, MA: Harvard University Press.

Michalec, Barret, Monica M Cuddy, Phillip Hafferty et al. 2018. "It's Happening Sooner Than You Think: Spotlighting the Pre-medical Realm." *Medical Education* 52 (4): 359–61.

Mick, Stephen S. 1978. "Understanding the Persistence of Human Resource Problems in Health." *Milbank Memorial Fund Quarterly—Health and Society* 56 (4) :463–99.

Mick, Stephen S. 1987. "Contradictory Policies for Foreign Medical Graduates." *Health Affairs* 6 (3): 5–18.

Mick, Stephen S. 1993. "Foreign Medical Graduates and United States Physician Supply—Old Issues and New Questions." *Health Policy* 24 (3): 213–25.

Mick, Stephen S., and Maureen E. Comfort. 1997. "The Quality of Care of International Medical Graduates: How Does It Compare to That of US Medical Graduates?" *Medical Care Research and Review* 54 (4): 379–413.

Miller, Stephen J. 1970. *Prescription for Leadership: Training for the Medical Elite.* Chicago: Aldine.

Moore, Richard A., and Eric J. Rhodenbaugh. 2002. "The Unkindest Cut of All: Are International Medical School Graduates Subjected to Discrimination by General Surgery Residency Programs?" *Current Surgery* 59 (2): 228–36.

Mounk, Yascha. 2014. "Is Harvard Unfair to Asian-Americans?" *New York Times.* https://www.nytimes.com/2014/11/25/opinion/is-harvard-unfair-to-asian-americans.html.

Mullan, Fitzhugh, Edward Salsberg, and Katie Weider. 2015. "Why a GME Squeeze Is Unlikely." *New England Journal of Medicine* 373 (25): 2397–99.

Mumford, Emily. 1970. *Interns: From Students to Physicians.* Cambridge, MA: Harvard University Press.

Muzio, Daniel, and Stephen Ackroyd. 2005. "On the Consequences of Defensive Professionalism: Recent Changes in the Legal Labour Process." *Journal of Law and Society* 32 (4): 615–42.

Naidoo, Rajani. 2004. "Fields and Institutional Strategy: Bourdieu on the Relationship Between Higher Education, Inequality and Society." *British Journal of Sociology of Education* 25 (4): 457–71.

Nasir, L. S. 1994. "Evidence of Discrimination Against International Medical Graduates Applying to Family Practice Residency Programs." *Family Medicine* 26 (10): 625–29.

National Board of Medical Examiners. 2015. "USMLE Score Interpretation Guidelines." http://www.usmle.org/pdfs/transcripts/USMLE_Step_Examination_Score_Interpretation_Guidelines.pdf.

National Resident Matching Program. n.d. "The Sveriges Riksbank Prize in Economic Sciences in Memory of Alfred Nobel." Accessed November 16, 2014. http://www.nrmp.org/wp-content/uploads/2013/08/The-Sveriges-Riksbank-Prize-in-Economic-Sciences-in-Memory-of-Alfred-Nobel1.pdf.

National Resident Matching Program. 1985. *Results and Data: 1985 Main Residency Match.* Washington, DC: National Resident Matching Program.

National Resident Matching Program. 2009. *Results and Data: 2009 Main Residency Match.* Washington, DC: National Resident Matching Program.

National Resident Matching Program. 2011. *Charting Outcomes in the Match.* 4th ed. Washington, DC: National Resident Matching Program.

National Resident Matching Program. 2014a. *Charting Outcomes in the Match.* 5th ed. Washington, DC: National Resident Matching Program.

National Resident Matching Program. 2014b. *Results and Data: 2014 Main Residency Match®.* Washington, DC: National Resident Matching Program.

National Resident Matching Program. 2014c. *Results and Data: Specialties Matching Service® 2014 Appointment Year.* Washington, DC.

National Resident Matching Program. 2015a. "How the Matching Algorithm Works." Accessed September 29, 2015. http://www.nrmp.org/match-process/match-algorithm/.

National Resident Matching Program. 2015b. "Match Commitment—What You Need to Know." Accessed April 6, 2015. http://www.nrmp.org/policies/the-match-commitment/.

National Resident Matching Program. 2015c. *Results and Data: 2015 Main Residency Match®*. Washington, DC: National Resident Matching Program.

National Resident Matching Program. 2015d. *Results and Data: Specialties Matching Service® 2015 Appointment Year*. Washington, DC: National Resident Matching Program.

National Resident Matching Program. 2016. *National Resident Matching Program, Results and Data: 2016 Main Residency Match®*. Washington, DC: National Resident Matching Program.

National Resident Matching Program. 2018a. "All In Policy: Main Residency Match." Accessed March 16. http://www.nrmp.org/all-in-policy/main-residency-match/.

National Resident Matching Program. 2018b. *Charting Outcomes in the Match: International Medical Graduates*. 2nd ed. Washington, DC: National Resident Matching Program.

National Resident Matching Program. 2018c. *Charting Outcomes in the Match: Senior Students of U.S. Osteopathic Medical Schools*. Washington, DC: National Resident Matching Program.

National Resident Matching Program. 2018d. *Charting Outcomes in the Match: U.S. Allopathic Seniors*. 2nd ed. Washington, DC: National Resident Matching Program.

National Resident Matching Program. 2018e. *Results and Data: 2018 Main Residency Match®*. Washington, DC: National Resident Matching Program.

National Resident Matching Program. 2019a. "About NRMP." Accessed January 21. http://www.nrmp.org/about-nrmp/.

National Resident Matching Program. 2019b. *Results and Data: 2019 Main Residency Match®*. Washington, DC: National Resident Matching Program.

National Resident Matching Program. 2019c. *Results and Data: Specialties Matching Service® 2019 Appointment Year*. Washington, DC: National Resident Matching Program.

Neckerman, Kathryn, and Joleen Kirschenman. 1991. "Hiring Strategies, Racial Bias, and Inner-City Workers." *Social Problems* 38 (4): 433–47.

Norcini, John J., J. R. Boulet, W. D. Dauphinee, A. Opalek, I. D. Krantz, and S. T. Anderson. 2010. "Evaluating the Quality of Care Provided by Graduates of International Medical Schools." *Health Affairs* 29 (8): 1461–68.

Norcini, John J., M. van Zanten, and John R. Boulet. 2008. "The Contribution of International Medical Graduates to Diversity in the US Physician Workforce: Graduate Medical Education." *Journal of Health Care for the Poor and Underserved* 19 (2): 493–99.

Oh, Hyeyoung, and Stefan Timmermans. 2013. "Can Physician Training and Fiscal Responsibility Coexist?" *Virtual Mentor* 15 (2): 131–35.

Olson, Elizabeth G. 2013. "Medical Students Confront a Residency Black Hole." *Fortune*. http://management.fortune.cnn.com/2013/04/01/medical-students-residencies/.

Palmer, Brian. 2011. "We Need More Doctors, Stat! Why Is It Taking So Long to Address the Physician Shortage?" *Slate*. http://www.slate.com/articles/news_and_politics/explainer/2011/06/we_need_more_doctors_stat.html.

Paolo, A. M., S. Stites, G. A. Bonaminio et al. 2006. "A Comparison of Students from Main and Alternate Admission Lists at One School: The Potential Impact on Student Performance of Increasing Enrollment." *Academic Medicine* 81 (9): 837–41.

Papadakis, M. A., A. Teherani, M. A. Banach et al. 2005. "Disciplinary Action by Medical Boards and Prior Behavior in Medical School." *New England Journal of Medicine* 353 (25): 2673–82.

Parkin, Frank. 1974. "Strategies of Social Closure in Class Formation." In *The Social Analysis of Class Structure*, ed. Frank Parkin, 1–18. London: Tavistock.

PASS Program. 2014. "PASS Program Guarantee." http://www.pass-program.com/pass-program -guarantee/.

Patel, Rikinkumar S., Ramya Bachu, Archana Adikey, Meryem Malik, and Mansi Shah. 2018. "Factors Related to Physician Burnout and Its Consequences: A Review." *Behavioral Sciences* (Multidisciplinary Digital Publishing Institute) 8 (11): 98.

Persell, Caroline Hodges, and Peter W. Cookson Jr. 1985. "Chartering and Bartering—Elite Education and Social Reproduction." *Social Problems* 33 (2): 114–29.

Petersen, Anne Helen. 2019. "How Millennials Became the Burnout Generation." BuzzFeed News. https://www.buzzfeednews.com/article/annehelenpetersen/millennials-burnout-generation -debt-work.

Petersen, T., I. Saporta, and M. D. L. Seidel. 2000. "Offering a Job: Meritocracy and Social Networks." *American Journal of Sociology* 106 (3): 763–816.

Pettigrew, Thomas F. 1998. "Intergroup Contact Theory." *Annual Review of Psychology* 49 (1): 65–85.

Phillips, Damon J., and Ezra W. Zuckerman. 2001. "Middle-Status Conformity: Theoretical Restatement and Empirical Demonstration in Two Markets." *American Journal of Sociology* 107 (2): 379–429.

Physicians Foundation. 2012. "A Survey of America's Physicians: Practice Patterns and Perspectives." http://www.physiciansfoundation.org/uploads/default/Physicians_Foundation_2012 _Biennial_Survey.pdf.

Pinsky, William W. 2017. "The Importance of International Medical Graduates in the United States." *Annals of Internal Medicine* 166 (11): 840–41.

Podolny, Joel M. 2005. *Status Signals: A Sociological Study of Market Competition.* Princeton, NJ: Princeton University Press.

Porter, J. L., T. Townley, K. Huggett, and R. Warrier. 2008. "An Acculturation Curriculum: Orienting International Medical Graduates to an Internal Medicine Residency Program." *Teaching and Learning in Medicine* 20 (1): 37–43.

Queensland Health. 2015. "Intern 2016 Priority Groups." http://www.health.qld.gov.au/medical /intern/Intern2016/Intern2016-Priority-Groups.pdf.

Reeves, Roy R., and Randy S. Burke. 2009. "Perception of Osteopathic Medicine Among Allopathic Physicians in the Deep Central Southern United States." *Journal of the American Osteopathic Association* 109 (6): 318–23.

Reich, Adam. 2014. *Selling Our Souls: The Commodification of Hospital Care in the United States.* Princeton, NJ: : Princeton University Press.

Reich, M., D. M. Gordon, and R. C. Edwards. 1973. "Theory of Labor Market Segmentation." *American Economic Review* 63 (2): 359–65.

Reskin, Barbara F. 1993. "Sex Segregation in the Workplace." *Annual Review of Sociology* 19: 241–70.

Reskin, Barbara F., Patricia Roos, Katharine M. Donato et al. 1990. *Job Queues, Gender Queues: Explaining Women's Inroads Into Male Occupations.* Philadelphia: Temple University Press.

Ridgeway, Cecilia L. 2014. "Why Status Matters for Inequality." *American Sociological Review* 79 (1): 1–16.

Ridgeway, Cecilia L., and Shelley Joyce Correll. 2006. "Consensus and the Creation of Status Beliefs." *Social Forces* 85 (1): 431–53.

Ridgeway, Cecilia L., and Kristan Glasgow Erickson. 2000. "Creating and Spreading Status Beliefs." *American Journal of Sociology* 106 (3): 579–615.

Ridgeway, Cecilia L., Kathy J. Kuipers, Elizabeth Heger Boyle, and Dawn T. Robinson. 1998. "How Do Status Beliefs Develop? The Role of Resources and Interactional Experience." *American Sociological Review* 63 (3): 331–50.

Rivera, Lauren. 2015. *Pedigree: How Elite Students Get Elite Jobs.* Princeton, NJ: Princeton University Press.

Roberts, John. 1996. "Too Many Doctors, and More on the Way." *BMJ* 312 (7035): 868.

Rotenstein, L. S., M. Torre, M. A. Ramos et al. 2018. "Prevalence of Burnout Among Physicians: A Systematic Review." *JAMA* 320 (11): 1131–50.

Roth, Alvin E. 2003. "The Origins, History, and Design of the Resident Match." *JAMA* 289 (7): 909–12.

Rothman, David. 1991. *Strangers at the Bedside: A History of How Law and Bioethics Transformed Medical Decision Making.* New York: Basic Books.

Sabharwal, Meghna. 2008. "Job Satisfaction of Foreign-Born Faculty in Science and Engineering by Citizenship Status." PhD diss., Arizona State University.

Sabharwal, Meghna. 2011a. "High-Skilled Immigrants: How Satisfied Are Foreign-Born Scientists and Engineers Employed at American Universities?" *Review of Public Personnel Administration* 31 (2): 143–70.

Sabharwal, Meghna. 2011b. "Job Satisfaction Patterns of Scientists and Engineers by Status of Birth." *Research Policy* 40 (6): 853–63.

Saideman, Steve. 2013. "Adjuncting Mystery." *Saideman's Semi-Spew* (blog). http://saideman.blogspot .ca/2013/04/adjuncting-mystery.html.

Saks, Mike. 2015. "Inequalities, Marginality and the Professions." *Current Sociology* 63 (6): 850–68.

Sánchez, Gloria, Theresa Nevarez, Werner Schink, and David E. Hayes-Bautista. 2015. "Latino Physicians in the United States, 1980–2010: A Thirty-Year Overview from the Censuses." *Academic Medicine* 90 (7): 906–12.

Sang, O. Rhee, Thomas Lyons, Beverly Payne, and Samuel Moskowitz. 1986. "USMGs Versus FMGs: Are There Performance Differences in the Ambulatory Care Setting?" *Medical Care* 24 (3): 248–58.

Saywell, R., Jr., J. Studnicki, J. A. Bean, and R. L. Ludke. 1979. "A Performance Comparison: USMG-FMG Attending Physicians." *American Journal of Public Health* 69 (1): 57–62.

Saywell, R., J.r, J. Studnicki, J. A. Bean, and R. L. Ludke. 1980. "A Performance Comparison: USMG-FMG House Staff Physicians." *American Journal of Public Health* 70 (1): 23–28.

Schatzman, Leonard, and A. Strauss. 1973. *Field Research: Strategies for a Natural Sociology.* Upper Saddle River, NJ: Prentice Hall.

National Navy UDT-SEAL Museum. 2019. "Ethos of the U.S. Navy SEALs." Accessed December 2, 2015. https://www.navysealmuseum.org/about-navy-seals/ethos-of-the-u-s-navy-seals.

Sennett, Richard, and Jonathan Cobb. 1972. *The Hidden Injuries of Class.* New York: Random House.

Silver, Julie K., Allison C. Bean, Chloe Slocum et al. 2019. "Physician Workforce Disparities and Patient Care: A Narrative Review." *Health Equity* 3 (1): 360–77.

Silverman, Lauren. 2015. "There Were Fewer Black Men in Medical School in 2014 Than in 1978." National Public Radio. http://www.npr.org/2015/10/24/449893318/there-were-fewer -black-men-in-medical-school-in-2014-than-in-1978.

Simon, Cecilia Capuzzi. 2012. "A Second Opinion: The Post-Baccalaureate." *New York Times*. http:// www.nytimes.com/2012/04/15/education/edlife/a-second-opinion-the-post-baccalaureate .html?pagewanted=all&_r=0.

Skrentny, John D., and Natalie Novick. 2018. "Research Universities and the Global Battle for the Brains." In *Education in a New Society: Renewing the Sociology of Education*, ed. Jal Mehta and Scott Davies, 271–96. Chicago: University of Chicago Press.

Smith, Harvey L. 1958. "Two Lines of Authority: The Hospital's Dilemma." In *Physicians, Patients and Illness*, ed. E. Gartly Jaco, 469–77. Glencoe, IL: Free Press.

Smith, R. Tyson. 2014. *Fighting for Recognition: Identity, Masculinity and the Act of Violence in Professional Wrestling*. Durham, NC: Duke University Press.

Sowell, Robert, Ting Zhang, Kenneth Redd, and The Council for Graduate Schools. 2008. *Ph.D. Completion and Attrition: Analysis of Baseline Program Data from the Ph.D. Completion Project*. Washington, DC: The Council of Graduate Schools.

Starr, Paul. 1982. *The Social Transformation of American Medicine*. New York: Basic Books.

Steele, C. M., and J. Aronson. 1995. "Stereotype Threat and the Intellectual Test Performance of African Americans." *Journal of Personality and Social Psychology* 69 (5): 797–811.

Stelling, Joan, and Rue Bucher. 1972. "Autonomy and Monitoring on Hospital Wards." *Sociological Quarterly* 13 (4): 431–46.

Stern, Alexandra Minna, and Howard Markel. 2004. "A Historical Perspective on the Changing Contours of Medical Residency Programs." *Journal of Pediatrics* 144: 1–2.

Stern, D. T. 1998. "In Search of the Informal Curriculum: When and Where Professional Values Are Taught." *Academic Medicine* 73 (10): S28–S30.

Swanson, A. G. 1973. "Graduate Education: Once for the Exceptional, Now Essential for All." *Journal of Medical Education* 48 (2): 183–85.

Swick, Herbert M. 2000. "Toward a Normative Definition of Medical Professionalism." *Academic Medicine* 75 (6): 612–16.

Szymczak, Julie E., and Charles L. Bosk. 2012. "Training for Efficiency: Work, Time, and Systems-Based Practice in Medical Residency." *Journal of Health and Social Behavior* 53 (3): 344–58.

Thomas, W. I., and Dorothy Swaine Thomas. 1928. *The Child in America: Behavior Problems and Programs*. New York: Knopf.

Thurow, Lester C. 1972. "Education and Economic Equality." *Public Interest* 28 (Summer): 66–81.

Timmermans, Stefan. 2008. "Oh Look, There Is a Doctor After All: About the Resilience of Professional Medicine: A Commentary on McKinlay and Marceau's 'When There Is No Doctor.'" *Social Science & Medicine* 67 (10): 1492–96.

Timmermans, Stefan, and Hyeyoung Oh. 2010. "The Continued Social Transformation of the Medical Profession." *Journal of Health and Social Behavior* 51: S94–S106.

Tolich, Martin. 2004. "Internal Confidentiality: When Confidentiality Assurances Fail Relational Informants." *Qualitative Sociology* 27: 101–6.

Tomlinson, J., D. Muzio, H. Sommerlad, L. Webley, and L. Duff. 2013. "Structure, Agency and Career Strategies of White Women and Black and Minority Ethnic Individuals in the Legal Profession." *Human Relations* 66 (2): 245–69.

Torche, Florencia. 2011. "Is a College Degree Still the Great Equalizer? Intergenerational Mobility across Levels of Schooling in the United States." *American Journal of Sociology* 117 (3): 763–807.

Tsugawa, Yusuke, Anupam Jena, John Orav, and Ashish Jha. 2017. "Quality of Care Delivered by General Internists in US Hospitals Who Graduated from Foreign Versus US Medical Schools: Observational Study. *BMJ* 356: j273.

Turner, Ralph H. 1960. "Sponsored and Contest Mobility and the School System." *American Sociological Review* 25 (6): 855–67.

Tyson, Karolyn, ed. 2011. *Integration Interrupted: Tracking, Black Students, and Acting White After Brown.* New York: Oxford University Press.

Underman, Kelly. 2015. "Playing Doctor: Simulation in Medical School as Affective Practice." *Social Science & Medicine,* 136: 180–88.

Underman, Kelly, and Laura E. Hirshfield. 2016. "Detached Concern? Emotional Socialization in Twenty-First Century Medical Education." *Social Science & Medicine* 160: 94–101.

U.S. Citizenship and Immigration Services. (2015). "Conrad 30 Waiver Program." http://www.uscis.gov/working-united-states/students-and-exchange-visitors/conrad-30-waiver-program

U.S. National Library of Medicine, Medline Plus. 2017. "Rhabdomyolysis." https://medlineplus.gov/ency/article/000473.htm.

Verghese, Abraham. 2009. *Cutting for Stone.* New York: Knopf.

Wacquant, Loic J. D. 1989. "Towards a Reflexive Sociology: A Workshop with Pierre Bourdieu." *Sociological Theory* 7: 26–63.

Waldinger, Roger, and Michael Lichter. 2003. *How the Other Half Works: Immigration and the Social Organization of Labor.* Berkeley: University of California Press.

Weber, Linda R., and Kevin B. Mathews. 2012. "Exploratory Study on the International Medical Graduate–Patient Relationship: Patients' Perceptions of the Quality of Care Delivered by His or Her Non-native Doctor." *Ethnicity and Disease* 22 (1): 79–84.

Weber, Max. 1968. "Political Communities." In *Economy and Society: An Outline of Interpretive Sociology,* ed. Guenther Roth and Claus Wittich, 901–40. New York: Bedminster Press.

West, Colin P., Tait D. Shanafelt, and Joseph C. Kolars. 2011. "Quality of Life, Burnout, Educational Debt, and Medical Knowledge Among Internal Medicine Residents." *JAMA* 306 (9): 952–60.

Whelan, G. P. 2006. "Coming to America: The Integration of International Medical Graduates Into the American Medical Culture." *Academic Medicine* 81 (2): 176–78.

Wu, Patrick, and Jonathan Siu. 2015. *A Brief Guide to Osteopathic Medicine for Students, by Students.* Chevy Chase, MD: American Association of Colleges of Osteopathic Medicine.

Young, Michael. 1958. *The Rise of the Meritocracy.* London: Thames and Hudson.

Young, Michael. 2001. "Down with Meritocracy: The Man Who Coined the Word Four Decades Ago Wishes Tony Blair Would Stop Using It." *The Guardian.* https://www.theguardian.com/politics/2001/jun/29/comment.

Zulla, R., M. O. Baerlocher, and S. Verma. 2008. "International Medical Graduates (IMGs) Needs Assessment Study: Comparison Between Current IMG Trainees and Program Directors." *BMC Medical Education* 8:42.

Zussman, Robert. 1992. *Intensive Care: Medical Ethics and the Medical Profession.* Chicago: University of Chicago Press.

Zussman, Robert. 1993. "Life in the Hospital: A Review." *Milbank Quarterly* 71 (1): 167–85.

Index

Page numbers in *italics* indicate figures or tables.

9 780231 189354